# ALIMENTARY TRACT IMAGING
A Teaching File

# Alimentary Tract Imaging
## A Teaching File

**C. DANIEL JOHNSON, M.D.**
*Consultant, Department of Diagnostic Radiology
Mayo Clinic and Mayo Foundation
Associate Professor of Radiology
Mayo Medical School
Rochester, Minnesota*

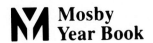

**Mosby
Year Book**

St. Louis    Baltimore    Boston    Chicago    London    Philadelphia    Sydney    Toronto

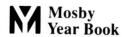

## Mosby
## Year Book

Dedicated to Publishing Excellence

Sponsoring Editor: Anne S. Patterson
Assistant Editor: Maura K. Leib
Assistant Director, Manuscript Services: Frances M. Perveiler
Production Supervisor: Carol A. Reynolds
Proofroom Manager: Barbara M. Kelly

1  2  3  4  5  6  7  8  9  0  CL  MV  97  96  95  94  93

**Library of Congress Cataloging-in-Publication Data**
Johnson, Charles Daniel.
    Alimentary tract imaging : a teaching file / C. Daniel Johnson.
       p.    cm.
    Includes bibliographical references and index.
    ISBN 0-8151-4927-1
    1. Alimentary canal—Diseases—Atlases.  2. Alimentary canal—
Radiography—Atlases.  I. Title.
    [DNLM: 1. Gastrointestinal System—radiography—atlases.  WI 17
J66a]
RC804.R6J64   1992
616.3'307572—dc20                                    92-22596
DNLM/DLC                                                  CIP
for Library of Congress

*To my wife, Therese,*
*my parents, Cliff and Ruth Johnson,*
*and my daughter, Kristina*

# PREFACE

The purpose in writing this book was to provide a pictorial presentation and overview of common abnormalities that affect the hollow viscera. This book is not intended to be an inclusive source of all diseases that affect the alimentary tract. Selected pediatric cases are included in the text primarily to provide a comparison case for a similar adult disease or to complete a discussion of a disease entity or group of abnormalities. The reader is referred to other textbooks for a comprehensive review of pediatric gastrointestinal disorders. Emphasis in this book is placed on common pathologic conditions; however, less common but important conditions are also included. The content is mainly directed to residents, particularly those studying for board examinations. Practicing radiologists wishing to review the spectrum of abnormalities affecting the hollow viscera may also find this book helpful.

The majority of the cases have been selected from our teaching file, and the radiographic techniques used are representative of our style of practice. We use both double- and single-contrast examinations, but we rely heavily on the fluoroscopic single-contrast examination. Regardless of the technique used, I hope that the reader will gain an understanding of the important lesions that affect the gastrointestinal tract and their radiologic presentations. Intraluminal contrast studies are the major focus of the text, but correlative computed tomography has been added to many cases when this technique has been shown to be helpful.

The text is divided into five chapters: esophagus, stomach, duodenum, small bowel, and colon. Each chapter begins with an outline and concludes with a list of differential considerations. Cross-reference notations are abundant throughout the text and among differential considerations. Each chapter has a list of selected readings which is organized in the same manner as the text. Readings that are cited in the text are noted by an asterisk for rapid identification.

I am deeply indebted to my many mentors and colleagues who have instructed me and given liberally of their time and case material. My resident training at the

Mayo Clinic was highly influenced by Dr. Harley C. Carlson, who early in my career convinced me of the fun and excitement that exists in gastrointestinal radiology. Drs. David H. Stephens and Robert L. MacCarty carefully guided me through the program and encouraged me to seek fellowship training at Duke University. Drs. Reed Rice and William Thompson are responsible for my eventual decision to choose a career in academic radiology. Reed's wonderful teaching style and interpersonal manner were exemplary and ignited my interest in resident education. Since I returned to the Mayo Clinic, Dr. Stephens has been my closest professional colleague. He approached me 3 years ago regarding the writing and publication of this book. He has been invaluable in answering questions, providing suggestions and insight, loaning case material, and reviewing the manuscript. I never would have started this book and surely would have given up if not for his genuine excitement and mastery of gastrointestinal radiology. I deeply appreciate all his help and his friendship.

There are, of course, many other people who have helped. I am grateful to my colleagues who have performed and loaned me many of the examinations used in the book: H.C. Carlson, D.H. Stephens, R.L. MacCarty, J.J. Gisvold, E.M. Ward, C.E. Bender, K.M. Dudiak, S.L. Coffey, and M.J. Smerud. The excellent technologists, headed by T.C. Kodet, and other paramedical personnel, headed by J.A. Klimpel, have always given willingly of their time, energies, and talents.

I also thank my secretary, Brenda L. Maxwell, who labored on the manuscript through many revisions. Her organizational skills and attention to detail were exemplary and greatly appreciated. Dr. Carol L. Kornblith, from the Section of Publications at Mayo, tirelessly edited the manuscript; Mary K. Horsman was the editorial assistant for the project; and Renee S. Van Vleet proofread the manuscript. Photographic Production, supervised by Thomas F. Flood, has performed a large volume of high-quality work, sometimes at breakneck speed, without complaints.

I am also grateful to the many residents in our program who have shown interest in many of these teaching cases. Their enthusiasm for learning has been a major impetus to write this book.

Finally, and most importantly, my wife Therese has without hesitation encouraged me the most to pursue this project from inception to completion. She has self-lessly given me unending support. There were many weekends and nights that I deserted my family to work on the book, and I shall not forget the sacrifices that they made.

*C. Daniel Johnson, M.D.*

# CONTENTS

# Esophagus

## Case 1

## NORMAL ESOPHAGUS

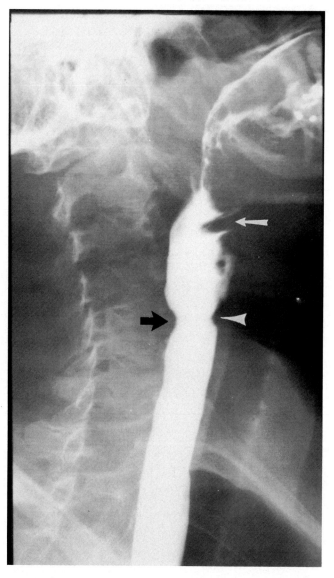

Single-contrast (full column) esophagram of the cervical and upper thoracic esophagus shows normal impressions on the esophagus from the cricopharyngeal muscle posteriorly *(black arrow)*, venous plexus anteriorly *(arrowhead)*, and epiglottis *(white arrow)*. The normal epiglottis can be seen as a linear filling defect in the barium pool.

The normal esophagus is a straight tube with smooth contours which begins at the level of the cricopharyngeal muscle (C-5 to C-6) and ends at the gastroesophageal junction. Normal impressions on the esophagus include the cricopharyngeal muscle posteriorly, the anterior venous plexus, the aortic arch, the left main-stem

bronchus, and occasionally the left atrium. Both full-column and double-contrast techniques can be used to evaluate the esophagus. Full-column examinations are particularly helpful in assessing for esophageal strictures and fistulae. Double-contrast techniques are useful in demonstrating subtle mucosal abnormalities. The cervical and upper thoracic esophagus can be difficult to evaluate fluoroscopically and by film examination because of the rapid transit time through this segment. Rapid sequence filming, video, and cineradiography may be helpful in evaluating patients with suspected abnormalities involving this region.

**Case 2**

# MUSCULAR RING

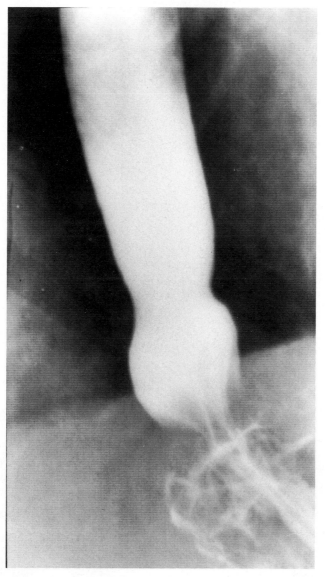

A muscular ring (A ring) is seen within the distal esophagus. At fluoroscopy, the ring was noted to be transient.

A muscular ring appears as a broad, smooth indentation in the lower esophagus, just superior to the esophageal vestibule. It is caused by a muscular thickening and can be observed to change shape and disappear at fluoroscopy. A prominent muscular ring is encountered more often in patients with a hiatal hernia or gastroesophageal reflux and in some esophageal motor disor-

ders. It is not known if these associations are significant. The esophageal vestibule roughly corresponds in location to the manometrically defined lower esophageal sphincter and should not be confused with a hiatal hernia. At fluoroscopy, a peristaltic wave can be seen to pass through this region. Often a mucosal ring (B ring) (Cases 82 and 83) will also be visible during the examination. The B line is a thin, fixed ring that does not change appearance and marks the location of the esophagogastric junction.

**Case 3**

## NORMAL ESOPHAGUS: TRIPHASIC ESOPHAGRAM

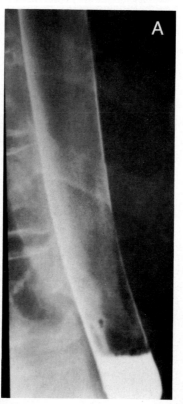

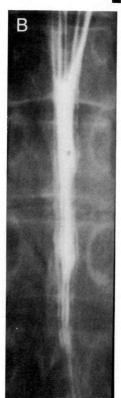

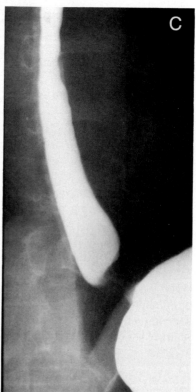

**A.** Normal air-contrast esophagram demonstrates smooth, straight wall contours and a featureless background.

**B.** Normal mucosal-relief esophagram demonstrates the collapsed esophagus with delicate, thin, and straight longitudinal folds.

**C.** Normal single-contrast (full column) esophagram demonstrates normal smooth contours of the esophageal mucosa without filling defects.

The triphasic esophagram is a useful technique for evaluating different types of esophageal diseases. The air-contrast phase best depicts mucosal abnormalities, whereas the mucosal-relief phase best displays abnormalities of fold thickness. The single-contrast phase often can depict abnormalities of distensibility and fistula(e) to best advantage. High density barium, with or without effervescent granules, is used in obtaining both the double-contrast and mucosal-relief films. "Thin" or lower density barium that can be penetrated by the x-ray beam is often used for the single-contrast phase.

## Case 4

### CT OF THE NORMAL ESOPHAGUS

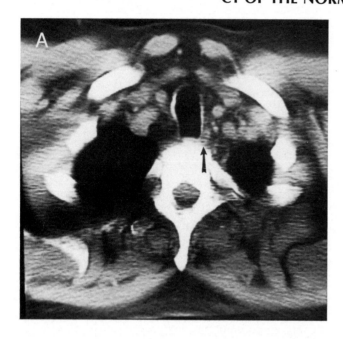

**A.** CT of the upper thoracic esophagus shows the collapsed esophageal lumen lying on the left side of the posterior wall of the trachea *(arrow)*.

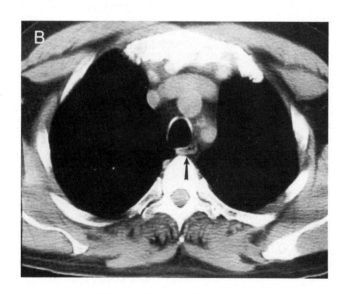

**B.** At a lower level, the esophagus lies nearly posterior to the trachea *(arrow)*. Esophageal wall thickness is only 2 to 3 mm normally.

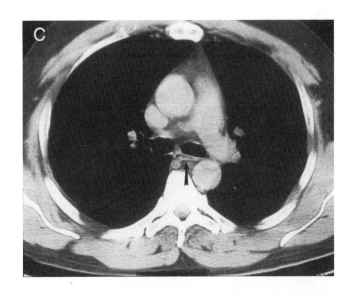

**C.** Normal esophagus *(arrow)* at the level of the carina lies posterior to the left main-stem bronchus.

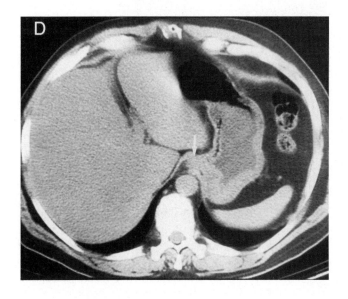

**D.** The normal gastroesophageal junction *(arrow)* is visible between the crura located anterior and posterior to the normal lower esophagus.

The normal esophagus is usually collapsed on CT, with a wall thickness of only 2 to 3 mm. In patients with ample mediastinal fat, the periesophageal fat is homogeneously dark. If wall thickening is questioned, patients can be given contrast material (paste or pudding consistency) that may be helpful in distending the lumen. Adjacent organs such as the trachea, bronchus, and aorta can be inspected also. These organs may be affected by adjacent esophageal disease.

**Case 5**

## ABERRANT RIGHT SUBCLAVIAN ARTERY

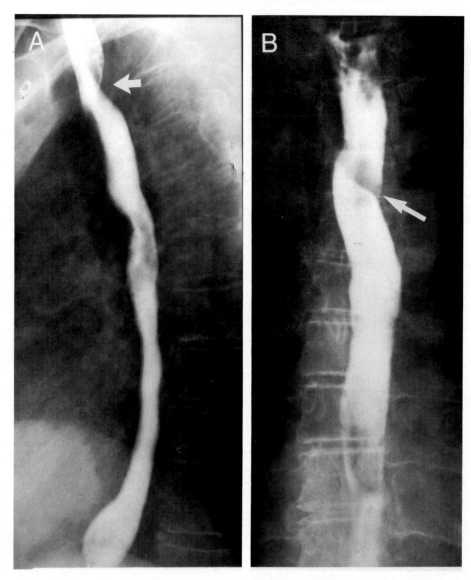

**A.** A smooth, extrinsic mass *(arrow)* impresses on the posterior wall of the upper thoracic esophagus.

**B.** The impression *(arrow)* has an oblique linear course, directed from the aortic knob toward the right shoulder. This is the characteristic appearance of an aberrant right subclavian artery.

An aberrant right subclavian artery is the most common nonaortic vascular lesion impressing on the esophagus. The aberrant right subclavian artery arises just distal to the normal left subclavian artery and traverses obliquely to the right, posterior to the esophagus. The impression is extramucosal and so typical of the abnormality that no further studies are required. The abnormality is rarely symptomatic and requires no treatment.

## Case 6

## FELINE ESOPHAGUS

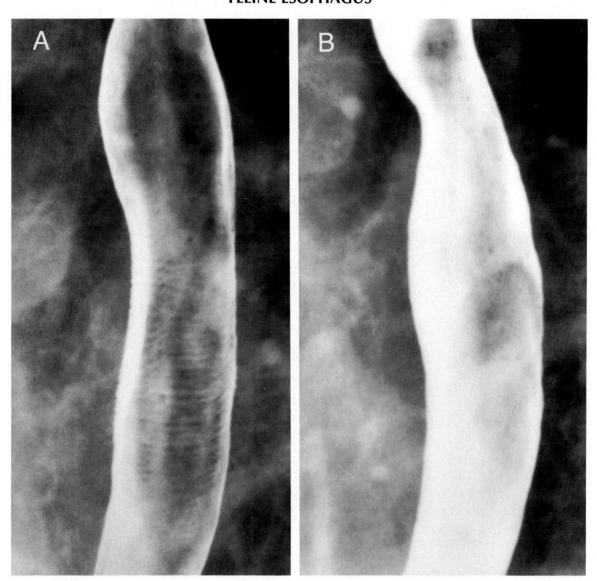

**A.** Multiple, thin, transverse folds are present in the lower esophagus.

**B.** An exposure taken a few seconds after *(A)* is normal and without evidence of the previously seen folds. Findings are characteristic of the feline esophagus.

The feline esophagus can be recognized by the presence of multiple transverse folds that are present transiently as the esophagus begins to collapse. The folds are fine and delicate in appearance, numerous, and symmetric. Their transient nature distinguishes them from the fixed, larger folds occasionally seen in patients with reflux esophagitis (Case 11).

The name is derived from the similar-appearing esophagram in cats. Often this finding is a normal variant that is due to contraction of the muscularis mucosae. Some investigators have suggested that this finding may be more common in patients with esophagitis (Laufer, 1982).

## Case 7

# MILD REFLUX ESOPHAGITIS: THICKENED FOLDS

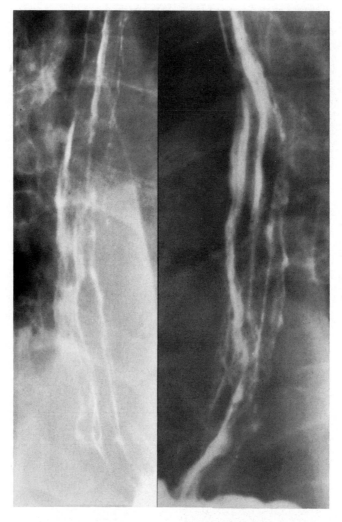

Thickened and somewhat nodular folds are seen in the distal esophagus. If this is the only finding visible on a triphasic esophagram, mild esophagitis commonly is encountered endoscopically. Folds are considered abnormal if they exceed 2 to 3 mm in diameter.

Reflux esophagitis usually is encountered during an upper gastrointestinal examination. Development of reflux esophagitis depends on several factors, including the acidity of the refluxed contents, the efficacy of esophageal clearance, and the frequency of reflux. These factors are particularly important in patients with Zollinger-Ellison syndrome and those with scleroderma, groups commonly affected with reflux esophagitis.

**Case 8**

## REFLUX ESOPHAGITIS: MODERATE SEVERITY

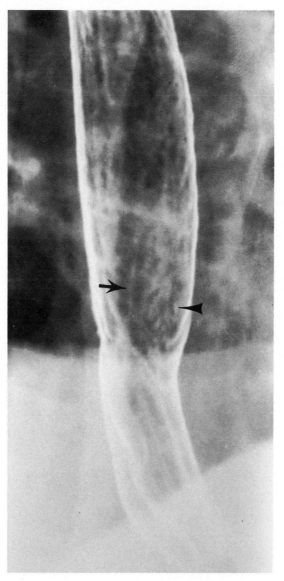

Linear erosions *(arrow)* and punctate superficial erosions *(arrowhead)* are present within a mildly nodular mucosal background. The esophagus is shortened and a small hiatal hernia is also present.

Moderate esophagitis usually is characterized by the presence of superficial erosions which may be either punctate or linear. Fold thickening (Case 7) and nodularity (Case 10) are also often present on the mucosal-relief phase films.

In patients with long-standing disease with esophageal intramural fibrosis, the esophagus shortens and pulls the stomach into an intrathoracic location. This type of "short esophagus" hiatal hernia is present in this patient.

## Case 9

# SEVERE ESOPHAGITIS: DEEP ULCER

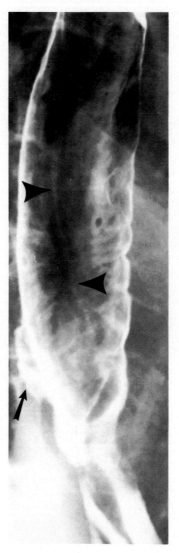

A large, flat ulcer is present in the distal esophagus *(arrow)* with associated diminished distensibility of the lower esophageal segment. There is also a long longitudinal ulcer *(arrowheads)* with a surrounding halo of edema and associated folds that radiate toward the linear crater.

Severe esophagitis usually is characterized by the presence of a moderate to large ulcer crater. These craters may be shallow or they may burrow deep into the esophageal wall. Typically, patients with severe esophagitis have superficial erosions (Case 8) and fold thickening (Case 7) in addition to the characteristic ulcer.

**Case 10**

## SEVERE ESOPHAGITIS: DEEP ULCERATION

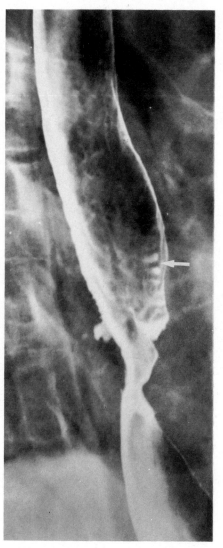

Mucosal nodularity is present throughout the distal esophagus. There is a deep ulcer as well as luminal narrowing distally. Transverse folds (Case 11) due to chronic scarring and buckling of the mucosa are also present *(arrow)*. Sharp spiculations are present just superior to the deep ulcer—these are due to transverse folds or tiny erosions seen in profile. Asymmetric scarring causes the distal deformity and narrowing. A short esophagus-type hiatal hernia is also present.

Patients with severe esophagitis usually have large ulcerations which may be deep or shallow. Histologically, acute inflammatory changes with accumulation of neutrophils and round cells in the lamina propria as well as basal cell hyperplasia of the squamous epithelium are seen in patients with reflux esophagitis.

## Case 11

## LINEAR ULCERATION WITH TRANSVERSE FOLDS

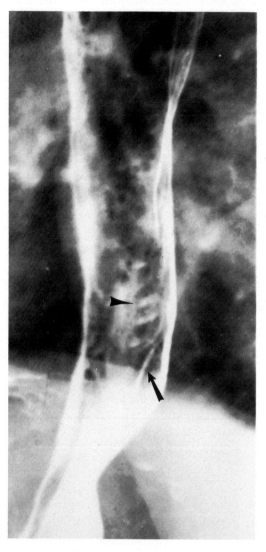

Transverse folds *(arrowhead)* develop as a result of scar formation within the longitudinal muscle layers of the distal esophagus. A linear ulcer *(arrow)* is also present. There are only a few transverse folds; they are well defined and do not span the entire esophageal lumen. It is believed these folds arise as a puckering of the mucosa after healing and scarring from a linear ul-

ceration (Levine and Goldstein, 1984). Transverse folds from esophagitis should be distinguished from the folds in "feline esophagus" (Case 6) because transverse folds are fixed, fewer in number, coarser, and shorter. Changes of both active and chronic disease commonly coexist (as seen in this case).

**Case 12**

# CHRONIC ESOPHAGITIS: CICATRICIAL STRICTURE

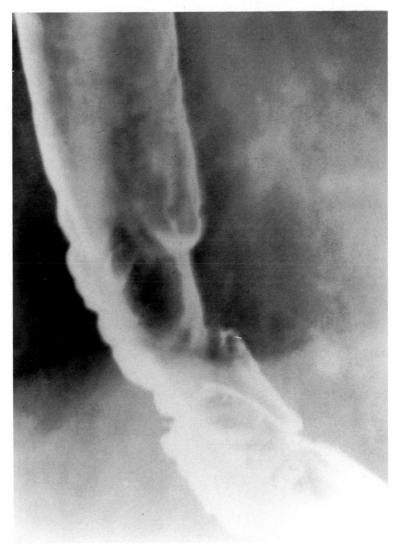

Luminal irregularity and narrowing with multiple sacculations of the distal esophagus resulted from scarring from reflux esophagitis. It may be impossible to exclude an active ulceration or carcinoma in patients with marked deformity. Endoscopy should be recommended for patients with such problematic findings.

**Case 13**

# CHRONIC ESOPHAGITIS: REFLUX STRICTURE

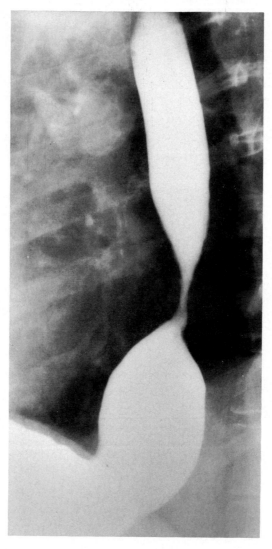

A moderate-sized hiatal hernia is present with esophageal shortening and narrowing beginning at the gastroesophageal junction. The margins of the stricture taper gradually. These findings are typical of a benign, reflux-induced esophageal stricture.

Stricture formation is the most frequent radiographic manifestation of chronic reflux esophagitis. The classic stricture begins at the level of the gastroesophageal junction and extends proximally a variable distance. Usually the margins are smooth and taper gradually.

Mild stricture may present as subtle regions of incomplete esophageal distension. Severe strictures that narrow the lumen to less than 1 cm are nearly always symptomatic—dysphagia is the most frequent complaint. Treatment of symptomatic strictures is usually by either balloon or bougie dilation. Surgical treatment is reserved for patients who do not respond to more conservative therapy. An antireflux operation may be performed at that time.

## Case 14

## CHRONIC ESOPHAGITIS: LONG STRICTURE

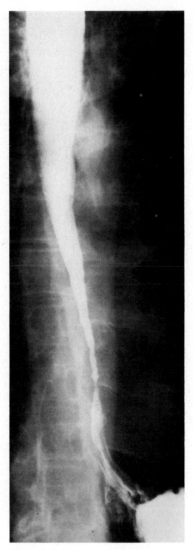

A long distal esophageal stricture is present with an associated hiatal hernia. This benign-appearing stricture is due to chronic reflux esophagitis. The smooth, tapered margins usually indicate a benign cause. Long strictures such as this are unusual for peptic esophagitis-induced strictures. Other conditions that should be considered include Zollinger-Ellison syndrome, prolonged vomiting, nasogastric intubation, and bile reflux after gastric resection.

**Case 15**

# BARRETT'S ESOPHAGUS

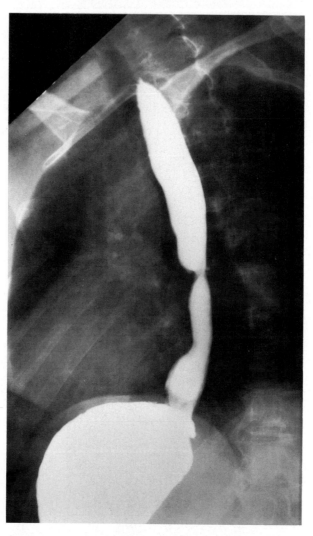

A short stricture is present in the mid-esophagus, with some luminal irregularity due to esophagitis at the level of the stricture. A short esophagus-type hiatal hernia is also visible due to long-standing reflux esophagitis. A focal esophageal stricture above the gastroesophageal junction is suggestive of Barrett's esophagus.

Barrett's esophagus is histologically described as metaplasia and replacement of the normal squamous epithelium with gastric-type adenomatous mucosa. Chronic reflux esophagitis is nearly always the underlying cause of this disease. Some authorities estimate that nearly 10% of patients with reflux esophagitis have some adenomatous transformation in their esophagus (Levine, 1989).

This case is a typical example of Barrett's esophagus. The short esophagus hiatal hernia indicates long-standing esophagitis. Usual reflux-induced strictures are located immediately above the gastroesophageal junction. Because adenomatous tissue is acid-resistant, strictures in Barrett's esophagus develop near the squamous-adenomatous transition zone. Barrett strictures commonly can be seen in the upper and mid-esophagus.

**Case 16**

## BARRETT'S ESOPHAGUS: TRANSITION ZONE

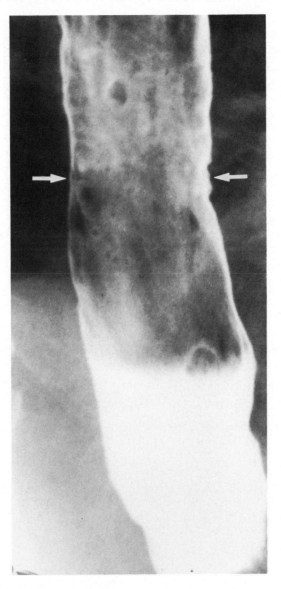

The normal featureless distal esophageal segment represents the region where acid-resistant adenomatous tissue is present. Above the featureless zone *(arrows)* are typical findings of active reflux esophagitis, including mucosal granularity and several superficial erosions.

It is important to recognize patients with Barrett's esophagus because the adenomatous tissue is at increased risk for malignant transformation. Some reports suggest adenocarcinoma may develop in up to 10% of these patients. In fact, 5% to 20% of all esophageal cancers (Cases 40, 42, and 43) develop in Barrett's mucosa (Levine et al., 1984).

Case 17

## BARRETT'S ESOPHAGUS: RETICULAR PATTERN

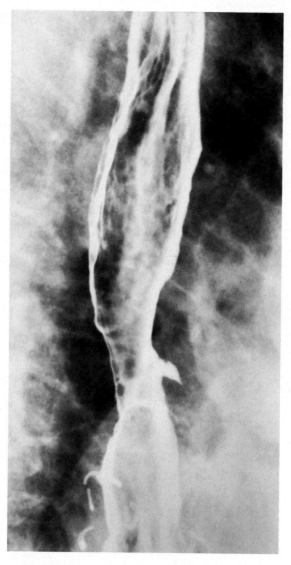

Subtle nodularity and reticularity are present in the esophagus of a patient with endoscopically proven Barrett's esophagus. There is a short esophagus-type hiatal hernia with a surgically induced deformity that mimics an ulcer crater. Notice also the moderately severe stricture of the distal esophagus due to chronic scarring from reflux esophagitis.

Reticular changes of Barrett's esophagus are often adjacent to an esophageal stricture. The nodularity and crevices may be smaller and more delicate than this example. Only 5% to 30% of patients with Barrett's esophagus will have these reticular changes (Levine et al., 1983). It is possible that the mucosal nodularity associated with usual reflux esophagitis (Case 10) without adenomatous transformation could have similar radiographic findings.

## Case 18

## BARRETT'S ESOPHAGUS: CT

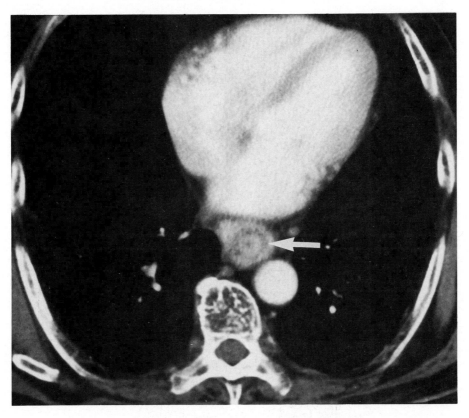

The esophageal wall is thickened and the esophagus resembles a target as a result of a hypodense circumferential ring in the esophageal wall. Barrett's esophagus was discovered at endoscopic biopsy.

The CT findings of mild to moderate esophagitis are often nonexistent or minimal, with only mild wall thickening. Occasionally, diffuse edema within the esophageal wall can be visualized at CT by detecting a low-density ring *(arrow)* within the thickened wall. This finding is nonspecific and could be due to any condition causing intramural edema.

## Case 19

# INTRAMURAL PSEUDODIVERTICULOSIS

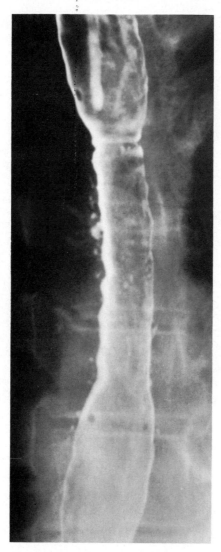

Multiple tiny outpouchings are seen within the mid-esophagus around a localized stricture.

Intramural esophageal pseudodiverticulosis is seen as multiple tiny outpouchings which either diffusely or segmentally affect the esophagus. Pathologically, these outpouchings are dilated submucosal glands, most commonly due to chronic reflux esophagitis. Elderly patients are most frequently affected and complain of progressive dysphagia due to the often-associated esophageal strictures. Dilatation of the stricture usually cures the symptoms. Their radiographic appearance is analogous to Rokitansky-Aschoff sinuses in the gallbladder and is virtually pathognomonic of this condition. *Candida* is frequently cultured from the esophagus in patients with this condition, but this is believed to be a secondary invader rather than a causative factor.

**Case 20**

# CANDIDIASIS

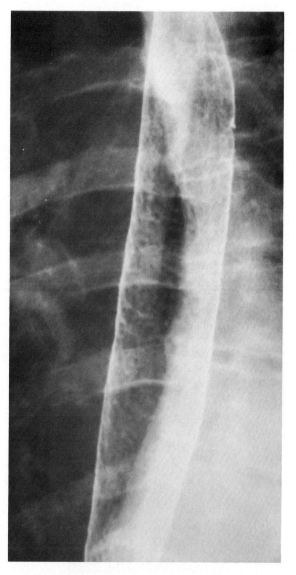

Multiple superficial erosions and mucosal nodularity are present throughout the esophagus. If these changes were confined to the lower esophagus it would be impossible to distinguish them from reflux esophagitis.

Infectious esophagitis is increasingly common today with the widespread use of immunosuppressants and with diseases that alter the immune status of the body. Patients with transplants, receiving chemotherapy or steroids, and with acquired immunodeficiency syndrome (AIDS) are most frequently affected.

Offending microorganisms that could cause these findings include *Candida* (*C. albicans* is the most common cause of infectious esophagitis), herpes simplex virus type 1, and cytomegalovirus. Regardless of the organism, most patients complain of odynophagia, dysphagia, and chest pain.

**Case 21**

# CANDIDIASIS

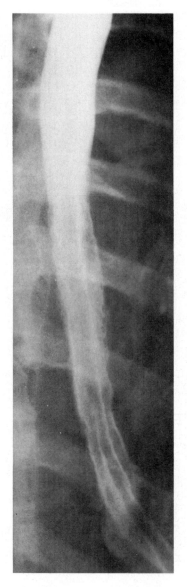

Enlarged, edematous folds are seen in the distal esophagus. This finding could be due to reflux esophagitis; however, the folds just above the gastroesophageal junction are smaller than those folds at a more proximal level. Usually, reflux esophagitis affects the esophagus just above the gastroesophageal junction "first and worst" (Case 7). Candidiasis was confirmed later.

## Case 22

### CANDIDIASIS

## Case 23

### ESOPHAGEAL CANDIDIASIS

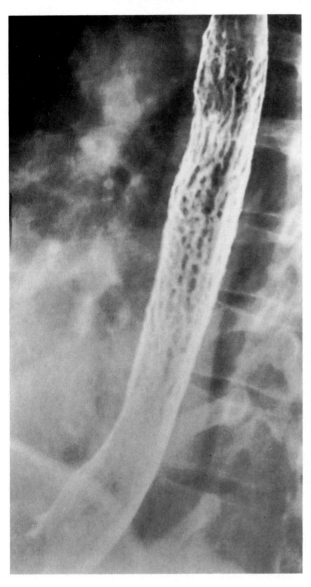

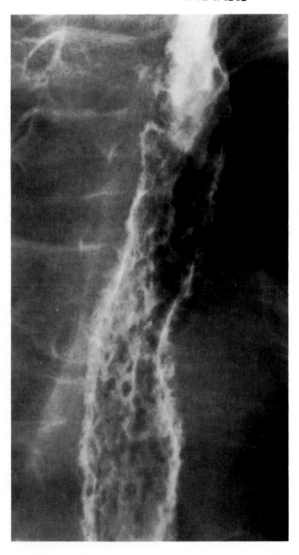

Multiple plaque-like filling defects are seen throughout the esophagus. This is the most frequently recognized manifestation of candidiasis.

There is a spectrum of radiographic findings associated with candidiasis. Patients may present early with findings only of dysmotility (atonicity and tertiary contractions). Discrete plaque-like lesions are the most common finding, ranging from a few to diffuse esophageal involvement. Nodularity, granularity (Case 20), and fold thickening (Case 21) may be seen as a result of mucosal inflammation and edema. More severe disease is manifested as a shaggy, irregular luminal surface (Case 23). Rarely, large filling defects can be seen due to giant plaques and fungus balls.

Shaggy, irregular luminal contours due to extensive plaque-like filling defects are present throughout the esophagus. *Candida albicans* was cultured and the patient was successfully treated.

Major differential considerations for multiple plaque-like filling defects in the esophagus include reflux esophagitis (Cases 8 and 10), other types of infections (herpes, cytomegalovirus), and glycogenic acanthosis (Case 77). Reflux esophagitis is usually confined to the lower esophagus and is rarely associated with well-defined plaques. Patients with glycogenic acanthosis are usually asymptomatic but could present with similar radiographic findings. Herpes esophagitis can occasionally present with multiple plaque-like filling defects, but ulcerations are more common.

## Case 24

# HERPES ESOPHAGITIS

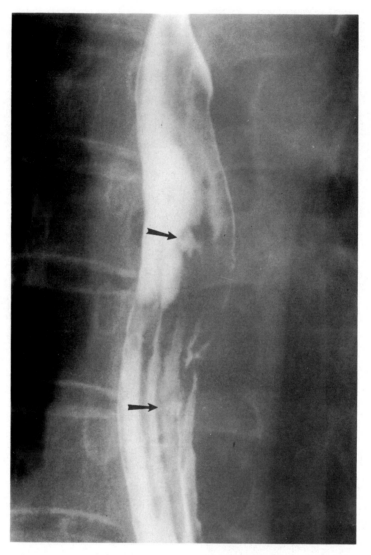

Multiple discrete ulcerations *(arrows)* are present on an otherwise normal esophageal background. In an immunosuppressed host, herpes esophagitis would be the most likely possibility.

Herpes simplex virus is an opportunistic infection usually found in immunosuppressed or debilitated patients. There are reports of this infection in otherwise healthy individuals (Deprew et al., 1977). Clinical findings are often indistinguishable from candidiasis. Definitive diagnosis is made from culture of the virus from esophageal brushings or biopsy specimens.

*From Levine MS, Laufer I, Kressel HY, Friedman HM. AJR 1981;136:863–866. By permission of the American Roentgen Ray Society.*

Radiographically, discrete ulcerations on an otherwise normal esophageal mucosal background are characteristic. Multiple plaque-like filling defects, with or without ulcerations, also can be seen.

Differential considerations include candidiasis, which usually presents with plaque-like filling defects (Case 22). Other members of the herpes virus group, including cytomegalovirus and varicella zoster, can present with identical radiographic findings. Cytomegalovirus infection often presents with large, solitary discrete ulcers (Cases 25 and 26). Ulcers from reflux esophagitis (Cases 9 and 10) are usually confined to the distal esophagus and associated with a hiatal hernia, reflux, and a lower esophageal stricture.

Case 25

# CYTOMEGALOVIRUS ESOPHAGITIS

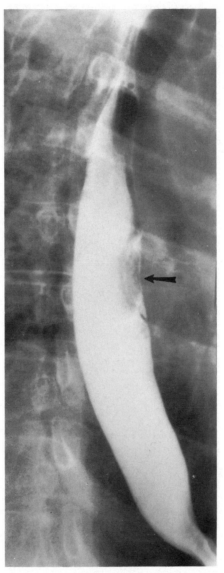

A large, flat ulceration *(arrow)* is present in the distal esophagus.

Cytomegalovirus infection is a disorder arising from the herpes virus family. Most patients with this opportunistic infection have AIDS. The small bowel and colon are most frequently affected. Diagnosis is usually made histologically by examining endoscopic brushings and biopsy specimens. Intranuclear inclusions are seen within endothelial cells or fibroblasts.

*Courtesy of Kyunghee C. Cho, M.D., The Bronx, New York.*

Radiographically, cytomegalovirus esophagitis may be indistinguishable from herpes simplex (Case 24) or human immunodeficiency virus (HIV) infection with multiple discrete ulcerations. Advanced disease may be associated with extensive ulceration. Giant ulcers can suggest cytomegalovirus or HIV infection rather than herpes esophagitis. These ulcers are often large, flat, and ovoid. Cytomegalovirus esophagitis should be considered in any patient with AIDS and esophageal ulcerations.

## Case 26

## CYTOMEGALOVIRUS ESOPHAGITIS

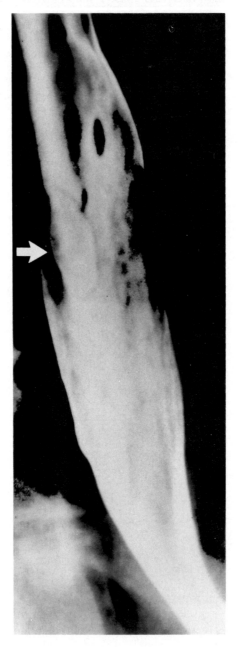

Multiple ulcerations are present in the distal esophagus. The largest ulcer *(arrow)* is large, flat, and ovoid.

There is a well-defined thin rim of edema surrounding the ulcer.

*From Levine MS.* Radiology of the esophagus. *Philadelphia: WB Saunders, **1989**:68. By permission of Kyunghee C. Cho, MD.*

Case 27

# MEDICATION-INDUCED ESOPHAGITIS

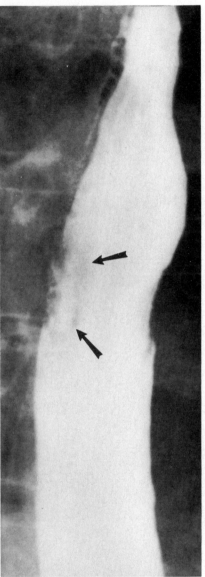

Single-contrast esophagram shows an irregular, linearly oriented ulceration with a surrounding soft tissue mass *(arrows)*. There is also a region of reduced distensibility on the opposite wall. Tiny ulcerations may be present within this area.

Localized inflammation secondary to medication lodged in the esophagus can lead to focal edema, ulceration, and stricture formation. Pills can stick anywhere within the esophagus, but usually they lodge at the level of the arch or within the distal esophagus. Tetracycline, quinidine, and potassium chloride are the usual offending drugs, but other medications including ascorbic acid, digitoxin, digoxin, and iron sulfate also have been implicated. Patients usually complain of odynophagia, dysphagia, and retrosternal pain.

Radiographic findings are usually those of single or multiple shallow ulcerations. Associated fold thickening also may be seen. Double-contrast examination of the esophagus has been shown to be sensitive in detecting these small subtle ulcers.

## Case 28

# LYE-INDUCED STRICTURE

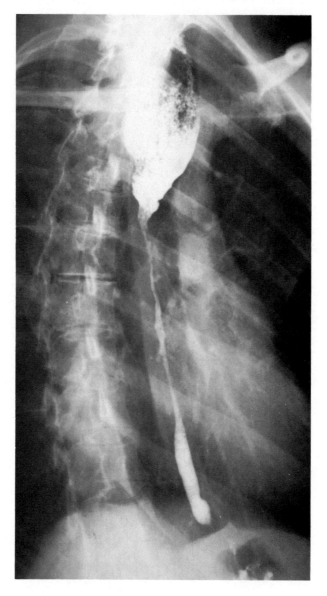

Beginning just below the level of the aortic arch, there is a long and narrow stricture involving the mid-esophagus and distal esophagus.

Caustic damage to the esophagus can occur from several agents, including alkali (lye), acid, phenols, ammonium chloride, and silver nitrate. In this country, lye ingestion is most often seen because of the availability of liquid drain cleaners. The extent of esophageal damage depends on the concentration of the agent, amount ingested, and duration of mucosal contact. Endoscopy is usually recommended to assess the severity of the esophageal "burn." Radiographic examinations are helpful in documenting the severity and extent of stricture formation.

Radiographic findings of acute caustic esophagitis include dysmotility, irregular margins, edema, ulcerations, plaques of sloughing mucosa, and occasionally intramural collection of contrast material. Esophageal strictures are usually seen about 1 to 3 months after the injury. The strictures may be focal and confined to the upper esophagus, or the esophagus may be diffusely involved with asymmetrical regions of narrowing and sacculations. Severe stricture formation will narrow the entire lumen, which may appear "threadlike."

The stomach also may be damaged and should routinely be examined. Acid ingestion commonly involves the stomach (Case 107) more than the esophagus, whereas lye ingestion results in gastric ulceration and narrowing in only about 20% of patients. These patients are also at significant risk (1% to 4%) of esophageal cancer in 20 to 40 years (Kiviranta, 1952).

## Case 29

## ESOPHAGEAL LEIOMYOMA

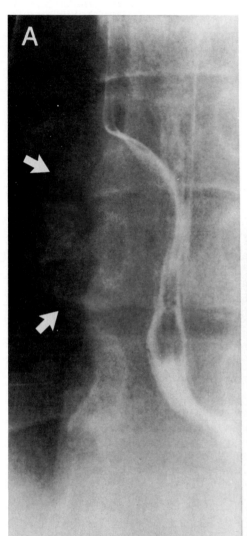

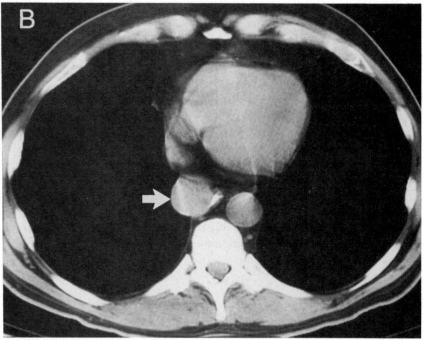

**A.** There is a smooth impression on the esophageal contour by a well-circumscribed mass. The lateral margins of the mass *(arrows)* can be seen to extend to the right of the spine. The location of the mass in relationship to the esophagus (its epicenter is in an intramural location), its smooth surface, and the obtuse angle between the mass and the esophageal lumen suggest a smooth muscle tumor.

**B.** The well-circumscribed, exophytic tumor *(arrow)* is seen at CT. A leiomyoma was surgically removed.

Leiomyomas are the most frequently occurring submucosal neoplasm of the esophagus—accounting for more than half of all benign esophageal tumors. They are more common in the mid-esophagus and distal esophagus—the segments where smooth muscle is most abundant. Approximately 3% to 4% of tumors will be multiple (Seremetis et al., 1976). Most leiomyomas are found incidentally. There has not been a reported case of sarcomatous degeneration of a leiomyoma (Glanz and Grünebaum, 1977). Most leiomyomas will present with findings that closely resemble this patient's tumor; however, rarely they can encase the esophagus as an annular lesion or present as an intraluminal mass. Leiomyomas are the only esophageal tumors that can calcify, with the exception of a single case report of a calcified leiomyosarcoma (Itai and Shimazu, 1978).

Differential considerations include other types of intramural tumors such as fibromas, neuromas, neurofibromas, lipomas, and hemangiomas. Enteric duplication cysts (Cases 79 and 80), solitary submucosal lymphomatous masses, or an isolated varix could have a similar appearance.

## Case 30

## ESOPHAGEAL ADENOMA

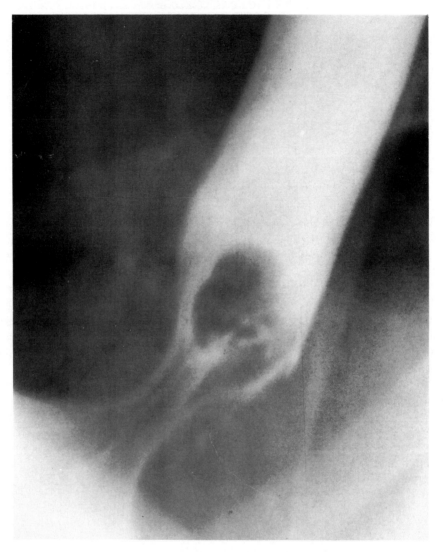

A lobulated filling defect is present in the distal esophagus.

Adenomas of the esophagus are rare lesions arising from adenomatous tissue in the distal esophagus, usually within Barrett's esophagus. Malignant degeneration has been reported in these lesions (Levine, 1989); therefore, endoscopic removal is recommended. Larger polyps are more likely to be malignant than smaller polyps.

Esophageal papillomas (fibrovascular excrescences that are covered with squamous epithelium) could have a similar radiographic appearance and are probably more common than previously believed because of their often small size. These polyps are usually removed endoscopically, but no malignant transformation has been reported in humans. Inflammatory esophagogastric polyps (Case 31) could also be confused with adenomas; however, these polypoid protuberances are usually foldlike and arise from the stomach.

Case 31

# INFLAMMATORY ESOPHAGOGASTRIC POLYP

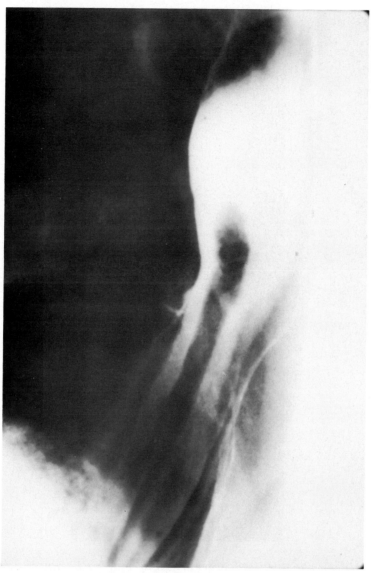

An enlarged polypoid fold extends from the stomach into the esophageal lumen. This is the characteristic appearance of an inflammatory esophagogastric polyp.

The inflammatory esophagogastric polyp is an enlarged gastric fold that projects into the lower esophagus. Inflammation is due to reflux esophagitis in these patients. These polyps have no malignant potential.

Usual radiographic features are a clubbed, bulbous fold that arises from the fundus of the stomach and projects into the lower esophagus. Occasionally, it may be difficult to differentiate an inflammatory esophagogastric polyp from papillomas or adenomas (Case 30). In these patients, endoscopy is recommended to exclude malignancy.

**Case 32**

# ULCERATIVE ESOPHAGEAL CARCINOMA

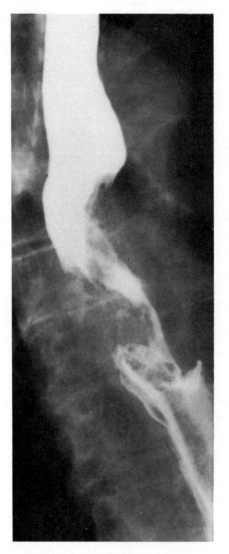

The central portion of this large mid-esophageal mass is ulcerated with a rim of tumor around it. A squamous cell carcinoma was removed surgically.

Esophageal carcinoma is a highly lethal disease that usually presents with chest pain or progressive dysphagia. Symptomatic tumors are often large and of advanced stage. Small tumors are usually discovered incidentally. Important risk factors in the development of esophageal cancer include tobacco and alcohol consumption (3- to 4-fold increase in males), race (twice as common in nonwhites), lye ingestion, achalasia, prior head and neck cancer, nontropical sprue, tylosis, Plummer-Vinson syndrome, and exposure to tannins and nitrosamines. Tobacco and alcohol consumption are the most important factors in the United States.

Squamous carcinomas are the most common histologic type. Squamous cell tumors do not usually cross the esophagogastric junction, whereas adenocarcinomas arising in Barrett's esophagus frequently will extend into the stomach (Cases 40–42). Most adenocarcinomas arise in Barrett's esophagus and, as expected, are usually located in the distal esophagus.

Case 33

# INFILTRATIVE ESOPHAGEAL CANCER

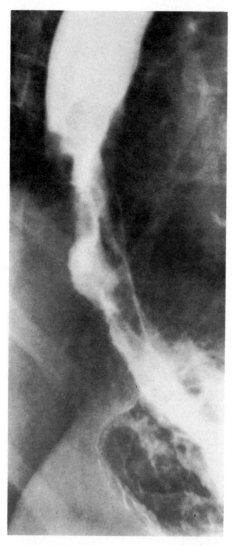

There is an irregular ulcerated mass in the distal esophagus typical of an infiltrative esophageal cancer. Adenocarcinoma was removed surgically.

Radiographically, most carcinomas appear as an irregular mass causing luminal narrowing. Surface ulceration often is present. Polypoid intraluminal masses (Case 35) and infiltrative tumors (Case 41) causing smoothly marginated strictures are seen less often. Radiographic features that suggest a malignant mass include surface irregularity and nodularity, abrupt and shelved margins, and fixed rigid masses that do not change shape or contour.

Case 34

# SMALL ESOPHAGEAL CARCINOMA

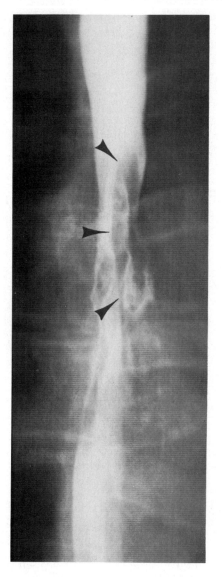

Small ulcerated mass *(arrows)* is present in the mid-esophagus. Squamous carcinoma was found at endoscopic biopsy. This cancer extended into but not through the muscularis. No lymph node metastases were found.

Unfortunately, most tumors detected in this country are of an advanced stage. The Japanese Society for Esophageal Diseases has adopted nomenclature for tumors that either are small or are early stage lesions. "Small" cancer refers to those less than 3.5 cm in diameter regardless of depth of invasion or nodal status. "Early" cancer is limited to the mucosa or submucosa without nodal metastases. "Superficial" cancer is confined to the mucosa or submucosa but lymph node metastases may be present. Prognosis is best determined by the presence of nodal metastases, which occur in nearly three-quarters of all patients. The esophagus has a rich intercommunicating lymphatic system. This allows metastatic deposits to implant anywhere within the esophagus or subdiaphragmatic region.

Case 35

# POLYPOID ESOPHAGEAL ADENOCARCINOMA

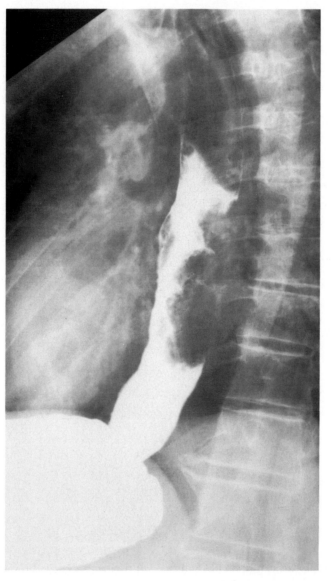

A large polypoid filling defect is present within the distal esophagus. This patient had an adenocarcinoma.

Squamous cell carcinomas rarely have this morphologic configuration. Adenocarcinomas and spindle cell carcinomas (carcinosarcoma) (Case 45) should be suspected when bulky polypoid tumors are present. Adenocarcinomas nearly always arise within Barrett's esophagus (Cases 15–18).

**Case 36**

## VARICOID ESOPHAGEAL CARCINOMA

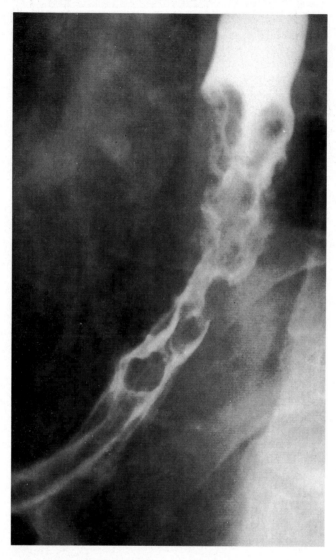

A large mass is present in the distal esophagus with associated thickened and nodular folds that resemble varices. Notice the abrupt edge forming the superior margin of the tumor. An adenocarcinoma was found at operation.

Most esophageal tumors do not have a varicoid appearance. These tumors have a substantial proportion of their mass extending within the submucosa, causing the distorted fold appearance. Tumors are fixed and rigid, unchanging with swallowing. Usually a peristaltic wave will not pass through such a diseased esophageal segment. Varices will change shape, especially with passage of a peristaltic stripping wave (Cases 52, 53, and 56).

**Case 37**

# ESOPHAGEAL CANCER WITH TRACHEOBRONCHIAL INVASION

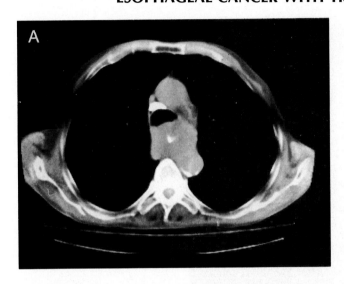

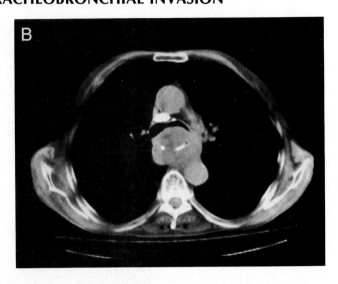

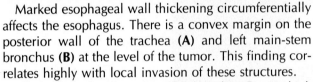

Marked esophageal wall thickening circumferentially affects the esophagus. There is a convex margin on the posterior wall of the trachea (**A**) and left main-stem bronchus (**B**) at the level of the tumor. This finding correlates highly with local invasion of these structures.

The normal esophageal wall is less than 3 mm thick (Halber et al., 1979). Wall thickening by itself is a nonspecific finding; both benign and malignant processes can have this appearance. Usually a barium swallow or endoscopy is necessary to determine the cause of the wall thickening. Detection of paraesophageal invasion can be difficult, especially if the patient is cachectic and has a paucity of mediastinal fat. Prior mediastinal operation or radiation therapy can also obliterate nor-

mal mediastinal fat planes. Intravenously administered contrast material may help display tissue boundaries better in some patients with questionable findings.

The posterior wall of the trachea and left main-stem bronchus is normally convex outward or flat (Case 4 B and C). Invasion by an adjacent esophageal mass should be suspected whenever there is inward bowing or a concavity of the trachea or left main-stem bronchus. Aortic invasion is rare (2% of patients at autopsy) (Postlethwait, 1979). Aortic invasion can be suspected if more than 90° of the periaortic fat is obliterated by the adjacent esophageal mass (Halvorsen and Thompson, 1984).

### Case 38

# ESOPHAGEAL CARCINOMA WITH PARAESOPHAGEAL LYMPHADENOPATHY

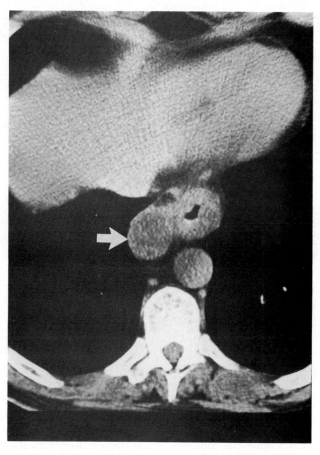

Marked esophageal wall thickening is present as a result of esophageal cancer. An enlarged lymph node *(arrow)* also is present and was found to contain metastases at operation.

Metastases often occur in microscopic quantities to normal-sized lymph nodes (often undetectable at CT).

The presence of enlarged nodes (1–1.5 cm) suggests metastases; however, the absence of adenopathy does not exclude disseminated disease. Even enlarged lymph nodes can be secondary to benign inflammatory disease.

**Case 39**

## METASTASES FROM ESOPHAGEAL CARCINOMA

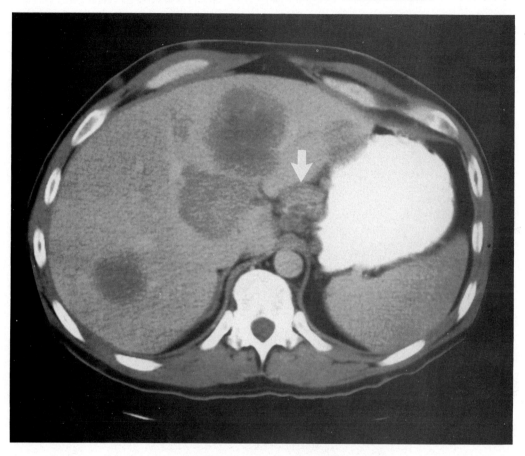

Multiple low-density liver metastases are present within all four segments of the liver. In addition, adenopathy *(arrow)* is present in the gastrohepatic ligament.

These are common locations for subdiaphragmatic metastases. Although distal esophageal tumors usually metastasize to sites below the diaphragm, tumors anywhere in the esophagus can metastasize to this region. The upper retroperitoneum about the celiac axis also is commonly affected by metastatic adenopathy. Complete CT staging of patients with esophageal carcinoma should include an examination of the upper abdomen enhanced with intravenously administered contrast material.

**Case 40**

## INFILTRATIVE ADENOCARCINOMA OF THE GASTROESOPHAGEAL JUNCTION

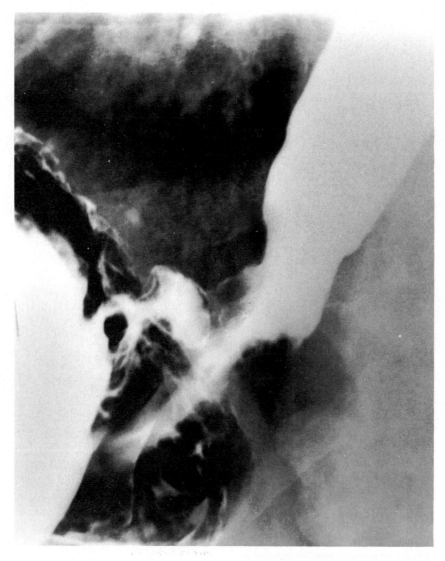

Irregular luminal narrowing is present, with nodularity of the distal esophagus. Adenocarcinoma was found at endoscopic biopsy.

Esophageal adenocarcinoma accounts for up to 20% of all esophageal malignancies (Levine et al., 1984). It is now believed that nearly all of these cancers either arise from Barrett's esophagus or from a fundal carcinoma that extends into the esophagus. The spread of adenocarcinoma resembles squamous carcinoma, except that there is a higher likelihood of involvement of the gastric cardia or fundus. There are some radiographic features that may suggest an adenocarcinoma rather than a squamous carcinoma: gastric invasion, distal esophageal location, and evidence of chronic reflux esophagitis (short esophagus hiatal hernia, reflux-induced stricture, significant history of reflux).

**Case 41**

# CARCINOMA OF THE ESOPHAGOGASTRIC JUNCTION: "SECONDARY ACHALASIA"

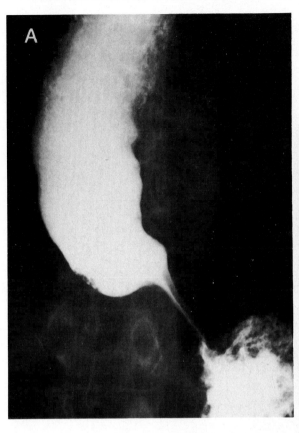

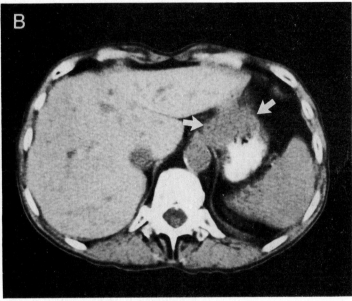

**A.** Fixed smooth narrowing is present in the distal esophagus. The proximal esophagus is dilated. At fluoroscopy the narrowing remained unchanged, even after the esophagus was half filled with contrast material.

**B.** A soft tissue mass *(arrows)* causing gastric wall thickening is present on the CT scan at the level of the gastroesophageal junction. The mass extended into the distal esophagus. Adenocarcinoma was found at operation.

Tumors such as this have predominantly submucosal growth and often arise from a gastric primary lesion. The radiographic findings can mimic achalasia. The terms "secondary achalasia" and "pseudoachalasia" have been used for such cases. Careful fluoroscopic observation of the cancerous esophagogastric junction during swallowing demonstrates a fixed, rigid stricture that never distends during esophageal emptying. The esophagogastric junction in achalasia (Case 60) opens transiently and distends when the hydrostatic barium column in the esophagus exceeds lower esophageal sphincter muscle tone. Peristalsis of the distal esophagus is absent in both conditions. The exact mechanism for this motor abnormality in patients with secondary achalasia is uncertain.

CT may be helpful in patients with equivocal findings because a soft tissue mass may be visible in patients with tumor.

Case 42

# VARICOID AND POLYPOID ADENOCARCINOMA OF THE ESOPHAGOGASTRIC JUNCTION

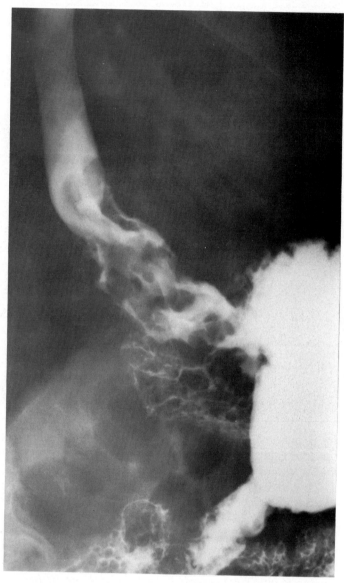

A lobulated, irregular mass is present within the distal esophagus. An adenocarcinoma was removed.

Most adenocarcinomas of the esophagus are infiltrative in appearance, but some have a polypoid component to them. Adenocarcinomas are more likely to appear polypoid than are squamous cancers. A varicoid appearance (Case 36) is due to submucosal infiltration by the tumor. Differentiation of submucosal tumor from varices is possible by observing that the neoplastic folds are fixed and unchanging, whereas varices (Cases 52 and 53) will empty and fill after a peristaltic stripping wave.

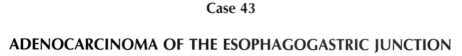

## Case 43

## ADENOCARCINOMA OF THE ESOPHAGOGASTRIC JUNCTION

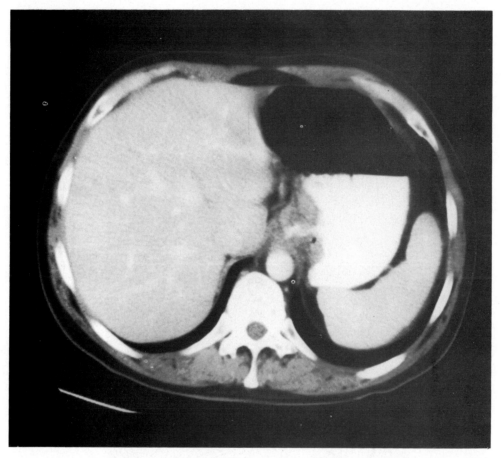

There is a circumferential soft tissue mass encasing the esophagogastric junction. At operation an adenocarcinoma was removed.

The normal gastric fundus can appear thickened if incompletely distended. Adequate distension of this region is necessary in order to detect masses about the esophagogastric junction and in the gastric cardia and fundus. Either positive orally administered contrast material or effervescent granules can be utilized. If effervescent granules are used, the patient may need to be scanned in the right lateral decubitus or prone position in order to achieve maximum gastric distension.

The exact role of CT in evaluating esophageal cancer is not yet clear. In some centers CT is used routinely in order to identify mediastinal invasion and subdiaphragmatic extent. These findings usually do not alter the surgical approach at our institution, but patient prognosis can be predicted if extensive metastases are present and radiation therapy can be planned. Tumors arising from the gastroesophageal junction are more often understaged by CT than are tumors located more proximally in the esophagus (Halvorsen and Thompson, 1984).

## Case 44

## RECURRENT ESOPHAGEAL CANCER

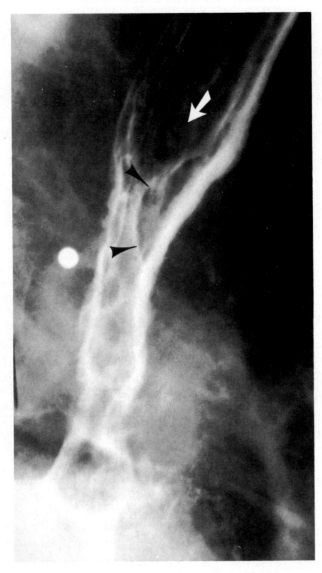

An esophagogastrectomy (Ivor-Lewis procedure) has been performed. The esophagus just above the anastomosis is narrowed with luminal irregularity, nodularity, mass effect *(arrowheads)*, and superficial ulceration *(arrow)*. Although these findings could be due to esophagitis, recurrent tumor should be excluded. Recurrent carcinoma was found at endoscopic biopsy.

The most frequent surgical procedure today for esophageal carcinoma is an esophagogastrectomy (Ivor-Lewis procedure or "gastric pull through"). This procedure has been associated with a lower complication rate than have jejunal or colon interposition grafts.

Complications occurring in the early postoperative period include anastomotic leaks and obstruction. Obstruction at the anastomosis is usually due to edema, hematoma, or, infrequently, spasm. Late complications include recurrent cancer, gastroesophageal reflux and esophagitis, and anastomotic strictures. Recurrent cancer should be suspected if a mass (usually > 1 cm) is identified, if there is eccentric narrowing of the lumen, or if there is nodularity or ulceration of the mucosa. Equivocal findings should be investigated further with endoscopy and biopsy.

**Case 45**

# CARCINOSARCOMA (SPINDLE CELL CARCINOMA)

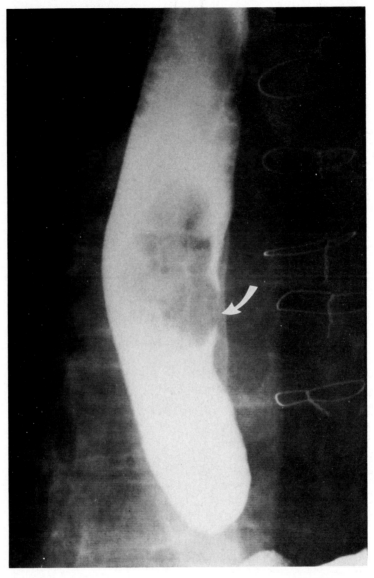

A large, bulky filling defect is seen within the distal esophagus. A pedicle *(arrow)* is seen attaching the tumor to the left side of the esophagus. Spindle cell carcinoma was diagnosed at operation.

Spindle cell carcinomas contain histologic elements of both carcinoma and sarcoma. In the past these tumors have been called carcinosarcomas. Patients usually present with dysphagia and weight loss. Radiologically, these tumors usually appear as bulky, polypoid intraluminal tumors. The mass may expand the esophageal lumen, but obstruction is rare.

Differential considerations include a pedunculated leiomyoma, lipoma, or fibrovascular polyp. Other sarcomatous tumors could also have this appearance.

## Case 46

## ESOPHAGEAL LYMPHOMA

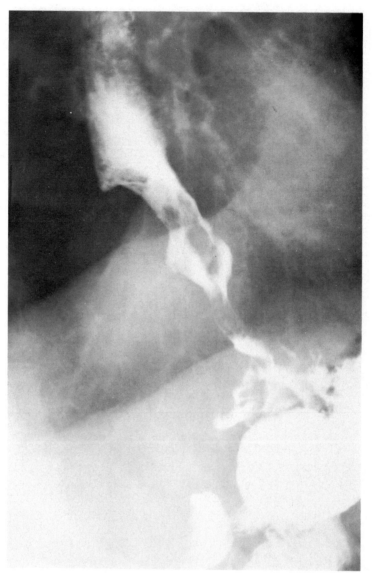

A large, lobulated, and ulcerated mass constricts the distal esophagus. This process resembles primary carcinoma of the esophagus, but lymphoma was proven pathologically.

The most common intrinsic manifestation of lym-phoma is a polypoid, ulcerative, or infiltrative mass—usually indistinguishable from primary esophageal cancer. Less frequently, submucosal infiltration of tumor will result in varicoid folds, discrete small submucosal masses, or diffuse nodular changes (Case 47).

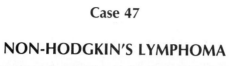

**Case 47**

# NON-HODGKIN'S LYMPHOMA

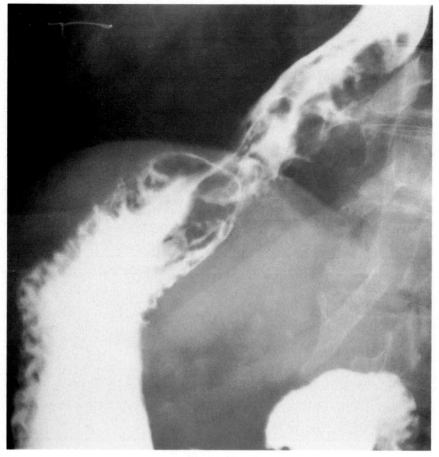

A polypoid mass is present in the distal esophagus. This has an appearance that suggests the more common adenocarcinoma. At operation, lymphoma was discovered.

**Case 48**

## NON-HODGKIN'S LYMPHOMA: TRACHEOESOPHAGEAL FISTULA

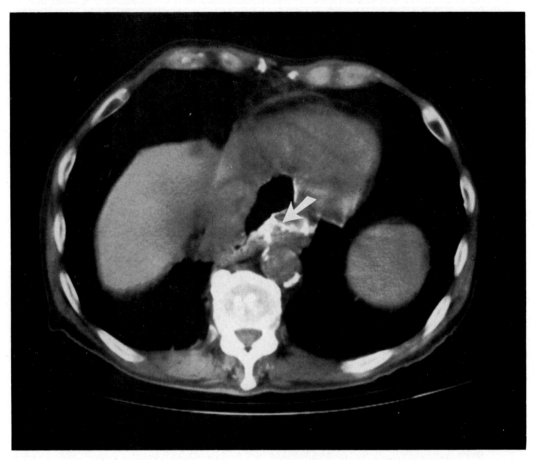

The wall of the esophagus is diffusely thickened. A fistulous communication *(arrow)* is opacified between the esophagus and a mediastinal cavity with orally administered contrast material. Esophageal lymphoma was confirmed pathologically.

Non-Hodgkin's lymphoma does not typically incite a host desmoplastic response about the tumor, as is often present with carcinomas. This lack of peritumoral fibrosis and containment probably is responsible for the relatively frequent occurrence of fistulae and perforation that is seen in patients with non-Hodgkin's lymphoma. Hodgkin's disease is often associated with a normal desmoplastic reaction, and fistulae and perforation are uncommon.

**Case 49**

## NON-HODGKIN'S LYMPHOMA: EXTRINSIC COMPRESSION

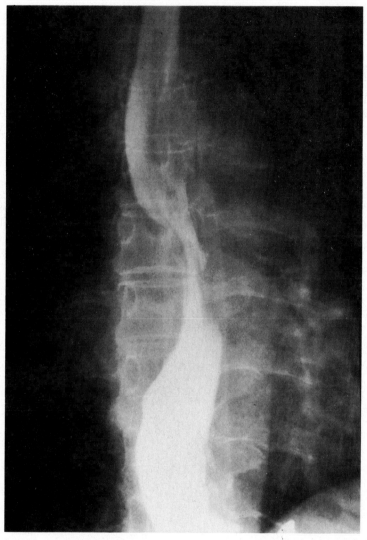

Extrinsic compression and narrowing is present involving the mid-esophagus from enlarged subcarinal lymph nodes. This patient had known lymphoma.

Lymphomatous involvement of the esophagus is unusual. Usually, patients have known generalized lymphoma before esophageal disease is discovered. This disease can affect the esophagus by mass effect or by direct spread from enlarged contiguous lymph nodes. Lymphomatous involvement of the stomach can spread directly to the esophagus or a lesion can develop in the esophagus simultaneous with disease elsewhere in the body.

## Case 50

# MEDIASTINAL LYMPHADENOPATHY WITH INVASION

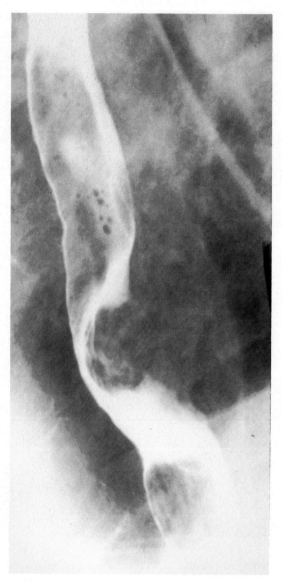

There is a polypoid, lobulated filling defect in the esophagus, with an associated extrinsic mass that displaces the esophagus posteriorly. This patient had a known small cell carcinoma of the lung. Extensive mediastinal lymphadenopathy causing the changes on the esophagram was present at CT.

Metastases to the esophagus usually arise from cancers of the stomach, lung, or breast. Most of these tumors metastasize to mediastinal lymph nodes, and with growth they can displace or directly invade the esoph-

agus. The surface of the esophagus will remain smooth (Case 51) if invasion and ulceration have not developed. In some patients the abnormality may resemble a primary esophageal cancer or present as a long, narrow stricture. Displacement of the lumen by nodal mass is common. The mid-esophagus is most commonly affected because subcarinal lymph nodes are most often affected. Hematogenous metastases to the esophagus are unusual.

## Case 51

## METASTATIC LYMPHADENOPATHY

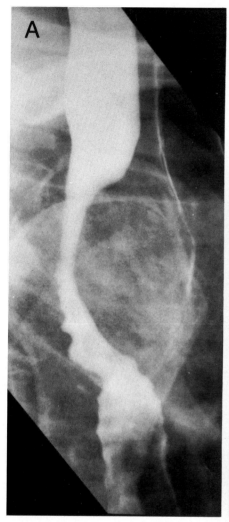

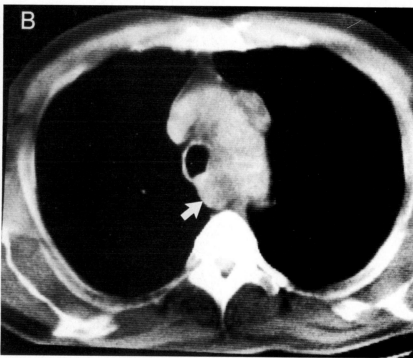

**A.** A smooth, extrinsic mass compresses and displaces the mid-esophagus.

**B.** Mediastinal lymphadenopathy *(arrow)* is present at CT.

This patient had an adenocarcinoma of the lung with metastatic lymphadenopathy. The enlarged metastatic lymph nodes are responsible for the changes in the esophagram.

Differential considerations for esophageal compression or displacement include benign tumors (most commonly a leiomyoma) (Case 29), enterogenous cysts (Cases 79 and 80), vascular anomalies or aneurysms, and pleural or mediastinal scarring. Mass lesions narrow the esophageal lumen, whereas pleural and pulmonary fibrosis often widens the lumen at the level of esophageal displacement.

## Case 52

## "UPHILL" VARICES

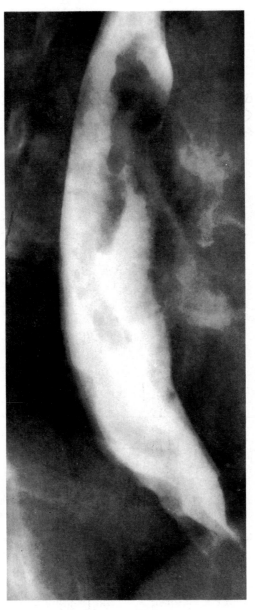

Multiple serpentine filling defects are present in the lower esophagus. This appearance is typical of varices.

Esophageal varices are dilated submucosal veins that develop as a result of portal venous hypertension. Hepatic cirrhosis is the most frequent cause of portal venous hypertension. Elevated portal venous pressure reverses normal venous blood flow so that flow occurs in an "uphill" fashion from portal vein to left gastric (coronary) vein to periesophageal venous plexus to azygous and hemiazygous collaterals that empty into the superior vena cava.

Varices almost never cause dysphagia but they can bleed and cause life-threatening hemorrhage. Variceal bleeding has been thought to cause one-third of the deaths and 90% of the bleeding in patients with cirrhosis (Dave et al., 1983).

**Case 53**

## ESOPHAGEAL VARICES

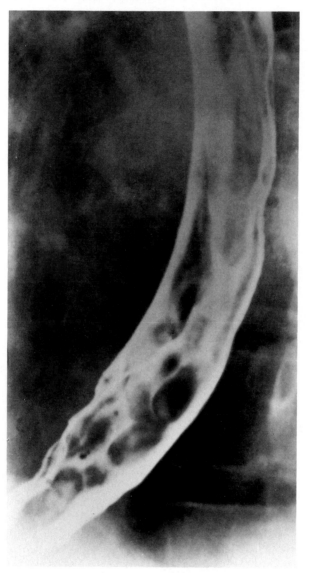

Double-contrast radiograph of the lower esophagus demonstrates multiple serpentine filling defects. These defects changed in size and shape during fluoroscopic observation and between radiographs. Varices were confirmed endoscopically.

The radiographic diagnosis of esophageal varices is most sensitive when the partially collapsed esophagus is examined. Varices can be obliterated by the filled distended esophagus as well as the collapsed esophagus immediately after a stripping peristaltic wave. Varices appear as linear, often serpentine filling defects with a scalloped esophageal contour. Uphill varices are more prominent in the distal esophagus. The changing nature of varices with esophageal distension, peristalsis, and respiratory effort is helpful in differentiating varices from a varicoid carcinoma (Case 36) that appears fixed, noncompliant, and often has shouldered margins. Reflux esophagitis can also cause thickened and irregular esophageal folds (Case 7). Usually patients have an associated hiatal hernia with gastroesophageal reflux and other radiographic signs of esophagitis.

## Case 54

# PORTAL VENOUS HYPERTENSION: LEFT GASTRIC AND ESOPHAGEAL VARICES

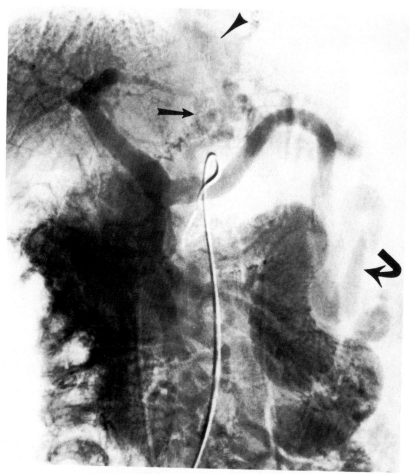

Subtraction mesenteric (superior mesenteric artery injection) arterial portogram in a patient with portal venous hypertension. Enlarged left gastric (coronary) veins *(straight arrow)* and esophageal varices *(arrowhead)* are visible as blood follows the lowest pressure venous channels—bypassing the high resistance portal circulation. The mesenteric veins appear mildly dilated, and large extraperitoneal collaterals *(curved arrow)* are also present along the left side of the abdomen.

## Case 55

## VARICES: CT

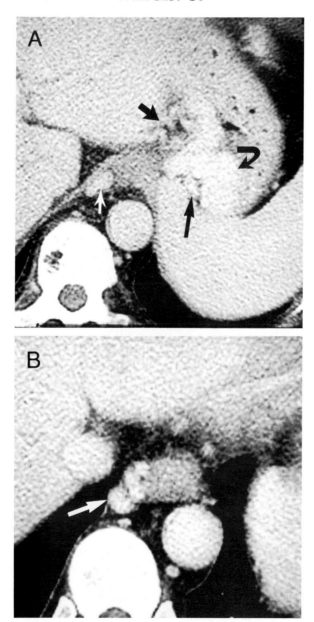

**A.** Multiple enhancing varices are present in the upper abdomen. Left gastric *(short, black arrow)*, short gastric *(long, black arrow)*, and esophageal varices *(white arrow)* can be identified. Gastric varices *(curved arrow)* are also visible by diffusely enhancing the gastric wall about the gastroesophageal junction.

**B.** Several esophageal varices *(arrow)* can be identified within the periesophageal tissues.

CT is an excellent technique for detecting upper abdominal varices and their distribution. In addition, morphologic changes of cirrhosis in the liver and enlargement of the spleen as well as patency of the portal and splenic veins can be assessed.

## Case 56

## DOWNHILL ESOPHAGEAL VARICES

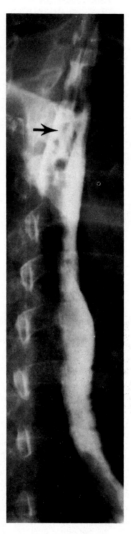

Tubular, thickened folds *(arrow)* are present in the upper thoracic esophagus due to endoscopically proven esophageal varices.

"Downhill" varices develop as a result of superior vena cava obstruction, most commonly due to bronchogenic carcinoma or lymphoma. Collaterals of the supreme intercostal vein, bronchial veins, inferior thyroidal veins, and other periesophageal collaterals will enlarge and may be visible on an esophagram in the upper one-third of the esophagus. Blood flows "down" (caudally) the azygous/hemiazygous system and reenters the systemic circulation via the left gastric and portal veins. Unlike uphill varices, which often cause gastrointestinal bleeding, downhill varices are usually asymptomatic. In fact, in clinical practice these varices are rarely encountered. In the absence of the "superior vena cava syndrome," other diagnostic considerations should be entertained, such as varicoid carcinoma (Case 36).

Rarely, a varix will be identified in patients without portal venous hypertension or superior vena cava obstruction. Varices in these patients are considered idiopathic. These varices will change size and shape (as will varices of any cause) with esophageal distension and after a peristaltic stripping wave. If the varix is thrombosed, it may be indistinguishable from a submucosal tumor.

## Case 57

# ESOPHAGEAL ULCERATION AFTER VARICEAL SCLEROTHERAPY

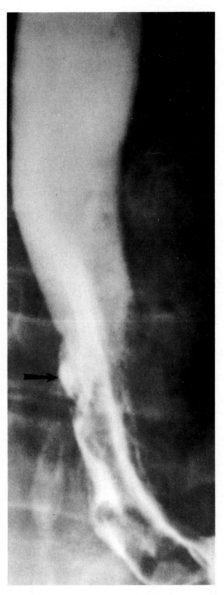

Nodular filling defects are present in the distal esophagus due to varices. A flat ulceration *(arrow)* is present at the site of injection after variceal sclerotherapy.

Endoscopic sclerotherapy for esophageal varices has been shown to be a useful treatment option in patients with portal venous hypertension. Obliteration of intraluminal varices is accomplished, decreasing the risk of recurrent variceal bleeding.

Acute complications after sclerotherapy include mucosal ulceration (as seen above), perforation, mediastinal abscess, and empyema. Chest pain and dysphagia are present transiently in many patients. Pleural effusions can be seen in about half of all patients. Chronically, an esophageal stricture may develop at the site of sclerosis.

## Case 58

## TERTIARY ESOPHAGEAL CONTRACTIONS

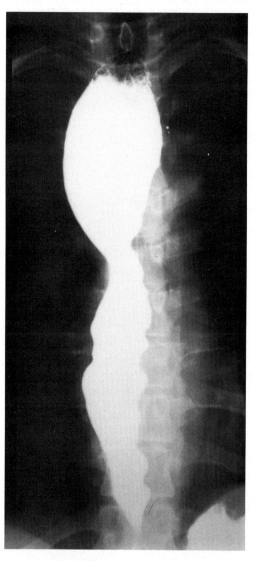

Multiple nonpropulsive contractions are present in the lower esophagus. These contractions are referred to as tertiary contractions and increase in frequency in aging individuals.

Esophageal contractions can be categorized as three separate types: primary, secondary, or tertiary. Primary esophageal peristalsis is initiated by a swallow and propagates a smooth continuous contraction the length of the esophagus. Secondary esophageal peristalsis appears fluoroscopically identical to a primary wave, except it is not initiated by a swallow but rather by a bolus within the esophagus or by intraesophageal disten-

sion. Tertiary esophageal contractions are nonpropulsive contractions that may be single or multiple, and they do not result in clearing of esophageal contents.

In addition to aging (presbyesophagus), tertiary contractions can be associated with many diseases such as diabetes, connective tissue disorders, chemical injuries to the esophagus, infections, metabolic disorders, neurologic disorders, muscular diseases, and vascular and neoplastic conditions. Incomplete relaxation of the lower esophageal sphincter can also be seen in some patients.

## Case 59

# DIFFUSE ESOPHAGEAL SPASM

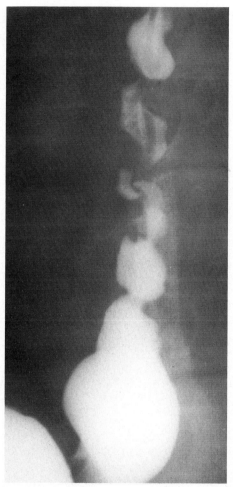

Numerous nonpropulsive contractions are present in the lower esophagus. This appearance has been likened to a "corkscrew."

Diffuse esophageal spasm is characterized by dysphagia or chest pain with at least 30% of swallows associated with vigorous, repetitive, nonpropulsive contractions (McNally and Katz, 1967; Cohen, 1979). Careful fluoroscopy eventually demonstrates a normal peristaltic sequence. Lower esophageal sphincter function may be normal; however, nearly a third of patients have impaired relaxation or increased resting pressures (DiMarino and Cohen, 1974). Various terms have been used to describe the radiologic appearance of the nonpropulsive contractions, including corkscrew, curling, rosary bead, and shish kebab esophagus.

The term "nutcracker esophagus" refers to a disorder characterized by the manometric findings of high amplitude (> 180 mm Hg) contractions in conjunction with chest discomfort. Radiographically, normal peristalsis is seen. Some authorities feel this disorder is a precursor to diffuse esophageal spasm.

The principal differential consideration is achalasia. Achalasia (Case 60) can be excluded by demonstrating a normal stripping wave in response to some swallows. Some patients will be symptomatic and others are not but have identical radiographic findings. It is important to exclude other causes of chest pain, especially coronary artery disease, before attributing it to the esophageal abnormalities.

## Case 60

## ACHALASIA

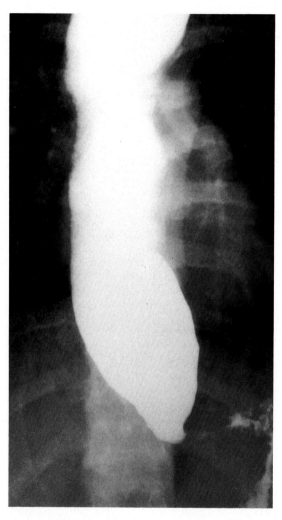

There is dilatation of the esophagus to the level of the lower esophageal sphincter. A "beaklike" deformity is present near the gastroesophageal junction. Aperistalsis of the smooth muscle portion (distal two-thirds) was observed fluoroscopically.

Achalasia is a motor disorder of the esophagus characterized by aperistalsis of the distal two-thirds (smooth muscle portion) of the esophagus and failure of the lower esophageal sphincter to relax. Patients usually complain of dysphagia, often with recumbent regurgitation and episodes of aspiration pneumonia.

Radiographically, the esophagus is often dilated and a standing column of contrast material is seen (the height of the column is proportional to the severity of lower esophageal obstruction). Periodic relaxation of the lower esophageal sphincter with continued drinking by the patient is a critical observation in distinguishing primary achalasia from secondary achalasia—most importantly due to carcinoma of the gastroesophageal junction (a fixed, nonrelaxing obstruction) (Case 41). Manometry is now considered the standard for diagnosing achalasia.

Treatment for achalasia depends on the severity of the lower esophageal obstruction. Medical treatment with smooth muscle relaxants, transesophageal balloon dilatation across the lower esophageal sphincter, or surgical incision of the lower esophageal muscle fibers (Heller myotomy) accounts for the majority of treatment options.

## Case 61

# VIGOROUS ACHALASIA

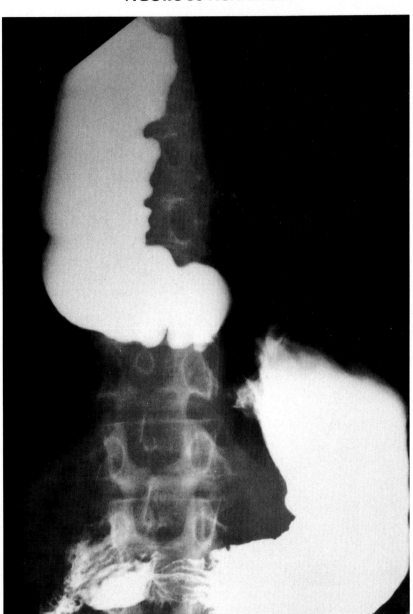

The esophagus is dilated to the gastroesophageal junction. Smooth, tapered narrowing of the lower esophageal segment was observed with intermittent, transient opening. In addition, multiple nonpropulsive contractions were present in the lower esophageal segment. No normal stripping wave was observed.

Vigorous achalasia is now considered a less severe or early form of achalasia with motor abnormalities similar to those of achalasia seen fluoroscopically, in addition to repetitive, simultaneous nonpropulsive contractions. These patients may have chest pain as well as typical dysphagia. Esophageal dilatation may be only minimal.

## Case 62

## ACHALASIA WITH ESOPHAGEAL CARCINOMA

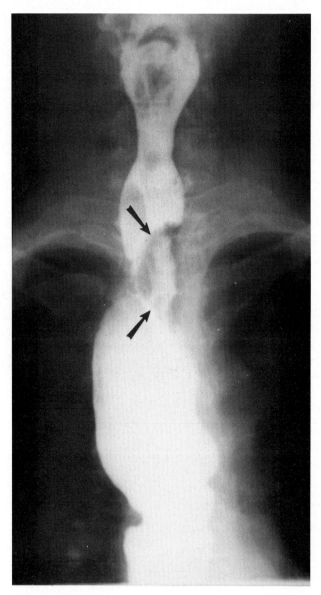

The esophagus is dilated. At the junction of the cervical and thoracic esophagus there is an ulcerated mass *(arrows)*. This was proved surgically to be a squamous cell carcinoma.

Complications from achalasia include carcinoma and *Candida* esophagitis. Carcinomas are nearly always squamous cell type, developing in a patient with long-standing (> 20 years) achalasia. The upper and mid-esophagus are common locations for these cancers.

Candidiasis (Cases 20–23) develops as a result of chronic stasis. Fine mucosal nodularity or a reticular pattern is a common finding. Occasionally, a fungus ball is present. These present as filling defects within the esophageal lumen. Esophageal lavage may be necessary to clear retained food and identify this abnormality.

## Case 63

# SCLERODERMA

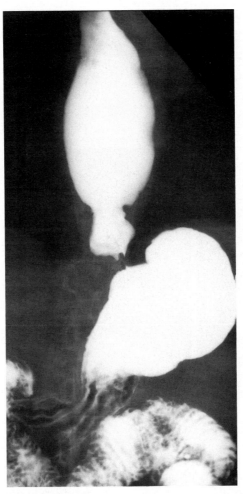

The lower esophagus is dilated above a lower esophageal benign ("peptic")-appearing stricture and small hiatal hernia. At fluoroscopy, peristalsis was absent below the level of the aortic arch. Scleroderma was later confirmed clinically.

Patients with scleroderma (progressive systemic sclerosis) often have changes that are recognized radiologically in the esophagus before the development of the characteristic skin changes. Pathologically, degeneration and atrophy of the smooth muscle are seen, with associated fibrosis within the distal two-thirds of the esophagus. Radiographic changes relate to decreased peristalsis or atony in the distal two-thirds of the esophagus, with a patulous and incompetent lower esophageal sphincter. Free gastroesophageal reflux and changes of active peptic esophagitis often can be ob-

served. Chronically, a lower esophageal stricture is often present. The stricture may be so severe as to cause high-grade obstruction of the distal esophagus, sometimes presenting with an esophageal air-fluid level on the chest radiograph.

Diminished esophageal clearance results in stasis and possible secondary esophageal candidiasis and aspiration pneumonitis. In addition, chronic reflux esophagitis can be complicated by Barrett's esophagus (Cases 15–17) and the associated risk of adenocarcinoma (Cases 33, 35, 36, and 40–42).

Interstitial fibrosis may be present in the lung bases as well as other changes of scleroderma in the small bowel, including diminished peristalsis, dilatation, sacculations, and closely spaced valvulae conniventes.

## Case 64

## SCLERODERMA

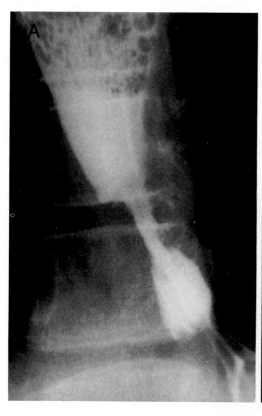

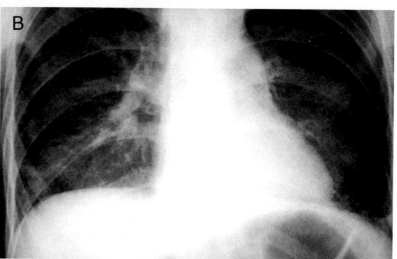

**A.** The lower esophagus is irregularly narrowed above a small esophageal hiatal hernia. The proximal esophagus is dilated, and spontaneous gastroesophageal reflux was observed at fluoroscopy with the patient in the recumbent position. The distal two-thirds of the esophagus was also observed to be aperistaltic.

**B.** A fine pattern of bilateral interstitial fibrosis is present in both lung bases. These findings are typical of scleroderma with associated pulmonary involvement.

The changes in the distal esophagus are due to active reflux esophagitis. The abrupt and shouldered margins of the stricture are worrisome for neoplasms and endoscopy was recommended to further evaluate this region.

Case 65

## ZENKER'S DIVERTICULUM

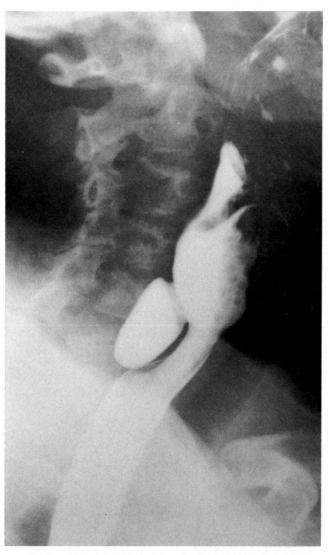

Zenker's diverticulum is a protrusion of the esophageal mucosa through an anatomically weak area in the posterior wall of the cervical esophagus. The site of weakness lies between the oblique and horizontal fibers of the esophageal wall known as Killian's dehiscence or triangle. The cricopharyngeus muscle is invariably prominent just caudal to the diverticulum.

Most authorities believe these diverticula result from abnormally increased pressure generated in the hypopharynx. This high pressure is due to failure of the cricopharyngeus muscle to relax after pharyngeal contraction during swallowing. The role of gastroesophageal reflux in abnormal cricopharyngeus muscle function is unclear. However, many patients with gastroesophageal reflux have a prominent cricopharyngeus muscle.

Retention of food and fluid within the diverticulum can be uncomfortable and socially embarrassing, and it can lead to aspiration when recumbent. Cricopharyngeal myotomy and either surgical diverticulopexy or diverticulectomy may be required to treat symptomatic diverticula.

## Case 66

## MID-ESOPHAGEAL DIVERTICULUM

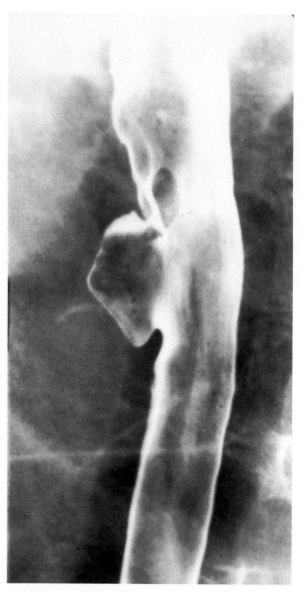

A wide-based outpouching arises from the mid-esophagus. The tip of this diverticulum is pointed and triangular. This particular shape is often found among traction diverticula as a result of fibrosis in periesophageal tissues. Tuberculosis with inflammatory mediastinal lymph nodes was implicated as an important cause of traction diverticula in the past. Today, most esophageal diverticula are pulsion in origin, developing as a result of esophageal motor disorders. Pulsion diverticula are usually rounded and fail to empty (they contain no muscle in their wall) with a peristaltic contraction.

Most mid-esophageal diverticula are asymptomatic. A large diverticulum can compress the esophagus and lead to dysphagia. If a diverticulum overflows into the esophagus, aspiration can occur. Inflammation and infection could lead to rare complications of perforation or fistulization.

**Case 67**

# EPIPHRENIC DIVERTICULUM

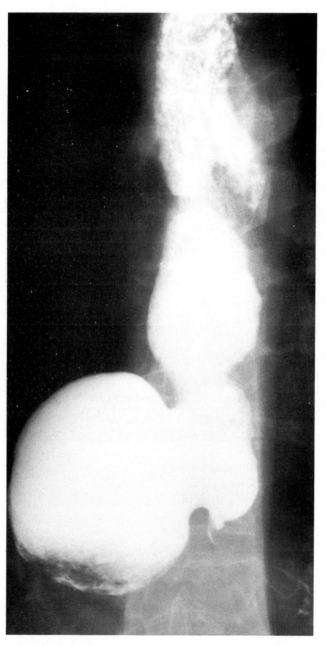

Diverticula arising in the distal esophagus just above the gastroesophageal junction are referred to as epiphrenic diverticula. These outpouchings are nearly always pulsion in origin. Achalasia or other motor abnormalities of the esophagus are often associated with this condition. This patient has achalasia.

## Case 68

## EPIPHRENIC DIVERTICULUM

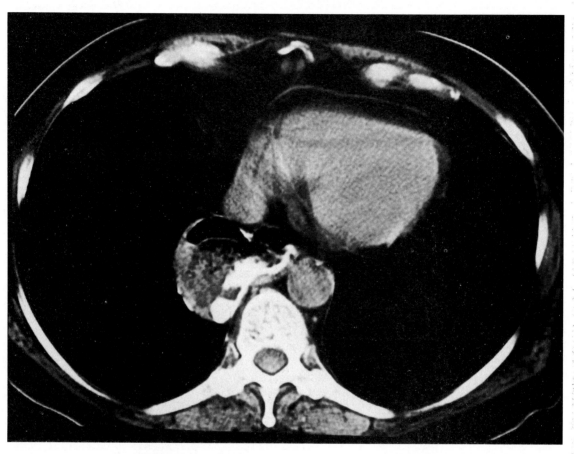

CT of the lower thorax shows a large thin-walled sac that communicates with the esophagus. Orally administered contrast material and food are seen within the diverticulum. Findings are typical of an epiphrenic diverticulum.

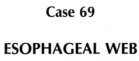

**Case 69**

# ESOPHAGEAL WEB

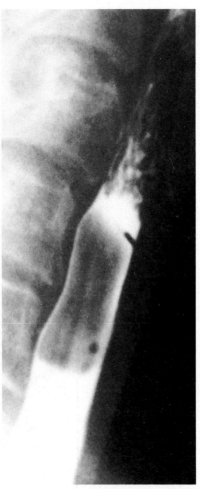

Esophageal webs are thin, delicate membranes that cause a shelflike impression on the anterior surface of the upper esophagus at the C5–6 level (usually at the pharyngoesophageal junction). Occasionally, webs may be multiple and more masslike in configuration.

Distinction of an esophageal web from the anteriorly located venous plexus (Case 1) may at times be difficult. Careful study of the venous plexus will demonstrate variability in its size, whereas a web remains fixed and unchanging from swallow to swallow.

Webs may cause dysphagia, depending on the degree of luminal narrowing. Clinically significant narrowing may present as a "jet phenomenon" whereby a narrow column of contrast material is seen distal to the obstruction.

In the past, many investigators attempted to associate cervical esophageal webs with other conditions. The Plummer-Vinson syndrome described patients with anemia and postcricoid dysphagia (Vinson, 1922). This same group of patients was also found to have atrophy of the tongue, pharynx, and esophagus (Kelly, 1919; Paterson, 1919). Later, the association of hypopharyngeal and cervical esophageal webs with iron deficiency anemia was described (Waldenström and Kjellberg, 1939). Subsequent reports have also suggested an association between webs and upper esophageal or pharyngeal carcinoma (Shamma'a and Benedict, 1958). Today, the association between esophageal webs and anemia is unclear. Most webs are an isolated finding, often incidentally discovered without an associated systemic disorder.

**Case 70**

## ESOPHAGEAL FOREIGN BODY

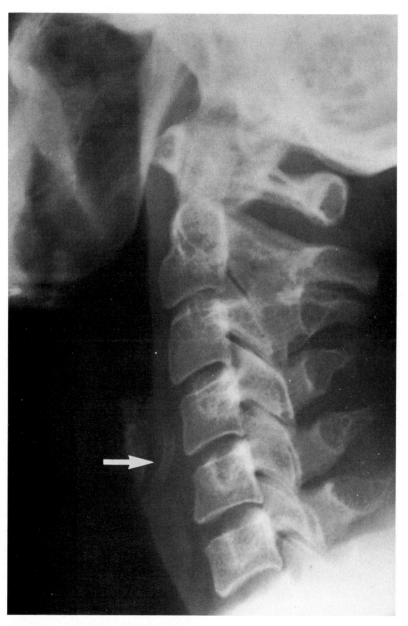

There is a bone fragment *(arrow)* in the region of the esophagus at the level of the C-4 interspace on this lateral plain film radiograph of the neck. The patient complained of food sticking and pain while eating chicken. A chicken bone was removed endoscopically.

Bony foreign bodies such as chicken or fish bones often lodge in the upper esophagus, whereas meat impactions (Case 71) most commonly occur at the gastroesophageal junction. Impacted bones are often best visualized on a lateral radiograph of the cervical region. Contrast material may obscure a small fragment. Esophageal perforation (Cases 73 and 74) is an unusual complication of impacted foreign bodies, but it occurs most frequently when the impaction persists more than 24 hours.

## Case 71

## ESOPHAGEAL FOREIGN BODY

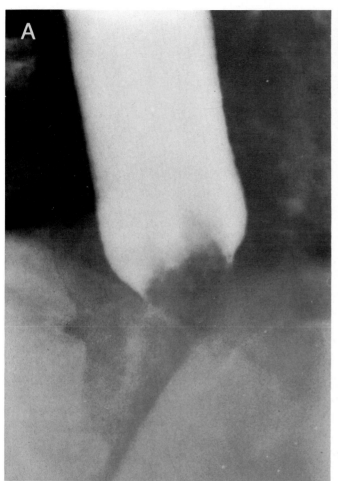

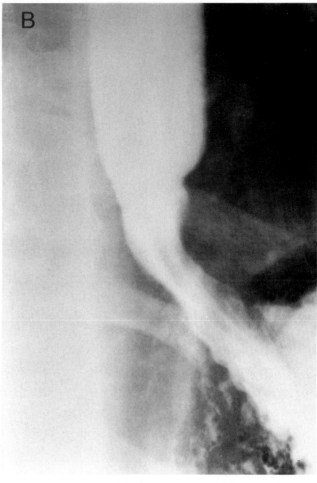

**A.** An intraluminal filling defect is present in the distal esophagus just above the gastroesophageal junction. This patient had a typical history of swallowing a large piece of meat and immediately experiencing odynophagia. Glucagon (1 mg) was given intravenously, and the meat bolus passed into the stomach.

**B.** Subsequent esophagram shows a small hiatal hernia and mild narrowing at the gastroesophageal junction.

Impacted food typically lodges above the gastroesophageal junction. Several techniques can be used to remove the food. Intravenously administered glucagon decreases the lower esophageal sphincter pressure and may facilitate passage of the food bolus into the stomach. Generally, if the bolus reaches the stomach, it will pass through the remainder of the alimentary tract without difficulty. Endoscopic retrieval is the traditional means of treatment. Baskets and balloon catheters also have been used successfully in extracting these foreign bodies. Effervescent granules and meat tenderizer have been used successfully by others but have not been used in our practice because of the possible risk of perforation by these methods. If an impaction has persisted for more than 24 hours, the risk of perforation increases due to possible transmural ischemia. Special care must be taken in these patients. It is important to examine the esophagus after the food bolus has been passed or removed in order to exclude an underlying lesion.

**Case 72**

## ESOPHAGEAL FOREIGN BODIES

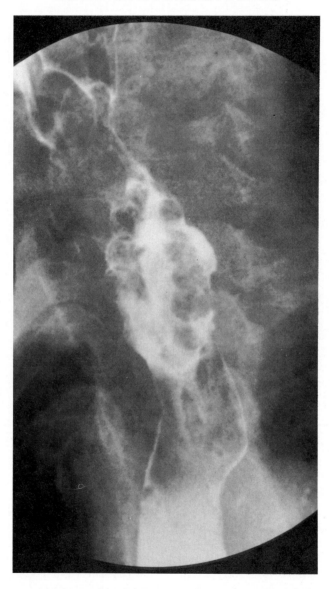

Multiple round foreign bodies (a rosary) are present in the upper esophagus.

Nonbony foreign bodies often require oral administration of contrast material to be visible. Barium is usually the best agent to use in patients with acute impactions and in the absence of signs of perforation. Barium is heavier per unit volume than water-soluble contrast material and may "push" a foreign body through the esophagus. Additionally, in the event of complete esophageal obstruction and aspiration, barium is less harmful than water-soluble agents. Careful fluoroscopic observation is important in assessing the proper amount of contrast material, in making the correct diagnosis, and in observing the passage or persistent impaction of the foreign body. Foreign bodies that will not spontaneously pass require endoscopic retrieval.

**Case 73**

## ESOPHAGEAL PERFORATION

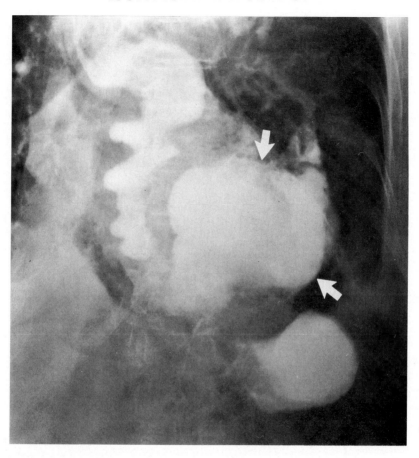

A large amount of contrast material has extravasated *(arrows)* into the mediastinum during the course of an esophagram with a water-soluble agent. This patient had a known history of achalasia, and pain developed after dilatation of the lower esophageal sphincter. Surgical repair was required.

Esophageal perforation is usually due to iatrogenic procedures (endoscopic perforations account for 75% to 80% of all esophageal leaks and occur in about 1 per 1,000 patients undergoing fiberoptic endoscopy) (Love and Berkow, 1978) or spontaneous perforation (Boerhaave's syndrome) from violent retching or vomiting. Most endoscopic perforations involve the cervical esophagus near the cricopharyngeal muscle. Spontaneous rupture nearly always occurs just above the gastroesophageal junction on the left. Early detection of these perforations is critical to patient survival. Small cervical esophageal leaks often can be treated conservatively, but larger leaks must be surgically repaired to

prevent development of a retropharyngeal abscess. Untreated thoracic esophageal perforations have at least a 70% mortality (due to mediastinitis) if the leak is undiscovered (O'Connell, 1967).

Esophageal perforations can be suspected from the chest radiograph by detection of pneumomediastinum, widening of the mediastinum, hydropneumothorax, pleural effusion(s), and subcutaneous emphysema. Suspected perforations on the basis of the chest radiograph or on clinical grounds should be confirmed by an esophagram with contrast material. A water-soluble contrast agent should be administered initially to assess for moderate to large leaks. Small leaks may be overlooked using water-soluble contrast agents and negative studies should be immediately followed by a barium esophagram, which is more sensitive in detecting smaller leaks (because of its higher density and better coating properties).

## Case 74

# ESOPHAGEAL PERFORATION

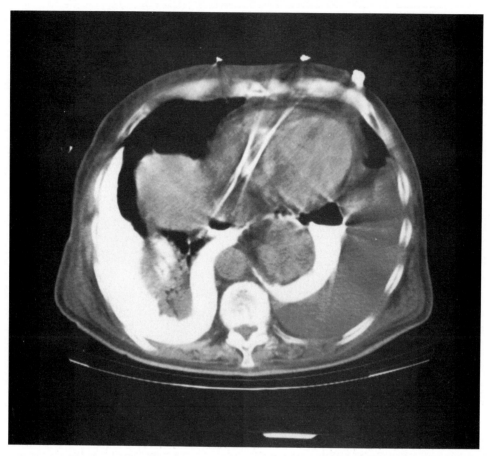

Orally administered contrast material is seen in the pleural spaces bilaterally. Air is also present within the mediastinum and pleural space. This patient had undergone endoscopy that resulted in a lower esophageal perforation. Emergent surgical drainage and diversion were required.

CT is an excellent modality for evaluating patients with suspected or known esophageal perforation. Small amounts of extravasated air (pneumomediastinum) or contrast material and its location within the chest can be identified readily. This information can be helpful in deciding if surgery will be necessary and the approach required.

**Case 75**

## LATERAL PHARYNGEAL POUCHES

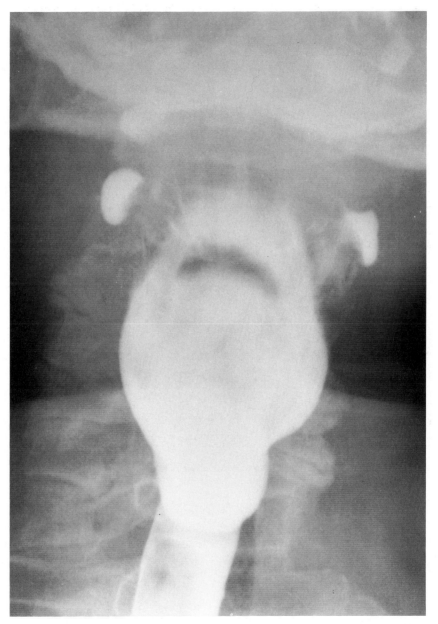

Small outpouchings are seen arising from both sides of the hypopharynx.

Lateral pharyngeal pouches arise from an unsupported "weak area" of the thyrohyoid membrane that does not contain a muscular covering. Pouches may be best demonstrated during the pharyngeal phase of swallowing or by asking a patient to blow through closed lips (modified Valsalva maneuver). These pouches are most commonly seen among glassblowers, wind instrument players, and the elderly. They usually do not cause symptoms but occasionally may reach several centimeters in diameter and be multiple.

## Case 76

## ESOPHAGEAL CROHN'S DISEASE

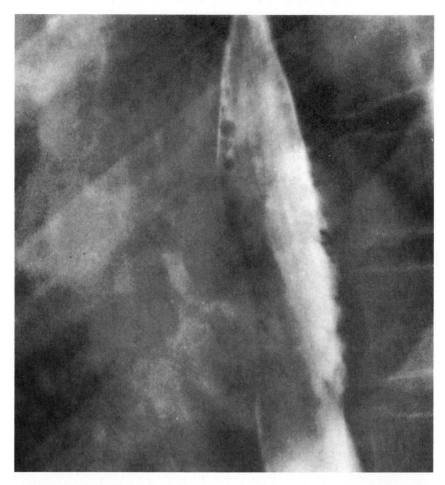

A segmental region of deep ulceration affects a non-circumferential portion of the mid-esophagus. These changes were due to Crohn's disease.

Crohn's disease rarely affects the esophagus, and when it does disease is almost always present in the small bowel and colon. Most patients seek medical attention because of symptoms from disease elsewhere in the alimentary tract or from an esophageal stricture that is causing dysphagia.

The usual radiographic finding is aphthous ulcers (discrete ulcers surrounded by a mound of edema) which usually require double-contrast radiography for detection. Confluent ulcerations and deep ulcers (as seen in this case) can be found in more severe disease. Transmural disease may lead to esophageal perforation and fistula formation. Progressive scarring can lead to stricture formation.

**Case 77**

# GLYCOGENIC ACANTHOSIS

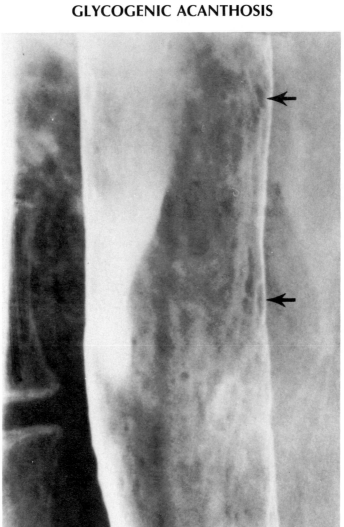

Multiple mildly elevated plaquelike defects *(arrows)* are seen within the esophagus. This elderly patient had no esophageal symptoms.

Glycogenic acanthosis is an incidental finding in older patients due to increased cytoplasmic glycogen within the squamous epithelial cells of the esophagus. Radiologically, nodular filling defects are seen which range in size from 1 to 15 mm (Bender et al., 1973). Rarely, nodules may coalesce to form larger plaques.

Often the margins of these lesions are hazy and fade peripherally.

Esophagitis (Cases 8 and 10) is the main differential consideration. Patients with glycogenic acanthosis are almost always asymptomatic. Conditions such as *Candida* esophagitis (Cases 20 and 22), superficial spreading carcinoma, and leukoplakia (Case 78) could have a similar appearance.

## Case 78

# ESOPHAGEAL LEUKOPLAKIA

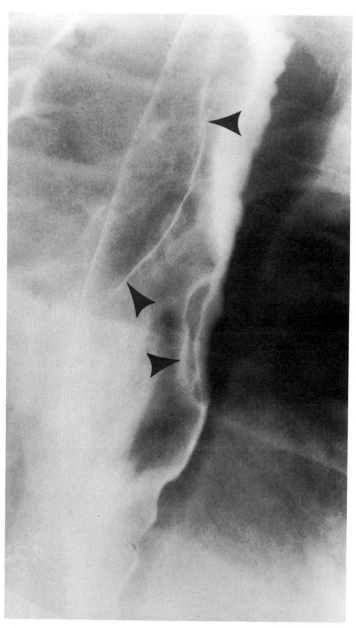

Two separate plaquelike filling defects *(arrowheads)* are present in the esophagus. These were due to leukoplakia proven endoscopically.

Leukoplakia is a rare condition in the esophagus; it is usually confined to the oral cavity. Oral leukoplakia is considered a premalignant condition, but there are no reports of esophageal leukoplakia becoming malignant.

Radiologically, a discrete mucosal plaque(s) is seen. It may be indistinguishable from glycogenic acanthosis radiologically (Case 77). Endoscopic biopsy is required to confirm the diagnosis.

**Case 79**

# ESOPHAGEAL DUPLICATION CYST

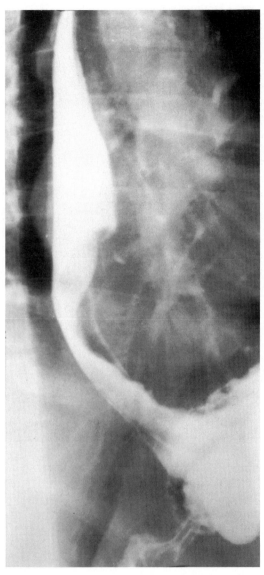

A large, extramucosal mass deforms the lumen of the distal esophagus. A duplication cyst (enterogenous or enteric cyst) was removed surgically.

Esophageal duplication cysts are a type of foregut cyst along with bronchogenic cysts and neurenteric cysts. Pathologically, esophageal duplication cysts are lined with squamous epithelium and have a smooth muscle wall. Bronchogenic cysts have respiratory epithelium and neurenteric cysts have associated vertebral body anomalies. Symptoms can occur from these cysts by compression on the adjacent esophagus or tracheobronchial tree or by infection of the cyst. If acid is secreted by the lining mucosa, peptic ulceration, perforation, and bleeding can occur on rare occasions.

Esophageal duplication cysts can be located anywhere in the posterior mediastinum. Contrast esophagraphy usually demonstrates an extramucosal (smooth, well-demarcated) mass, which is often impossible to differentiate from a leiomyoma (Case 29) or other mass arising from the esophageal wall.

**Case 80**

## ESOPHAGEAL DUPLICATION CYST

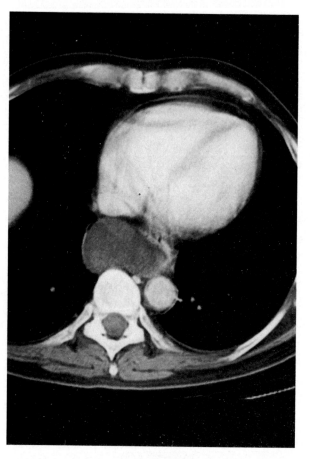

A paraesophageal mass the density of water is located in the lower mediastinum. An esophageal duplication cyst was removed surgically.

The CT findings of a duplication cyst include a sharply defined, homogeneous paraesophageal mass that is usually the density of water. Communication with the normal esophageal lumen is unusual. CT can be helpful in distinguishing a leiomyoma (density of soft tissue) (Case 29 B) from a duplication cyst (density of water).

Case 81

## SLIDING HIATAL HERNIA

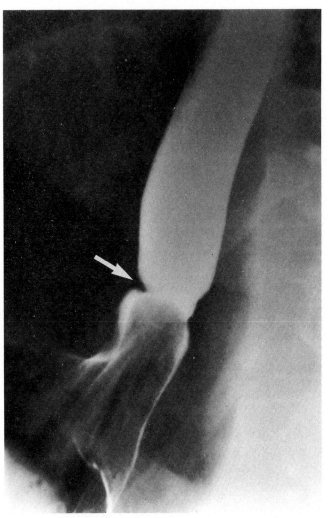

A sliding esophageal hiatal hernia is present, with a portion of the gastric cardia protruding through the esophageal hiatus into the thorax. Gastric rugae can often be seen within the hernia sac. A lower esophageal mucosal ring *(arrow)* (B ring or Schatzki's ring) demarcates the gastroesophageal junction. Identification of this ring at least 2 cm above the diaphragm allows the diagnosis of a hiatal hernia to be made with confidence.

The significance of esophageal hiatal hernias is controversial. Usual symptoms are from gastroesophageal reflux: heartburn, chest pain, and water brash. Occasionally, larger hernias can be associated with aspiration, respiratory distress, and compromised lung excursion. A hiatal hernia as a single radiographic finding is a poor predictor of gastroesophageal reflux or reflux esophagitis. Most patients with significant reflux esophagitis, however, have a hiatal hernia.

A lower esophageal ring has little clinical relevance unless there is significant compromise of the esophageal lumen. Some patients experience dysphagia if the luminal diameter is between 10 and 15 mm, whereas virtually all patients are symptomatic if the diameter is 10 mm or less. Pneumatic dilatation of the mucosal ring is often successful in treating symptomatic patients.

## Case 82

# MUCOSAL RING

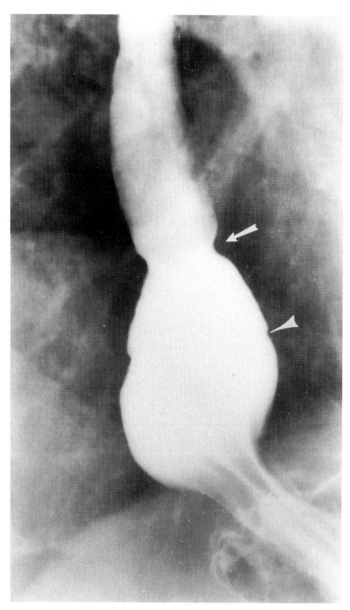

Both a muscular "A" ring *(arrow)* and a mucosal "B" ring *(arrowhead)* are seen in the lower esophagus.

The portion of the esophagus between the "A" ring and "B" ring is referred to as the vestibule. A muscular ring is a transient phenomenon that occurs from muscular contraction of the esophagus. The mucosal ring or "B" ring is a thin, web-like, fixed region of narrowing that denotes the location of the gastroesophageal junction. Mucosal rings can be identified in about 10% of patients if a prone, full-column technique is used (Keyting et al., 1960). They are unusual in patients less than age 30 years. Most mucosal rings have a diameter in excess of 20 mm and are asymptomatic. If the ring significantly narrows the esophageal lumen, dysphagia can occur. A symptomatic mucosal ring is referred to as a Schatzki ring (Case 83).

## Case 83

# SCHATZKI RING

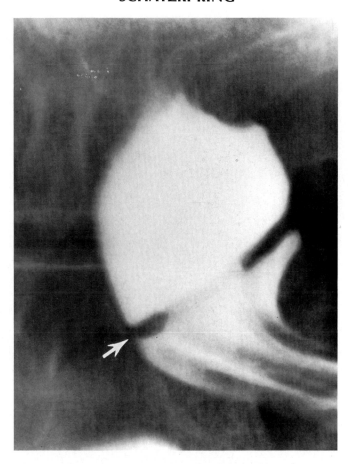

A Schatzki ring *(arrow)* and associated hiatal hernia are seen on the esophagram.

A Schatzki ring refers to a symptomatic, thin constricting ring at the level of the gastroesophageal junction. The pathogenesis of this condition is unknown. Most patients complain of dysphagia with solid foods. Large pieces of meat are often most troublesome. Treatment varies from instructions on eating and chewing more carefully to mechanically disrupting the ring with bougie, endoscopic rupture, or pneumatic dilatation.

Radiographically, a thin, web-like constriction is present at the gastroesophageal junction. A hiatal hernia is invariably present. Some patients experience dysphagia if the luminal diameter is between 10 and 15 mm at the level of the ring. Virtually all patients are symptomatic if the ring narrows to 10 mm or less.

The term "lower esophageal ring" denotes a visible "B" ring (Case 2) that is asymptomatic. A Schatzki ring has such a characteristic appearance, and other conditions are rarely mistaken for it.

## Case 84

## HIATAL HERNIA: SLING FIBERS IMPRESSION

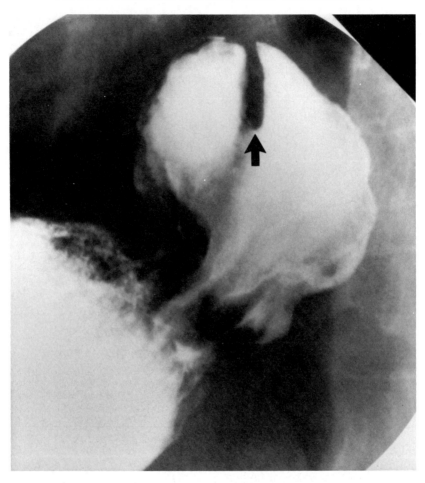

A moderate-sized hiatal hernia is present with a notch *(arrow)* on its superior aspect.

Moderate to large hiatal hernias may contain a characteristic diagonal notch due to crossing gastric sling fibers looping around the gastroesophageal junction. This appearance should not be mistaken for a para-esophageal hernia (Case 89)—a condition in which the esophagogastric junction is normally positioned at the diaphragmatic hiatus. The diaphragmatic hiatus can be identified in this case where the stomach narrows and appears pinched by the muscular fibers of the diaphragm.

**Case 85**

## LARGE HIATAL HERNIA

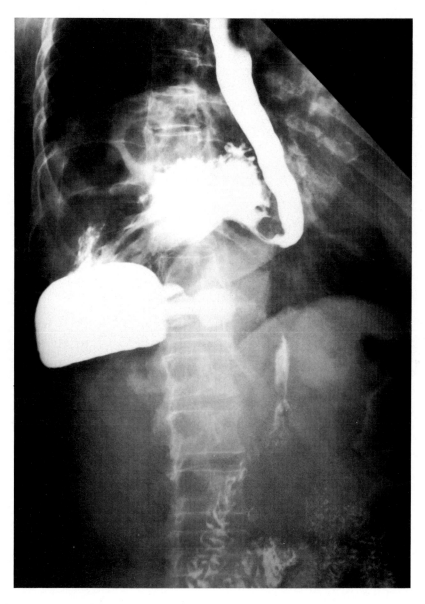

The entire stomach is in an intrathoracic location. In addition, a gas-filled transverse colon can be seen in the chest. The diagnosis of a hiatal hernia can be made with assurance because the gastroesophageal junction is clearly in an intrathoracic location. If the diaphragmatic hiatus is large enough, other intra-abdominal organs can enter the chest cavity—e.g., colon, small bowel, omentum, liver, and spleen.

Large hernias can twist and a volvulus can develop, but this is an unusual event that is seen more frequently among paraesophageal hernias. Mucosal ulcerations also can develop within the stomach at the level of the hiatal orifice. It is believed that repeated trauma from the stomach sliding over the diaphragmatic ridges is the cause of these "riding" ulcers.

## Case 86

# HIATAL HERNIA: CT

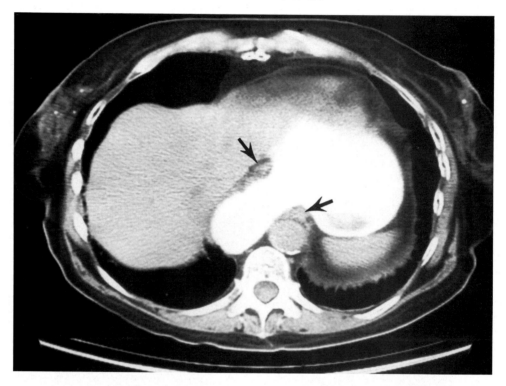

This CT scan is at the level of the esophageal hiatus. The esophageal hiatus can be located by identifying the diaphragmatic crura *(arrows)*. The stomach can be seen to extend from the abdominal cavity through the hiatus and into the chest as a hiatal hernia.

**Case 87**

## HIATAL HERNIA AND PROMINENT DIAPHRAGMATIC CRUS

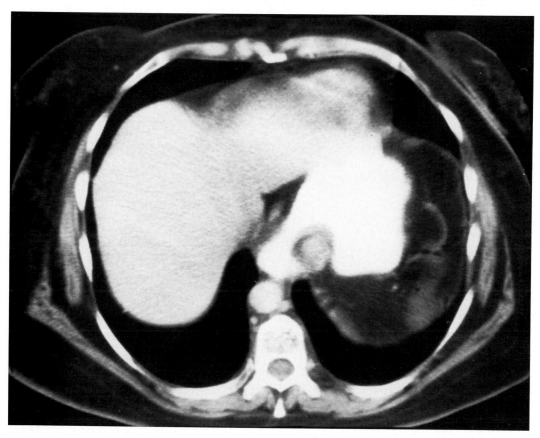

Prominent left diaphragmatic crus at the level of the esophagogastric junction can simulate a mass. Note the rim of fat around the crus. Adjacent sections showed that this region was indeed a portion of the diaphragm. A small hiatal hernia is also present.

**Case 88**

# HIATAL HERNIA CONTAINING OMENTUM

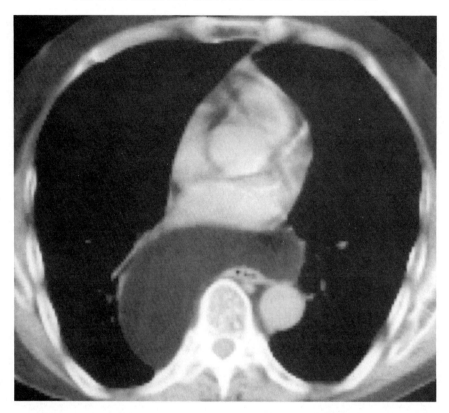

CT scan in the lower chest demonstrates a mass the density of fat that is posterior to the heart and in a right paravertebral location. On lower sections this mass originated from the abdomen and entered the thorax through the esophageal hiatus. This is characteristic of herniated omentum through the esophageal hiatus.

Usually the stomach is the organ that herniates through the esophageal hiatus, but potentially any intraperitoneal upper abdominal organ(s) could migrate into the thorax. Omental herniation does not usually cause any symptoms and may be discovered incidentally on a routine chest radiograph as an abnormal soft tissue mass behind the heart.

**Case 89**

# PARAESOPHAGEAL HERNIA

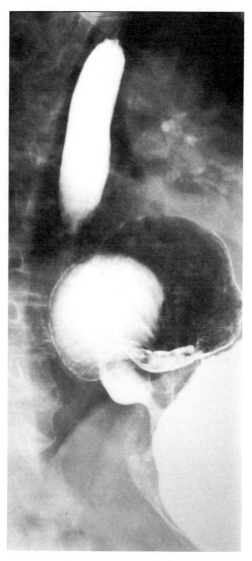

The gastroesophageal junction is normally positioned, with a portion of the stomach herniating into the thorax via the esophageal diaphragmatic hiatus. This is a typical appearance of a paraesophageal hernia.

These hernias are more prone to complication than usual esophageal hiatal hernias. Complications include gastritis and bleeding in the hernia (secondary to edematous and hemorrhagic rugal folds from venous and lymphatic obstruction), gastric ulcers at the level of the diaphragmatic hiatus, and strangulation of the hernia sac.

Radiologic diagnosis is dependent on identifying a normally positioned esophageal junction with the stomach passing through the esophageal hiatus anteriorly. Hiatal hernias (Case 85) can at times mimic a paraesophageal hernia, but in these patients the esophageal junction is always abnormally located within the thoracic cavity. Most paraesophageal hernias undergo surgical repair because a high mortality is associated with strangulation—a complication that may occur in up to 30% of patients (Hill, 1973).

**Case 90**

## PARAESOPHAGEAL HERNIA

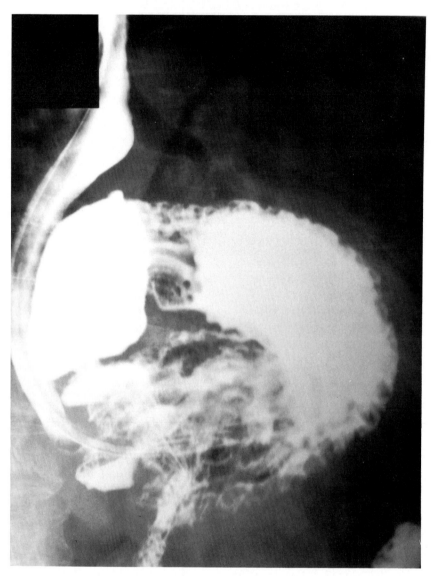

Nearly the entire stomach and proximal duodenum are located within the chest (upside down intrathoracic stomach). The gastroesophageal junction is in a normal location. Findings are those of a large paraesophageal hernia. Because the vascular pedicle supplying the stomach, distal esophagus, and duodenum all pass through the same diaphragmatic hiatus, it is understandable how twisting of the stomach could result in gastric ischemia/infarction and obstruction. Large her-

nias such as this one are at a higher risk for incarceration and strangulation than are small hernias. In some hernias, contrast material will not fill the entire stomach because of obstruction. Similarly, it may be impossible to pass a nasogastric tube into the stomach to decompress it. These patients require urgent surgical repair and have a higher morbidity and mortality than do patients in whom nasogastric decompression is possible.

| DIFFERENTIAL DIAGNOSES | CASE NUMBER |
|---|---|
| **FILLING DEFECTS** | |
| Tumors | |
|   Malignant | |
|     Carcinoma | 32−36, 40, 42, 44, 62 |
|     Metastases | 50 |
|     Lymphoma | 46, 47 |
|     Spindle cell tumor | 45 |
|     Leiomyosarcoma | 29 |
|   Benign | |
|     Leiomyoma | 29 |
|     Adenoma | 30 |
|     Inflammatory polyp | 31 |
| Nontumorous conditions | |
|   Esophagitis | |
|     Peptic | |
|       Thickened, nodular folds | 7 |
|     Infectious | |
|       Monilial plaques | 20−23 |
|   Varices | 52−56 |
|   Food bolus | 71 |
|   Aberrant right subclavian artery | 5 |
|   Glycogenic acanthosis | 77 |
|   Duplication cyst | 79, 80 |
|   Foreign body | 70−72 |
|   Venous plexus/ cricopharyngeus muscle | 1 |
|   Web(s) | 69 |
|   Schatzki ring | 82, 83 |
| **ENLARGED FOLDS** | |
| Esophagitis | 7, 11, 21, 24 |
| Varices | 52−56 |
| Varicoid carcinoma | 36 |
| Lymphoma | 46, 47 |
| **LUMINAL NARROWING** | |
| Tumor | |
|   Carcinoma | 32−43 |
|   Lymphoma | 46, 49 |
|   Adenopathy | 49−51 |
|   Metastases | 50, 51 |
|   Benign neoplasm | 29−31 |
| Stricture | |
|   Peptic | 12−15, 17, 63, 64 |
|   Corrosive ingestion (including nasogastric tube) | 28 |
| Achalasia | 60, 61 |

| DIFFERENTIAL DIAGNOSES | CASE NUMBER |
|---|---|
| Motor abnormalities | |
|   Esophageal spasm/ tertiary contractions | 58, 59 |
|   Prominent cricopharyngeus muscle | 65 |
| *ULCERATION* | |
| Esophagitis | |
|   Peptic | 8–11, 16 |
|   Infectious | 20, 24–26 |
|   Other types | 27, 57, 76 |
| Tumor | |
|   Carcinoma | 32–34, 62 |
|   Lymphoma | 46 |
|   Metastases | 50 |
|   Iatrogenic | 57 |

## SELECTED READINGS

### Normal Anatomy and Variants

Laufer I. Technique and normal anatomy. In: Levine MS, ed. *Radiology of the esophagus*. Philadelphia: WB Saunders, 1989:1–14

Stewart JR, Kincaid OW, Edwards JE. *An atlas of vascular rings and related malformations of the aortic arch system*. Springfield, IL: Charles C Thomas, 1964

### Reflux Esophagitis

Brühlmann WF, Zollikofer CL, Maranta E, et al. Intramural pseudodiverticulosis of the esophagus: report of seven cases and literature review. *Gastrointest Radiol* 1981;6:199–208

Gilchrist AM, Levine MS, Carr RF, et al. Barrett's esophagus: diagnosis by double-contrast esophagography. *AJR* 1988;150:97–102

Kressel HY, Glick SN, Laufer I, Banner M. Radiologic features of esophagitis. *Gastrointest Radiol* 1981;6:103–108

*Laufer I. Radiology of esophagitis. *Radiol Clin North Am* 1982 Dec;20:687–699

Levine MS. Barrett's esophagus: a radiologic diagnosis? *AJR* 1988;151:433–438

*Levine MS. Reflux esophagitis. In: Levine MS, ed. *Radiology of the esophagus*. Philadelphia: WB Saunders, 1989:15–48

*Levine MS, Caroline D, Thompson JJ, Kressel HY, Laufer I, Herlinger H. Adenocarcinoma of the esophagus: relationship to Barrett mucosa. *Radiology* 1984;150:305–309

*Levine MS, Goldstein HM. Fixed transverse folds in the esophagus: a sign of reflux esophagitis. *AJR* 1984;143:275–278

*Levine MS, Kressel HY, Caroline D, Laufer I, Herlinger H, Thompson JJ. Barrett esophagus: reticular pattern of the mucosa. *Radiology* 1983;147:663–667

Levine MS, Moolten DN, Herlinger H, Laufer I. Esophageal intramural pseudodiverticulosis: a reevaluation. *AJR* 1986;147:1165–1170

Mendl K, McKay JM, Tanner CH. Intramural diverticulosis of the oesophagus and Rokitansky-Aschoff sinuses of the gall-bladder. *Br J Radiol* 1960;33:496–501

Ott DJ, Chen YM, Gelfand DW, Munitz HA, Wu WC. Analysis of a multiphasic radiographic examination for detecting reflux esophagitis. *Gastrointest Radiol* 1986;11:1–6

Ott DJ, Gelfand DW, Lane TG, Wu WC. Radiologic detection and spectrum of appearances of peptic esophageal strictures. *J Clin Gastroenterol* 1982;4:11–15

Ott DJ, Gelfand DW, Wu WC, Castell DO. Esophagogastric region and its rings. *AJR* 1984;142:281–287

### Infectious Esophagitis

DeGaeta L, Levine MS, Guglielmi GE, Raffensperger EC, Laufer I. Herpes esophagitis in an otherwise healthy patient. *AJR* 1985;144:1205–1206

*Deprew WT, Prentice RSA, Beck IT, Blakeman JM, DaCosta LR. Herpes simplex ulcerative esophagitis in a healthy subject. *Am J Gastroenterol* 1977;68:381–385

Laufer I. Radiology of esophagitis. *Radiol Clin North Am* 1982 Dec;20:687–699

Levine MS, Laufer I, Kressel HY, Friedman HM. Herpes esophagitis. *AJR* 1981;136:863–866

Levine MS, Loercher G, Katzka DA, Herlinger H, Rubesin SE, Laufer I. Giant, human immunodeficiency virus-related ulcers in the esophagus. *Radiology* 1991;180:323–326

Levine MS, Loevner LA, Saul SH, Rubesin SE, Herlinger H, Laufer I. Herpes esophagitis: sensitivity of double-contrast esophagography. *AJR* 1988;151:57–62

Roberts L Jr, Gibbons R, Gibbons G, Rice RP, Thompson WM. Adult esophageal candidiasis: a radiographic spectrum. *Radiographics* 1987;7:289–307

### Caustic/Medication-Induced Esophagitis

Appelqvist P, Salmo M. Lye corrosion carcinoma of the esophagus: a review of 63 cases. *Cancer* 1980;45:2655–2658

Bova JG, Dutton NE, Goldstein HM, Hoberman LJ. Medication-induced esophagitis: diagnosis by double-contrast esophagography. *AJR* 1987;148:731–732

Creteur V, Laufer I, Kressel HY, et al. Drug-induced esophagitis detected by double-contrast radiography. *Radiology* 1983;147:365–368

Goldman LP, Weigert JM. Corrosive substance ingestion: a review. *Am J Gastroenterol* 1984;79:85–90

*Kiviranta UK. Corrosion carcinoma of the esophagus: 381 cases of corrosion and nine cases of corrosion carcinoma. *Acta Otolaryngol (Stockh)* 1952;42:89–95

Martel W. Radiologic features of esophagastritis secondary to extremely caustic agents. *Radiology* 1972;103:31–36

*Cited in text.

## Benign Tumors

Ghahremani GG, Meyers MA, Port RB. Calcified primary tumors of the gastrointestinal tract. *Gastrointest Radiol* 1978;2:331–339

*Glanz I, Grünebaum M. The radiological approach to leiomyoma of the oesophagus with a long-term follow-up. *Clin Radiol* 1977;28:197–200

*Itai Y, Shimazu H. Leiomyosarcoma of the oesophagus with dense calcification. *Br J Radiol* 1978; 51:469–471

*Levine MS. Benign tumors. In: Levine MS, ed. *Radiology of the esophagus*. Philadelphia: WB Saunders, 1989:121–124

McDonald GB, Brand DL, Thorning DR. Multiple adenomatous neoplasms arising in columnar-lined (Barrett's) esophagus. *Gastroenterology* 1977;72:1317–1321

*Seremetis MG, Lyons WS, deGuzman VC, Peabody JW Jr. Leiomyomata of the esophagus: an analysis of 838 cases. *Cancer* 1976;38:2166–2177

Shaffer HA. Multiple leiomyomas of the esophagus. *Radiology* 1976;118:29–34

Spin FP. Adenomas of the esophagus: a case report and review of the literature. *Gastrointest Endosc* 1973;20:26–27

## Esophageal Carcinoma

Agha FP. Barrett carcinoma of the esophagus: clinical and radiographic analysis of 34 cases. *AJR* 1985;145:41–46

Correa P. Precursors of gastric and esophageal cancer. *Cancer* 1982;50:2554–2565

Gloyna RE, Zornoza J, Goldstein HM. Primary ulcerative carcinoma of the esophagus. *Am J Roentgenol* 1977;129:599–600

*Halber MD, Daffner RH, Thompson WM. CT of the esophagus: I. Normal appearance. *AJR* 1979;133:1047–1050

*Halvorsen RA, Thompson WM. Computed tomographic evaluation of esophageal carcinoma. *Semin Oncol* 1984;11:113–126

Itai Y, Kogure T, Okuyama Y, Akiyama H. Superficial esophageal carcinoma: radiologic findings in double-contrast studies. *Radiology* 1978;126:597–601

Japanese Society for Esophageal Diseases. Guide lines for the clinical and pathologic studies on carcinoma of the esophagus. *Jpn J Surg* 1976 June;6:69–78

Laufer I, Yamada A. Tumors of the esophagus. In: Laufer I, ed. *Double contrast gastrointestinal radiology with endoscopic correlation*. Philadelphia: WB Saunders, 1979:129–153

Lawson TL, Dodds WJ, Sheft DJ. Carcinoma of the esophagus simulating varices. *Am J Roentgenol* 1969;107:83–85

Levine MS, Dillon EC, Saul SH, Laufer I. Early esophageal cancer. *AJR* 1986;146:507–512

Moss AA, Koehler RE, Margulis AR. Initial accuracy of esophagograms in detection of small esophageal carcinoma. *Am J Roentgenol* 1976;127:909–913

Picus D, Balfe DM, Koehler RE, Roper CL, Owen JW. Computed tomography in the staging of esophageal carcinoma. *Radiology* 1983;146:433–438

*Postlethwait RW. *Surgery of the esophagus*. New York: Appleton-Century-Crofts, 1979:341–414

Quint LE, Glazer GM, Orringer MB, Gross BH. Esophageal carcinoma: CT findings. *Radiology* 1985;155:171–175

Raphael HA, Ellis FH Jr, Dockerty MB. Primary adenocarcinoma of the esophagus: 18-year review and review of the literature. *Ann Surg* 1966;164:785–796

Silver TM, Goldstein HM. Varicoid carcinoma of the esophagus. *Am J Dig Dis* 1974;19:56–58

Soga J, Tanaka O, Sasaki K, Kawaguchi M, Muto T. Superficial spreading carcinoma of the esophagus. *Cancer* 1982;50:1641–1645

Thompson WM, Halvorsen RA, Foster WL, Williford ME, Postlethwait RW, Korobkin M. Computed tomography for staging esophageal and gastroesophageal cancer: reevaluation. *AJR* 1983;141:951–958

Wynder EL, Mabuchi K. Cancer of the esophagus. Etiological and environmental factors. *JAMA* 1973;226:1546–1548

Yates CW Jr, LeVine MA, Jensen KM. Varicoid carcinoma of the esophagus. *Radiology* 1977;122:605–608

Zornoza J, Lindell MM Jr. Radiologic evaluation of small esophageal carcinoma. *Gastrointest Radiol* 1980;5:107–111

## Gastroesophageal Junction and Recurrent Carcinoma

Agha FP, Orringer MB, Amendola MA. Gastric interposition following transhiatal esophagectomy: radiographic evaluation. *Gastrointest Radiol* 1985;10:17–24

Carlson HC. Carcinoma at the esophagogastric junction. In: Marshak RH, Lindner AE, Maklansky D, eds. *Radiology of the stomach*. Philadelphia: WB Saunders, 1983:172–204

Freeny PC, Marks WM. Adenocarcinoma of the gastroesophageal junction: barium and CT examination. *AJR* 1982;138:1077–1084

*Halvorsen RA, Thompson WM. Computed tomography of the gastroesophageal junction. *Crit Rev Diagn Imag* 1984;21(no. 3):183–228

Kalish RJ, Clancy PE, Orringer MB, Appelman HD. Clinical, epidemiologic, and morphologic comparison between adenocarcinomas arising in Barrett's esophageal mucosa and in the gastric cardia. *Gastroenterology* 1984;86:461–467

Lawson TL, Dodds WJ. Infiltrating carcinoma simulating achalasia. *Gastrointest Radiol* 1976;1:245–248

*Levine MS, Caroline D, Thompson JJ, Kressel HY, Laufer I, Herlinger H. Adenocarcinoma of the esophagus: relationship to Barrett mucosa. *Radiology* 1984;150:305–309

McCallum RW. Esophageal achalasia secondary to gastric carcinoma: report of a case and review of the literature. *Am J Gastroenterol* 1979;71:24–29

Owen JW, Balfe DM, Koehler RE, Roper CL, Weyman PJ. Radiologic evaluation of complications after esophagogastrectomy. *AJR* 1983;140:1163-1169

Sarr MG, Hamilton SR, Marrone GC, Cameron JL. Barrett's esophagus: its prevalence and association with adenocarcinoma in patients with symptoms of gastroesophageal reflux. *Am J Surg* 1985;149:187–192

### Other Malignant Tumors

Agha FP. Secondary neoplasms of the esophagus. *Gastrointest Radiol* 1987;12:187–193

Agha FP, Keren DF. Spindle-cell squamous carcinoma of the esophagus: a tumor with biphasic morphology. *AJR* 1985;145:541–545

Anderson MF, Harell GS. Secondary esophageal tumors. *AJR* 1980;135:1243–1246

Carnovale RL, Goldstein HM, Zornoza J, Dodd GD. Radiologic manifestations of esophageal lymphoma. *Am J Roentgenol* 1977;128:751–754

Caruso RD, Berk RN. Lymphoma of the esophagus. *Radiology* 1970;95:381–382

Kirsch HL, Cronin DW, Stein GN, Latour F, Herrera AF. Esophageal perforation: an unusual presentation of esophageal lymphoma. *Dig Dis Sci* 1983;28:371–374

Lambert A. Malignant tracheoesophageal fistula secondary to Hodgkin's disease: successful surgical treatment with free fascia-muscle graft and left colon bypass. *J Thorac Cardiovasc Surg* 1975;69:820–826

Levine MS, Gilchrist AM. Esophageal deviation: pushed or pulled? *AJR* 1987;149:513–514

Olmsted WW, Lichtenstein JE, Hyams VJ. Polypoid epithelial malignancies of the esophagus. *AJR* 1983;140:921–925

Osamura RY, Shimamura K, Hata J, et al. Polypoid carcinoma of the esophagus: a unifying term for "carcinosarcoma" and "pseudosarcoma." *Am J Surg Pathol* 1978;2:201–208

### Varices

Agha FP. The esophagus after endoscopic injection sclerotherapy: acute and chronic changes. *Radiology* 1984;153:37–42

Balthazar EJ, Megibow A, Naidich D, Lefleur RS. Computed tomographic recognition of gastric varices. *AJR* 1984;142:1121–1125

Balthazar EJ, Naidich DP, Megibow AJ, Lefleur RS. CT evaluation of esophageal varices. *AJR* 1987;148:131–135

Clark KE, Foley WD, Lawson TL, Berland LL, Maddison FE. CT evaluation of esophageal and upper abdominal varices. *J Comput Assist Tomogr* 1980;4:510–515

*Dave P, Romeu J, Messer J. Upper gastrointestinal bleeding in patients with portal hypertension: a reappraisal. *J Clin Gastroenterol* 1983;5:113–115

Felson B, Lessure AP. "Downhill" varices of the esophagus. *Dis Chest* 1964;46:740–746

Johnson LS, Kinnear DG, Brown RA, Mulder DS. "Downhill" esophageal varices: a rare cause of upper gastrointestinal bleeding. *Arch Surg* 1978;113:1463–1464

Kirsh IE, Blackwell CC, Bennett HD. Roentgen diagnosis of esophageal varices: comparison of roentgen and esophagoscopic findings in 502 cases. *Am J Roentgenol* 1955;74:477–485

Mikkelsen WJ. Varices of the upper esophagus in superior vena cava obstruction. *Radiology* 1963;81:945–948

Schatzki R. Roentgen demonstration of esophageal varices: its clinical importance. *Arch Surg* 1940;41:1084–1100

Tihansky DP, Reilly JJ, Schade RR, Van Thiel DH. The esophagus after injection sclerotherapy of varices: immediate postoperative changes. *Radiology* 1984;153:43–47

### Motor Abnormalities

Bruggeman LL, Seaman WB. Epiphrenic diverticula: an analysis of 80 cases. *Am J Roentgenol* 1973;119:266–276

*Cohen S. Motor disorders of the esophagus. *N Engl J Med* 1979;301:184–192

Debas HT, Payne WS, Cameron AJ, Carlson HC. Physiopathology of lower esophageal diverticulum and its implications for treatment. *Surg Gynecol Obstet* **1980;**151:593–600

*DiMarino AJ Jr, Cohen S. Characteristics of lower esophageal sphincter function in symptomatic diffuse esophageal spasm. *Gastroenterology* **1974;**66:1–6

Dohlman G, Mattsson O. The role of the cricopharyngeal muscle in cases of hypopharyngeal diverticula: a cineroentgenographic study. *Am J Roentgenol* **1959;**81:561–569

Gefter WB, Laufer I, Edell S, Gohel VK. Candidiasis in the obstructed esophagus. *Radiology* **1981;**138:25–28

Hankins JR, McLaughlin JS. The association of carcinoma of the esophagus with achalasia. *J Thorac Cardiovasc Surg* **1975;**69:355–360

Kaye MD. Oesophageal motor dysfunction in patients with diverticula of the mid-thoracic oesophagus. *Thorax* **1974;**29:666–672

*McNally EF, Katz I. The roentgen diagnosis of diffuse esophageal spasm. *Am J Roentgenol* **1967;**99:218–222

Ott DJ, Richter JE, Wu WC, Chen YM, Gelfand DW, Castell DO. Radiologic and manometric correlation in "nutcracker esophagus." *AJR* **1986;**147:692–695

Recht MP, Levine MS, Katzka DA, Reynolds JC, Saul SH. Barrett's esophagus in scleroderma: increased prevalence and radiographic findings. *Gastrointest Radiol* **1988;**13:1–5

Saladin TA, French AB, Zarafonetis CJD, Pollard HM. Esophageal motor abnormalities in scleroderma and related diseases. *Am J Dig Dis* **1966;**11:522–535

Stewart ET. Radiographic evaluation of the esophagus and its motor disorders. *Med Clin North Am* **1981** Nov;65:1173–1194

Vantrappen G, Janssens J, Hellemans J, Coremans G. Achalasia, diffuse esophageal spasm, and related motility disorders. *Gastroenterology* **1979;**76:450–457

### Miscellaneous Disorders

Bachman AL, Seaman WB, Macken KL. Lateral pharyngeal diverticula. *Radiology* **1968;**91:774–782

*Bender MD, Allison J, Cuartas F, Montgomery C. Glycogenic acanthosis of the esophagus: a form of benign epithelial hyperplasia. *Gastroenterology* **1973;**65:373–380

Berliner L, Redmond P, Horowitz L, Ruoff M. Glycogen plaques (glycogenic acanthosis) of the esophagus. *Radiology* **1981;**141:607–610

Campbell JB, Davis WS. Catheter technique for extraction of blunt esophageal foreign bodies. *Radiology* **1973;**108:438–440

Clements JL Jr, Cox GW, Torres WE, Weens HS. Cervical esophageal webs—a roentgen-anatomic correlation: observations on the pharyngoesophagus. *Am J Roentgenol* **1974;**121:221–231

Ghahremani GG, Gore RM, Breuer RI, Larson RH. Esophageal manifestations of Crohn's disease. *Gastrointest Radiol* **1982;**7:199–203

Glick SN, Teplick SK, Goldstein J, Stead JA, Zitomer N. Glycogenic acanthosis of the esophagus. *AJR* **1982;**139:683–688

Gohel V, Long BW, Richter G. Aphthous ulcers in the esophagus with Crohn colitis. *AJR* **1981;**137:872–873

Holsinger JW Jr, Fuson RL, Sealy WC. Esophageal perforation following meat inpaction and papain ingestion. *JAMA* **1968;**204:734–735

Herschman BR, Uppaputhangkule V, Maas L, Gelzayd E. Esophageal leukoplakia: a rare entity. *JAMA* **1978;**239:2021

*Kelly AB. Spasm at the entrance to the oesophagus. *J Laryngol Otol* **1919;**34:285–289

*Love L, Berkow AE. Trauma to the esophagus. *Gastrointest Radiol* **1978;**2:305–321

Nandi P, Ong GB. Foreign bodies in the oesophagus: review of 2394 cases. *Br J Surg* **1978;**65:5–9

Nosher JL, Campbell WL, Seaman WB. The clinical significance of cervical esophageal and hypopharyngeal webs. *Radiology* **1975;**117:45–47

*O'Connell ND. Spontaneous rupture of the esophagus. *Am J Roentgenol* **1967;**99:186–203

*Paterson DR. A clinical type of dysphagia. *J Laryngol Otol* **1919;**34:289–291

Rywlin AM, Ortega R. Glycogenic acanthosis of the esophagus. *Arch Pathol* **1970;**90:439–443

*Shamma'a MH, Benedict EB. Esophageal webs. A report of 58 cases and an attempt at classification. *N Engl J Med* **1958;**259:378–384

Thompson NW, Ernst CB, Fry WJ. The spectrum of emetogenic injury to the esophagus and stomach. *Am J Surg* **1967;**113:13–25

Trenker SW, Maglinte DDT, Lehman GA, Chernish SM, Miller RE, Johnson CW. Esophageal food impaction: treatment with glucagon. *Radiology* **1983;**149:401–403

*Vinson PP. Hysterical dysphagia. *Minn Med* **1922;**5:107–108

Vithesponge P, Blank S. Ciliated epithelial esophageal cyst. *Am J Gastroenterol* **1971;**56:436–440

*Waldenström J, Kjellberg SR. The roentgenological

diagnosis of sideropenic dysphagia. *Acta Radiol* **1939**;20:618–638

Whitaker JA, Deffenbaugh LD, Cooke AR. Esophageal duplication cyst. *Am J Gastroenterol* **1980**;73:329–332

### Diaphragmatic Hernias

Fataar S, Schulman A. Diagnosis of diaphragmatic tears. *Br J Radiol* **1979**;52:375–381

*Hill LD. Incarcerated paraesophageal hernia. A surgical emergency. *Am J Surg* **1973**;126:286–290

Hood RM. Traumatic diaphragmatic hernia. *Ann Thorac Surg* **1971**;12:311–324

*Keyting WS, Baker GM, McCarver RR, Daywitt AL. The lower esophagus. *Am J Roentgenol* **1960**;84:1070–1075

Reed JO, Lang EF. Diaphragmatic hernia in infancy. *Am J Roentgenol* **1959**;82:437–449

Skinner DB. Hernias (hiatal, traumatic, and congenital). In: Berk JE, Haubrich WS, Kalser MH, Roth JLA, Schaffner F, eds. *Bockus gastroenterology*, 4th ed, vol 2. Philadelphia: WB Saunders, **1985**:705–716

Stein GN, Finkelstein A. Hiatal hernia: roentgen incidence and diagnosis. *Am J Dig Dis* **1960**;5:77–87

Whittaker LD Jr, Lynn HB, Dawson B, Chaves E. Hernias of the foramen of Bochdalek in children. *Mayo Clin Proc* **1968**;43:580–591

# CHAPTER 2

# Stomach

## Case 91

## NORMAL STOMACH

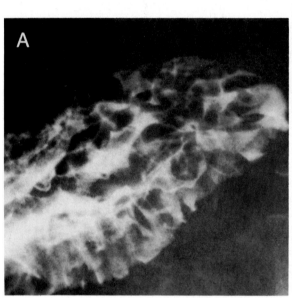

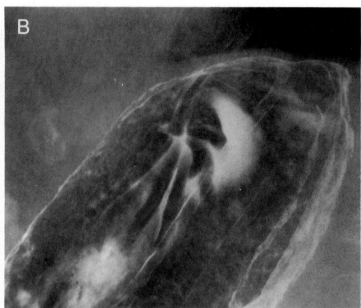

**A.** There are multiple, prominent folds in the gastric fundus and cardia.

**B.** Distension of the proximal stomach after orally administered effervescent granules shows normal-caliber gastric folds and the normal-appearing "rosette" of the esophagogastric junction.

The normal gastric cardia and fundus are composed of smooth rugal folds, which may vary considerably in size, and the esophagogastric junction. Distension of the stomach may entirely obliterate normal rugal folds, and the use of high density barium and effervescent granules is a useful technique if a fundal abnormality is questioned. The appearance of the esophagogastric junction varies depending on the ligamentous laxity about the cardia and the presence of a hiatal hernia. Usually a "rosette" is seen due to the folds converging toward the esophageal lumen. Several long folds often radiate from the esophagogastric junction toward the distal stomach.

**Case 92**

## NORMAL STOMACH: CT

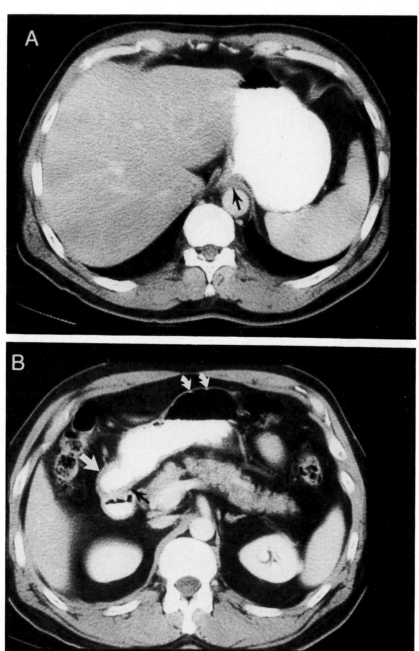

**A.** Complete distension of the gastric fundus and cardia with orally administered contrast material demonstrates the normal gastroesophageal junction *(arrow)* and gastric wall. Normally, the gastric wall is not more than 3 mm thick (Komaki, 1982). The wall of the stomach at the esophagogastric junction is often thicker than the remainder of the stomach.

**B.** The gastric antrum *(straight arrows)* may also appear thicker than the more proximal stomach. The wall thickness of this antrum is within normal limits. Note the normal gastric rugal folds *(curved arrows)*.

Case 93

# FUNDAL PSEUDOTUMOR

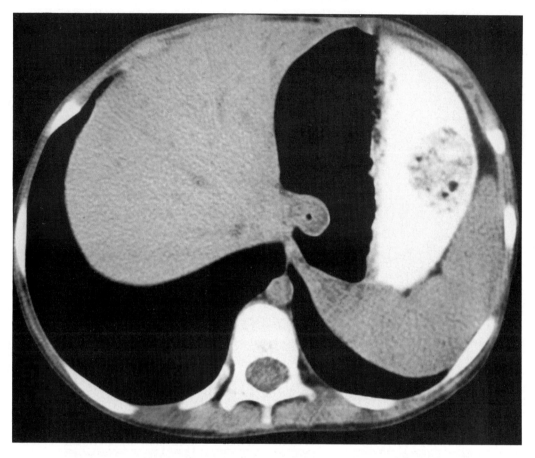

The distal esophagus at the level of the gastroesophageal junction is protruding into the gastric lumen. This "pseudotumor" can be shown to be esophageal in origin by its contiguity with the esophagus in (more cephalad) CT sections. In addition, the air in its lumen and its round shape confirm its esophageal nature. This scan was obtained with the patient in the left lateral decubitus position.

## Case 94

## NORMAL STOMACH

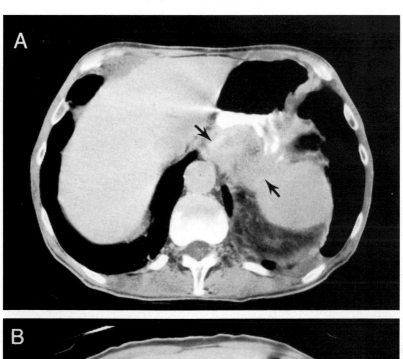

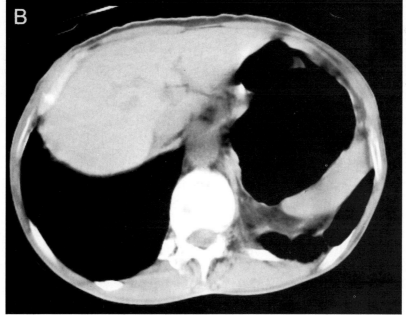

**A.** Masslike thickening of the gastric fundus *(arrows)* is present near the esophagogastric junction.

**B.** After the administration of effervescent granules, the apparent mass is no longer seen.

The gastric fundus nearly always appears thickened in an incompletely distended stomach. This region is particularly prominent in this patient. The gastric wall around the esophagogastric junction is most commonly "pseudothickened," especially posteriorly. Adequate fundal distension either with positive orally administered contrast material or with gas usually helps exclude a mass in this region. If the patient is in the prone or right posterior oblique position, this may help to ensure adequate fundal distension if effervescent granules were administered.

Case 95

## ACUTE EROSIVE GASTRITIS

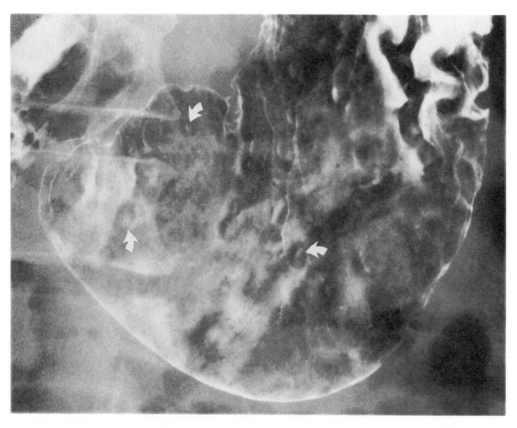

Multiple *(arrows)* small, round filling defects (mounds of edema) containing a small central collection of barium (erosion or tiny ulceration) are present in the gastric antrum and body. Findings are typical of acute erosive gastritis.

Acute gastritis often presents with symptoms mimicking peptic ulcer disease. This disorder has many causes, including stress reactions, alcohol, aspirin, synthetic anti-inflammatory agents, chemotherapeutic agents, and several other medications. In our practice, aspirin and anti-inflammatory agents are the most common causes.

Typically, multiple small elevated mounds of edema with central ulcerations are identified, often in line with a rugal fold. These typical erosions are often referred to as varioliform erosions. Incomplete erosions appear as linear streaks or dots that may or may not have a surrounding mound of edema. These are more difficult to detect radiologically.

It is important not to mistake barium precipitates for punctate erosions. Precipitates never have a surrounding mound of edema and are often randomly oriented —not along the crest of a rugal fold as often seen with true erosions. The early aphthous ulcerations found in Crohn's disease (Case 108), gastric candidiasis (Cronan et al., 1980), or viral infections may be indistinguishable from erosive gastritis. Erosions are almost always multiple, and caution should be used if only a solitary lesion is seen. Single lesions may represent an artifact or a small submucosal process (pancreatic rest [Case 124], leiomyoma [Case 119], or metastases [Case 145]).

Case 96

# BENIGN GASTRIC ULCER

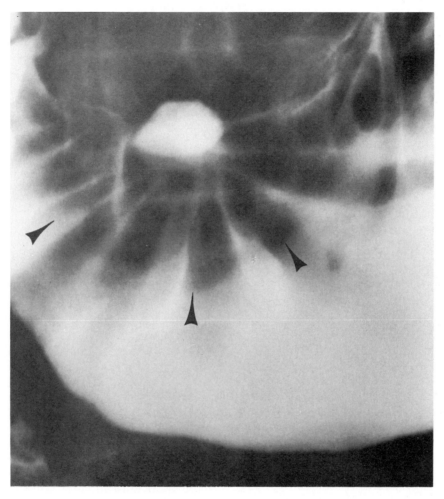

An ulcer crater is located along the lesser curvature of the gastric antrum. Symmetric and smoothly contoured folds radiate to the crater. The mound of edema *(arrowheads)* is smooth in contour, and the crater is located centrally within the mound.

This ulcer illustrates some of the typical signs of benignity: a round or oval crater, folds that cross the mound of surrounding edema and extend up to the crater, a symmetric and smooth filling defect (edema) about the crater, and radiating gastric folds that are smooth and symmetric (without nodularity or clubbing). Most benign ulcers occur in the gastric antrum or body. The anterior wall is affected least often. The greater curvature is a somewhat unusual location for benign ulcers; ulcers there are often associated with ingestion of aspirin-containing medication (Case 99) (Kottler and Tuft, 1981).

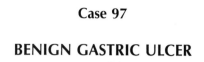

Case 97

# BENIGN GASTRIC ULCER

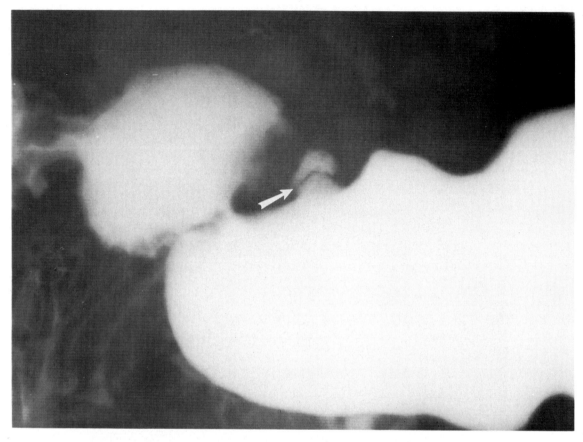

An ulcer crater is seen on this tangential view of the gastric antrum. Hampton's line *(arrow)* is seen at the base of the crater.

Gastric ulcers are common abnormalities today, in large part as a result of the widespread use of anti-inflammatory agents. The radiographic examination is a reliable method for distinguishing benign from malignant ulcers (Levine et al., 1987). Characteristics of a benign ulcer on the tangential view include a Hampton line (as seen in this case) or a smooth and symmetric

ulcer "collar" or mound. Hampton's line represents the nonulcerated mucosa surrounding the crater that is more "acid resistant" than is the undermined submucosal tissues. An ulcer "collar" represents edematous submucosal tissue that surrounds the ulcer tract. A "collar" is always wider than the thin, delicate Hampton line. Ulcers with typical features of benignity are nearly always benign and can be followed radiographically until complete healing has occurred.

## Case 98

## BENIGN LINEAR ULCER

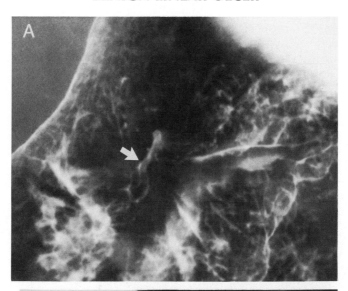

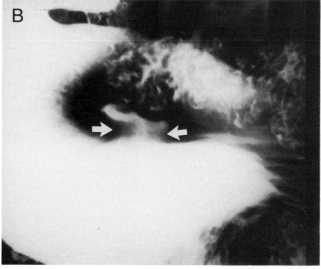

**A.** A linear ulcer *(arrow)* is visible on this *en face* view of the gastric body. Several folds radiate to the edge of the crater.

**B.** The elongated ulcer crater and ulcer collar *(arrows)* are seen on the lesser curvature.

An ulcer "collar" represents edematous mucosa about the ulcer crater. The crater extends linearly within the submucosa because this tissue is not as "acid resistant" as the mucosa. The linear configuration of the crater is often seen in patients with a healing ulcer. These ulcers may be asymmetric or "split" into two smaller craters as reepithelialization occurs. The average time required for healing of an ulcer is 8 weeks.

Large ulcers require more time to heal than do smaller ones. For this reason, follow-up studies should probably not be performed less than 6 to 8 weeks after the initial diagnosis (Levine et al., 1987). Most ulcers leave a scar after healing has occurred. Scars often appear as a depression or pit on the mucosal surface. Radiating folds often can be seen to radiate up to the depression. Retraction (as a result of intramural fibrosis) of the adjacent gastric wall is also commonly encountered. The finding of areae gastricae covering the scarred region confirms ulcer healing; however, this is only rarely encountered on double-contrast examinations.

**111**

## Case 99

## BENIGN GASTRIC "SUMP" ULCER

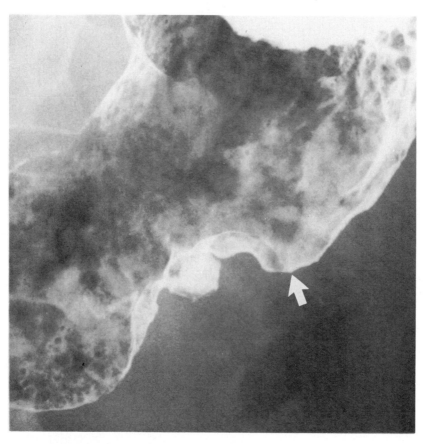

An ulcer crater is present on the greater curvature of the stomach. There is a smooth mound of edema surrounding the centrally located ulcer. The crater does not extend beyond the normal gastric lumen contour.

Benign greater curvature ulcers may not have all of the usual radiographic features associated with benignity. The location of an ulcer is generally not a reliable predictor of benignity or malignancy. As a general rule, benign ulcers are rarely located in the proximal half of the stomach along the greater curvature (Gelfand et al., 1984). It is not uncommon for gastric ulcers to be found in the proximal stomach along the lesser curvature in elderly patients (Amberg and Zboralske, 1966).

Many of the ulcers in the distal stomach are benign and medication-induced. Aspirin-induced ulcers often develop along the greater curvature because it is a dependent location where pills collect and directly cause mucosal injury. Sometimes they are referred to as "sump" ulcers (as in this case). Usually the mound of edema surrounding a benign ulcer is smooth surfaced and tapers gradually, merging imperceptibly with the normal gastric wall. In this particular patient, the surrounding mass of edema has rather abrupt margins *(arrow)* with the normal gastric wall. Endoscopy is often necessary to exclude malignancy if equivocal or worrisome findings are present.

## Case 100

## CIRCUMFERENTIAL GASTRIC ULCER

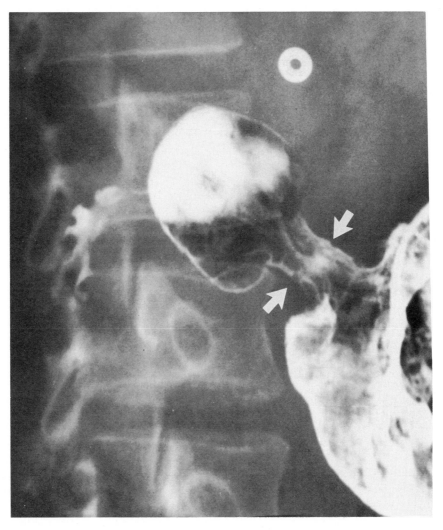

Circumferential narrowing *(arrows)* is present within the gastric antrum. The margins are abruptly shouldered with the normal gastric wall. An annular neoplasm was suspected, but a benign circumferential ulcer extending through the pylorus was found at endoscopic biopsy.

## Case 101

# GIANT GASTRIC ULCER

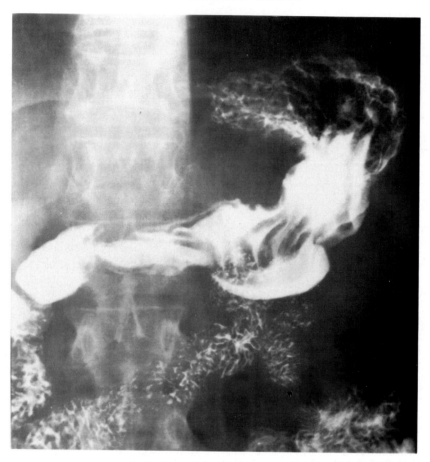

A large ulcer is present along the greater curvature of the stomach. Gastric folds can be seen to extend up to the crater. A benign chronic peptic ulcer was later proved.

Giant ulcers are defined as those larger than 3 cm in diameter. The size of the crater has no bearing on its benign or malignant nature. They are commonly associated with contained perforations. Usually, a large mass is visible in patients with giant malignant ulcers (Case 127). Multiple ulcerations are also unusual but can be seen in 12% to 20% of patients with benign gastric ulcers (Boyle, 1971). Multiplicity favors a benign cause, but each ulcer should be evaluated individually. It is unusual to see concurrent gastric and duodenal ulcers.

## Case 102

## BENIGN GASTRIC ULCER

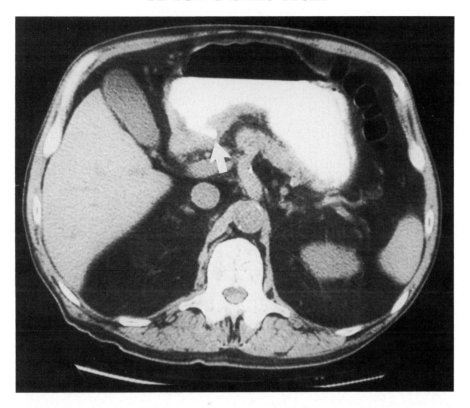

The posterior wall of the gastric antrum is thickened. A small collection of contrast material *(arrow)* fills a defect (ulceration) within the thickened wall. A benign peptic ulcer was found endoscopically.

CT does not have a primary role in the diagnosis of peptic ulcer disease. As in this patient, the disease may be encountered incidentally at CT. Complications of peptic ulcer disease—including pancreatitis, pancreatic abscess, and localized perforations—can be demonstrated well at CT (Case 104).

## Case 103

# GASTROCOLIC FISTULA SECONDARY TO A BENIGN GASTRIC ULCER

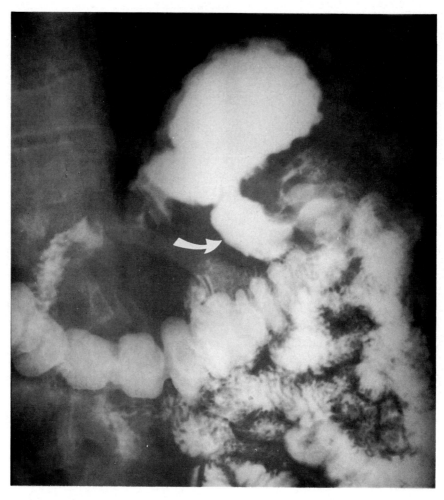

A large fistulous communication *(arrow)* exists between the greater curvature of the stomach and the left transverse colon. A penetrating benign gastric ulcer was found at operation.

Major complications of gastric ulcers include bleeding, perforation, obstruction, and penetration. Bleeding is the most frequent complication, occurring in 10% to 24% of patients with peptic ulcer disease (Pulvertaft, 1968). Most actively bleeding ulcers are assessed endoscopically. An ulcer can penetrate into any adjacent organ or tissue. Common sites include the pancreas, omentum, biliary tract, liver, and colon. Most gastrocolic fistulas are secondary to primary carcinomas or lymphomas arising from either the stomach or colon. Offending ulcers are usually located along the greater curvature, and offending benign ulcers are usually seen in patients on aspirin or steroid therapy, or both. Penetration of an ulcer into the pancreas may present as typical pancreatitis or as a pancreatic abscess (Case 104). Gastric-outlet obstruction is nearly always secondary to ulcerations in the prepyloric or pyloric region, with narrowing due to edema or fibrotic scarring.

**Case 104**

## PERFORATED GASTRIC ULCER

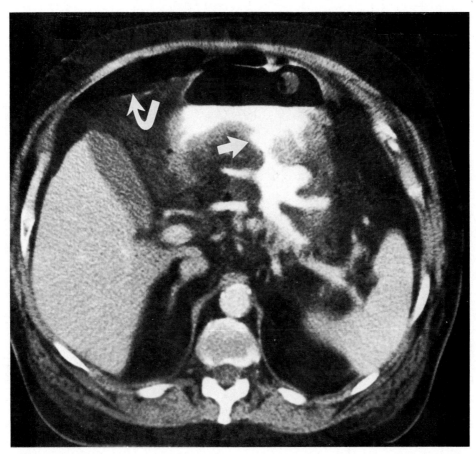

Orally administered contrast material is seen within the body of the stomach and within an ulcer crater *(straight arrow)* in the posterior gastric wall. There is a fistulous communication from the ulcer into the lesser sac. Pneumoperitoneum *(curved arrow)* is seen anteriorly within the peritoneal cavity (postoperative in origin).

CT can be helpful in determining the extraluminal extent of disease in a patient with a known or suspected penetrating ulcer. This information can be very helpful for preoperative planning and in the assessment of possible percutaneous drainage.

## Case 105

## ZOLLINGER-ELLISON SYNDROME

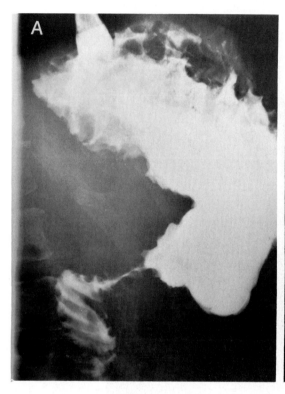

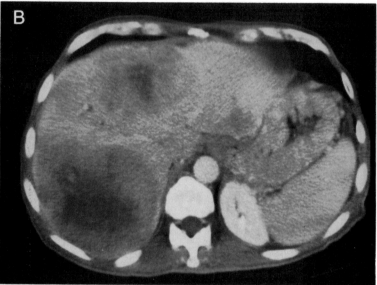

**A.** Enlarged rugal folds are present in the gastric fundus. Thickened folds are also present in the duodenum.

**B.** The gastric wall is markedly thickened. Multiple liver metastases with central necrosis are also present. These findings are consistent with the diagnosis of Zollinger-Ellison syndrome.

Zollinger-Ellison syndrome is a disease caused by a gastrin-secreting, islet cell neoplasm of the pancreas that results in marked gastric hypersecretion of hydrochloric acid and severe peptic ulcer disease. At least half of these tumors are malignant, metastasizing to regional lymph nodes and liver. Approximately one-fourth of patients have the multiple endocrine neoplasia syndrome, Type I (parathyroid adenomas, pituitary adenoma, pheochromocytomas) (Jensen et al., 1983). Patients are usually middle-aged and present with intractable peptic ulcer disease, often with associated malabsorption (secondary to inactivation of lipase and bile salt precipitation from hyperacidity). Serum gastrin levels are always elevated, and a paradoxical increase

in gastrin levels occurs after an injection of secretin. This latter test distinguishes Zollinger-Ellison syndrome from other diseases with elevated serum gastrin levels, i.e., retained gastric antrum, antral G-cell hyperplasia, short bowel syndrome, and uremia.

Upper gastrointestinal radiographic findings include enlarged rugal folds, hypersecretion, peptic ulcers, and thickened folds in the proximal small bowel. At CT, gastric and duodenal wall thickening and hypersecretion may be seen. The primary tumor in the pancreas and evidence of extrapancreatic metastases may also be visible.

Small pancreatic tumors without evidence of metastases are surgically resected. Advanced lesions are treated with a combination of $H_2$ blockers, chemotherapy, and hepatic artery embolization. CT and MRI are most commonly used in the identification of the primary tumor and in the follow-up imaging studies of these patients.

## Case 106

## ZOLLINGER-ELLISON SYNDROME

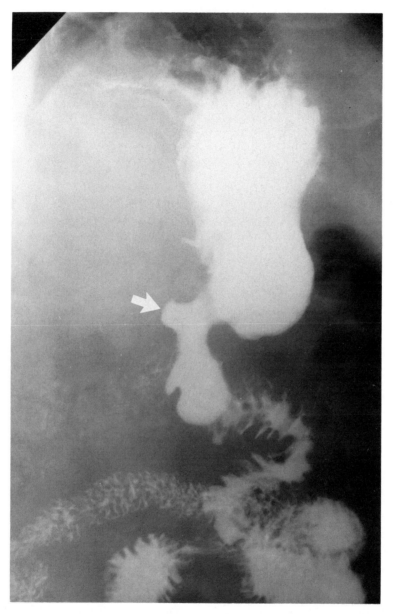

A Billroth II gastroenterostomy is present with a large ulceration *(arrow)* near the anastomosis (marginal ulcer). This patient had Zollinger-Ellison syndrome.

Three conditions are commonly considered in patients with marginal ulcers: Zollinger-Ellison syndrome (Case 105), retained gastric antrum (retained parietal cells), and incomplete vagotomy. A majority of these patients have no identifiable cause for their ulcer.

Large, rapidly developing anastomotic ulcers should be highly suspect for Zollinger-Ellison syndrome. These ulcers can rapidly penetrate, perforate, and bleed. Hypersecretion is also often encountered in Zollinger-Ellison syndrome. This can be identified by noting excess fluid in the stomach and poor mucosal coating and dilution of barium in the proximal small bowel.

## Case 107

# CAUSTIC STRICTURE OF THE GASTRIC ANTRUM

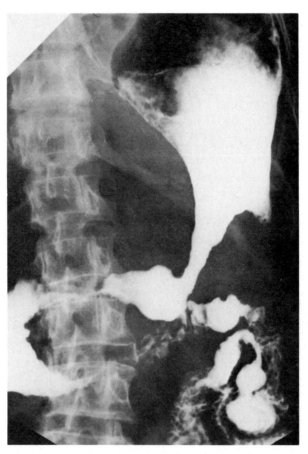

The antrum of the stomach is irregularly narrowed. There is an abrupt margin at the junction of the antrum and body along the greater curvature. These findings are compatible with a history of ingesting a corrosive agent, but an annular carcinoma also could have this appearance. This patient had a history of ammonia ingestion.

Caustic injury to the stomach from acid, alkali, or other chemicals usually affects the antrum more severely than the proximal stomach. The amount of gastric damage depends on the depth of the burn. Mucosal damage (first degree burn) alone will heal without sequelae. Second degree burns involve the submucosa and muscular layers of the stomach. Healing occurs with fibrosis and stricture formation. The secretory and peristaltic functions of the stomach may also be inhibited depending on the amount of damage. Third degree burns involve transmural damage, usually resulting in inflammation in the surrounding affected tissues. Hemorrhage, sepsis, and shock can occur.

Abdominal plain films taken soon after the initial injury usually demonstrate that the stomach is air-filled with thickened rugal folds. Mediastinal widening on the chest radiograph often indicates mediastinitis. Mediastinal emphysema, gastric emphysema, or pneumoperitoneum commonly accompanies third degree burns. Ulceration of the stomach and duodenum can be seen 2 to 3 days after ingestion. Subsequent changes include large intraluminal filling defects from hematomas, contraction of the distal stomach with atony, rigidity, and contour irregularity. Late changes include antral stenosis (as seen in this case). Abrupt annular narrowing of the gastric lumen can be confused with a carcinoma (Case 132). Associated lesions in the esophagus and duodenum, in addition to a history of caustic ingestion, can help differentiate this lesion from cancer.

## Case 108

## CROHN'S DISEASE

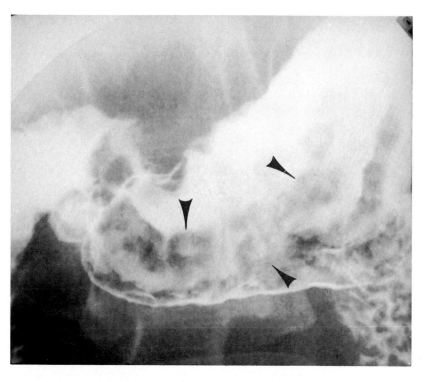

Multiple erosions *(arrowheads)* are present in the gastric antrum. Crohn's disease was proved by endoscopic biopsy (chronic inflammation and granulomas).

Crohn's disease (regional enteritis) of the stomach is uncommon, but when present it is usually associated with disease in either or both the small bowel and the colon. The earliest changes from Crohn's disease include aphthous ulcers and fold thickening (as seen in this case). Continued inflammation results in confluent ulcers, cobblestoning, denuded mucosa, fibrosis, and strictures (Case 109). The distal half of the stomach is usually affected, often with concomitant duodenal involvement (Cases 207 and 208).

The finding of "aphthous" ulcerations (superficial erosions) is nonspecific and could be secondary to peptic ulcer disease or medication-induced gastritis (i.e., aspirin). Endoscopy and histologic examination are often nonspecific as well.

## Case 109

## CROHN'S DISEASE

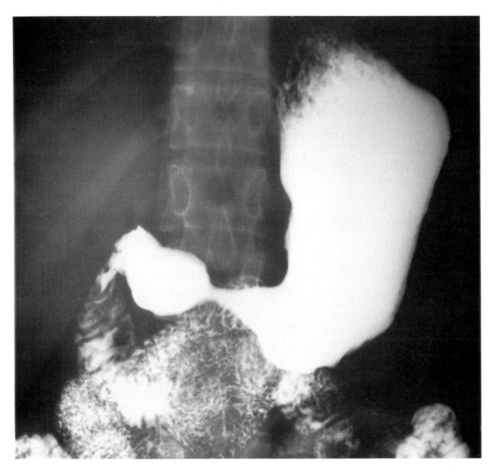

Symmetric tapered narrowing of the gastric antrum is present in this patient with known Crohn's disease.

Chronic changes of Crohn's disease are usually due to previous intramural inflammation and subsequent fibrosis. Because the distal stomach is most commonly involved, diffuse narrowing of this region often results in a tubular configuration resembling a "ram's horn" (Farman et al., 1975) or "pseudo-Billroth I" appearance. The scarring may not affect the circumference of the antrum evenly, resulting in irregular deformity of the antrum and proximal duodenum. Fistula formation and mass effect are less frequently encountered in the stomach than in the small bowel or colon. Differential considerations for the radiographic changes seen in this case include scarring from previous peptic ulcer disease, scirrhous carcinoma, eosinophilic gastroenteritis, and other granulomatous diseases (sarcoidosis [Case 112], tuberculosis, syphilis).

Case 110

# MÉNÉTRIER'S DISEASE

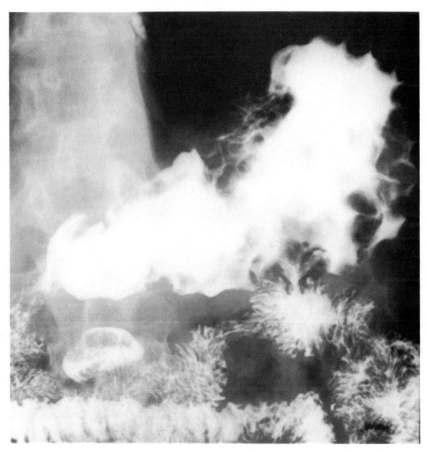

Markedly enlarged gastric folds are present within the proximal half of the stomach. A diverticulum is present involving the third portion of the duodenum.

Ménétrier's disease is a disorder of unknown cause, sometimes referred to as a hypertrophic gastropathy. Pathologically, hyperplasia of surface epithelial cells is present with abundant mucous cells and mucoid secretions. Parietal cells may be replaced by the epithelial cells, causing achlorhydria. The process is not primarily inflammatory, but inflammatory cells may be present. Erosions and hemorrhage may cause anemia. Carcinoma has been reported in patients with this disorder but it is unknown if it predisposes to malignancy (Fieber and Rickert, 1981). Treatment (antisecretory drugs and occasionally gastrectomy) is often not necessary unless pain, bleeding, or protein loss is severe.

Radiologic findings are usually those of enlarged rugal folds, often sparing the antrum. The folds are pliable, with a distensible stomach. Folds are enlarged but organized and follow the distribution of normal rugae. Occasionally, segmental rugal enlargement is seen and presents as a polypoid mass.

Gastric folds may be enlarged without any associated clinical disorder. These folds can nearly always be effaced with adequate distension of the gastric fundus. Enlarged folds in patients with lymphoma are usually disorganized and can be nodular and irregular (Cases 137 and 139). Zollinger-Ellison syndrome with enlarged gastric folds is often associated with hypersecretion, peptic ulcers, a dilated duodenum, and thickened folds in the proximal small bowel (Case 105). Patients with pseudolymphoma (Case 113) usually have localized thickened gastric folds and an associated chronic ulcer. Eosinophilic gastritis patients have thickened folds within the stomach and small bowel as well as an allergic history. *Campylobacter pyloris* gastritis has been reported to be associated with enlarged gastric folds.

## Case 111

## MÉNÉTRIER'S DISEASE

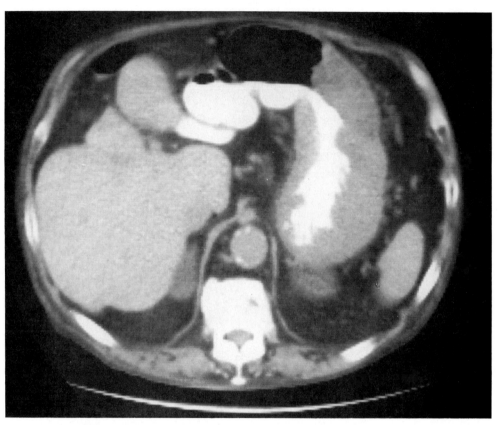

The wall of the gastric fundus and body is markedly thickened, especially along the greater curvature. The antral wall is of normal thickness. Bilateral adrenal masses are present. Findings of chronic gastritis consistent with Ménétrier's disease were confirmed pathologically after an endoscopic biopsy.

The CT appearance of Ménétrier's disease is nonspecific. The bulky wall thickening could be due to lymphoma (Case 140). This amount of wall thickness is unusual in patients with gastric adenocarcinoma. Zollinger-Ellison syndrome (Case 105 **B**) is usually associated with enlarged rugal folds with normal or near-normal intervening gastric wall thickness.

**Case 112**

# GRANULOMATOUS GASTRITIS (SARCOID)

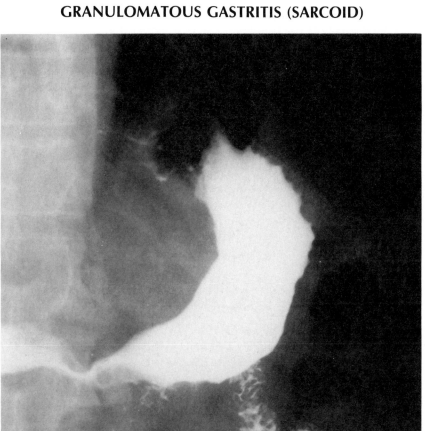

The distal third of the stomach is narrowed, tapered, and nondistensible.

The most frequent cause of granulomatous gastritis is Crohn's disease (Case 109). Most patients with Crohn's disease have concomitant disease in the small bowel. Sarcoidosis involving the stomach nearly always presents in association with disseminated disease. In fact, disease in other organs usually is critical in distinguishing sarcoidosis from the other granulomatous diseases.

Isolated granulomatous gastritis does not antedate the development of Crohn's disease or sarcoidosis. Other diseases that can present with similar radiographic findings include tuberculosis, syphilis, and histoplasmosis. There are no specific radiologic findings that are helpful in differentiating these entities. Gastric carcinoma (Case 125), metastatic breast cancer (Case 144), and scarring from corrosive ingestion (Case 107) could have similar radiographic changes.

# Case 113

## PSEUDOLYMPHOMA

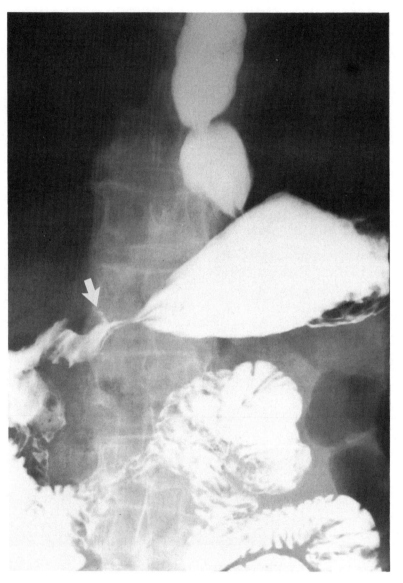

The distal stomach is narrowed and poorly distensible. An ulcer crater *(arrow)* is seen along the lesser curvature. Thickened gastric folds are present in the prepyloric region. At operation, pseudolymphoma was found. An incidental esophageal hiatal hernia is also present.

Pseudolymphoma is an inflammatory disease of the stomach, often secondary to a chronic gastric ulcer. Histologically, multiple inflammatory cell types are present (lymphocytes, histiocytes, fibroblasts, and plasma cells), whereas lymphomas are composed of a single cell line. There is no malignant potential.

No typical radiographic appearance has been reported. An ulcerated mass with associated folds that are enlarged either about the mass or throughout the stomach is considered the most common presentation. Infiltrating constricting lesions with ulceration, well-defined solitary ulcers, and enlarged rugal folds have also been described (Martel et al., 1976). Ulcers can appear radiographically benign or malignant, and associated submucosal infiltration can resemble lymphoma.

### Case 114

## GASTRIC POLYPS

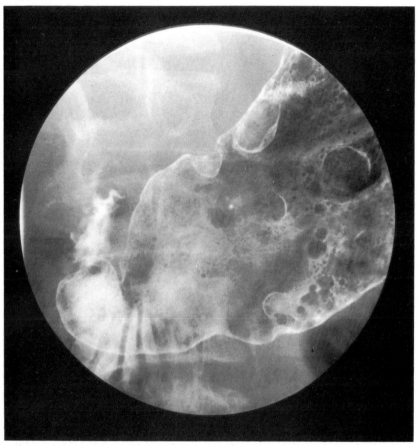

Multiple polypoid filling defects are present in the stomach. These were found to be hyperplastic polyps at endoscopic biopsy.

Gastric polyps occur in about 2% of the population (Feczko, 1989). Most polyps are either hyperplastic or adenomatous histologically. Hyperplastic polyps develop as a reactive change to chronic inflammation with mucosal proliferation and cystic dilatation of gastric glands. Some authors refer to them as regenerative or inflammatory polyps. They are often multiple and usually small (<1 cm in diameter). They have a propensity to develop in the fundus of the stomach, but they may be found anywhere. Hyperplastic polyps are believed to be benign, without malignant potential; however, rare malignant transformation has been reported (Feczko et al., 1985).

Adenomatous polyps are infrequent, often solitary lesions, with diameters exceeding 1 cm. These polyps can develop into carcinomas, but this is an unusual occurrence generally encountered among large (>2 cm) lesions (Feczko, 1989). Some studies have reported an increased incidence of gastric carcinoma in patients with adenomatous polyps. Overall, development of a cancer from gastric polyps is a rare event, perhaps occurring in 1% to 2% of patients. Endoscopic biopsy and polypectomy are safe and should be considered for solitary polyps 2 cm or more in diameter.

## Case 115

## GASTRIC POLYPS

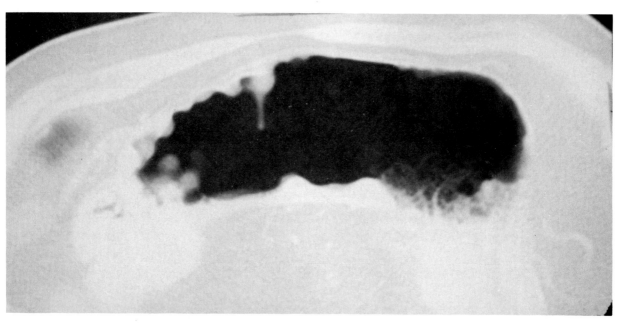

Multiple polyps arise from the anterior and posterior walls of the stomach. A drop of contrast material (stalactite phenomenon) hangs from a polyp on the nondependent (anterior) gastric wall.

Multiple polyps are usually hyperplastic histologically.

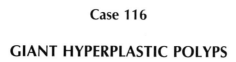

## Case 116

## GIANT HYPERPLASTIC POLYPS

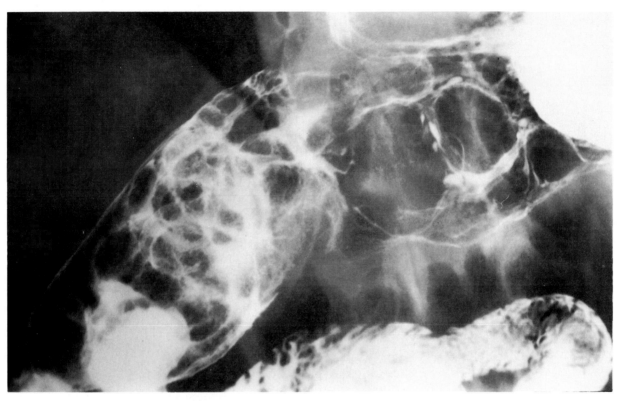

Multiple, large, lobulated filling defects are present within the stomach. Multiple hyperplastic polyps were confirmed at endoscopic biopsy.

In the literature, the histologic description of gastric polyps is confusing. At one time all gastric polyps were referred to as adenomas. Even today, agreement on the nomenclature of these polyps is not possible. Generally, polyps can be regarded as adenomatous and hyperplastic. Hyperplastic polyps are more often multiple than are adenomatous polyps. Polyp size is not always a helpful criterion in distinguishing adenomatous from hyperplastic polyps. Some studies report a compound-type polyp that contains both hyperplastic and adenomatous elements (Smith and Lee, 1983). This type of polyp may account for the discrepancy in classification that can occur from tissue obtained at endoscopic biopsy and at surgical polypectomy. To be safe, polyps larger than 2 cm in diameter should be removed.

## Case 117

## GASTRIC POLYPS: GARDNER'S SYNDROME

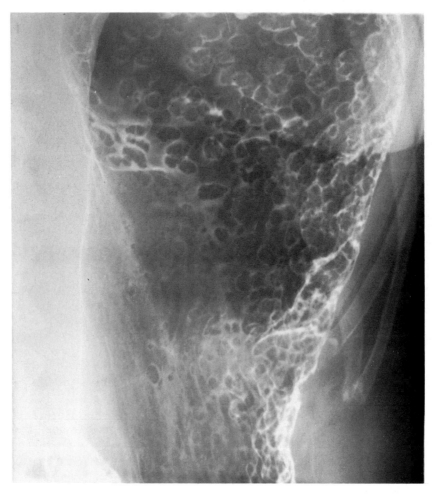

Innumerable small polyps are present throughout the stomach. They are most numerous within the fundus. This patient had known Gardner's syndrome.

Gastric polyps in patients with familial polyposis or Gardner's syndrome are usually hyperplastic, whereas polyps elsewhere in the intestines are adenomatous. Gastric adenomatous polyps are uncommon, but when they occur in these patients they are usually located in the antrum and may be multiple (Feczko, 1989). Gastric polyps developing in the other polyposis syndromes (Peutz-Jeghers syndrome, juvenile polyposis, and Canada-Cronkhite syndrome) are classified as hamartomas (Feczko, 1989).

**Case 118**

## INTUSSUSCEPTED GASTRIC POLYP

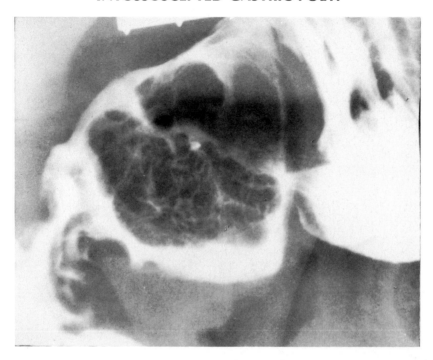

A polypoid filling defect is seen within the duodenal bulb. At fluoroscopy, this could be seen to move freely between the stomach and duodenum with a gastric attachment. The surface of the polyp is lobulated and has some villous features (barium fills many small interstices on its surface). At removal, the polyp was hyperplastic histologically.

## Case 119

# GASTRIC LEIOMYOMA

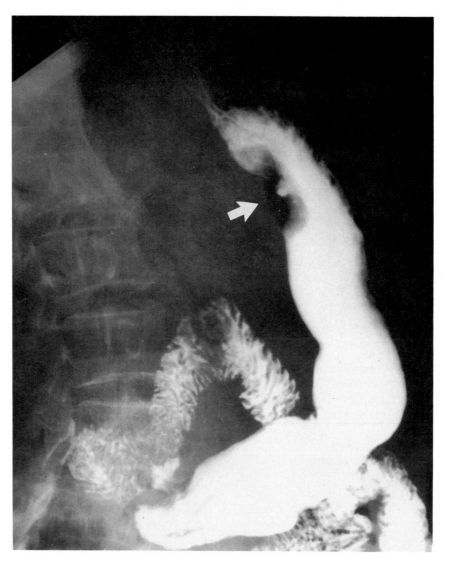

A well-demarcated, smooth-surfaced mass *(arrow)* is present along the lesser curvature of the gastric fundus. A central ulceration is present.

Leiomyomas are the most common submucosal gastric tumor. They can occur anywhere within the stomach. Depending on their growth characteristics, they can occupy an intramural location (as in this case), extend intraluminally (Case 120), or extend as an exophytic mass from the stomach (Case 122). The smooth surface is characteristic of a submucosal tumor. A 90° angle is often formed between the edges of the mass and the normal gastric wall.

Leiomyomas are often asymptomatic lesions that are discovered incidentally. Bleeding and melena are common complaints in patients with symptomatic lesions. Abdominal pain and obstruction can also occur.

Any tumor arising from the cellular elements of the submucosa could have similar radiographic features. These neoplasms include fibromas, lipomas (Case 123), neurogenic tumors, leiomyosarcomas (Case 142), vascular tumors, and carcinoids.

## Case 120

## LEIOMYOMA: INTRALUMINAL

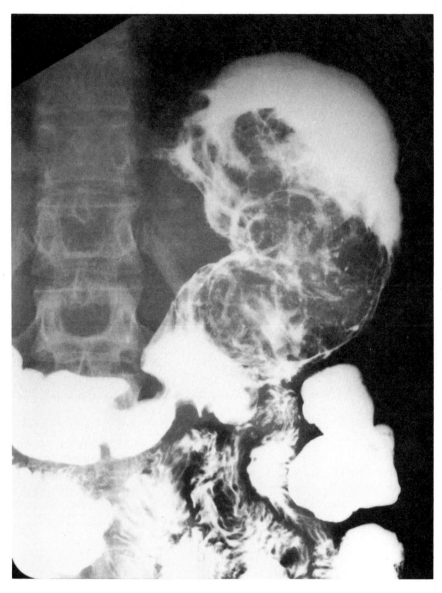

A large intraluminal mass is present within the stomach. A large leiomyoma was removed surgically.

Some smooth muscle tumors will grow intraluminally and resemble a polypoid neoplasm (carcinoma or lymphoma) (Cases 129, 130, and 136) or a foreign body (bezoar) (Case 169). Large tumors such as this may cause gastric obstruction.

It is often difficult to differentiate leiomyomas from leiomyosarcomas either radiographically or histologically. The behavior of the tumor best determines its biologic aggressiveness. Metastases and recurrence are features of malignant tumors. In addition, large size, surface lobulations, surface irregularity, and ulceration are all worrisome radiographic features for a leiomyosarcoma (Case 142).

## Case 121

## LEIOMYOMA: INTRALUMINAL, ULCERATED

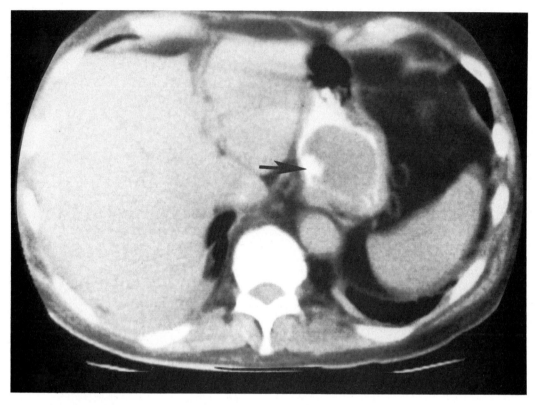

A mass is present within the gastric fundus. An ulcer crater *(arrow)* can be seen within the mass. At operation a leiomyoma was removed.

CT may be helpful in patients with a known or suspected smooth muscle tumor, especially if sarcomatous degeneration is likely. The origin and extent of exophytic tumors can be delineated at CT. The malignant nature of these tumors can also be suggested at CT. Malignant tumors (leiomyosarcomas) tend to be larger (often >10 cm diameter) than their benign counterparts, have an irregular shape, and are often inhomogeneous with regions of central necrosis (Case 142). The presence of distant metastases and adjacent organ invasion can also be assessed at CT.

**Case 122**

## EXOPHYTIC LEIOMYOBLASTOMA

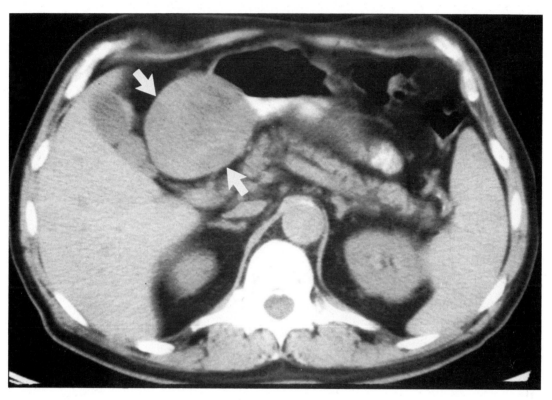

A well-marginated, inhomogeneous mass *(arrows)* is present adjacent to the gastric antrum. At operation, an exophytic leiomyoblastoma was removed.

Leiomyoblastomas have identical radiographic features of other smooth muscle tumors in the alimentary tract. They are distinguished from leiomyomas by the distinctive smooth muscle cells seen microscopically. Approximately 10% of these tumors are malignant—the same proportion as for leiomyomas.

## Case 123

## GASTRIC LIPOMA

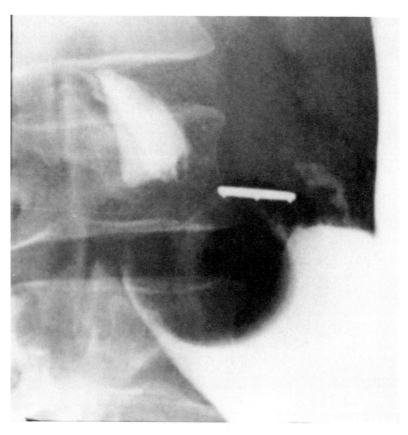

A well-circumscribed, round filling defect fills the distal gastric antrum. The mass has a smooth surface due to the intact overlying mucosa. The appearance is typical of a submucosal tumor. A 2-cm metallic marker attached to a compression device is visible adjacent to the mass.

Gastric lipomas may be radiologically indistinguishable from leiomyomas. Lipomas usually present as solitary intraluminal masses within the antrum and may change shape during peristalsis or compression. These tumors may be pedunculated and can prolapse into the duodenum or, rarely, obstruct the pylorus. The surface of these tumors may ulcerate. CT of these lesions is diagnostic if the typical fatty density is identified within the tumor (Cases 226, 312, and 407).

## Case 124

# ECTOPIC PANCREAS

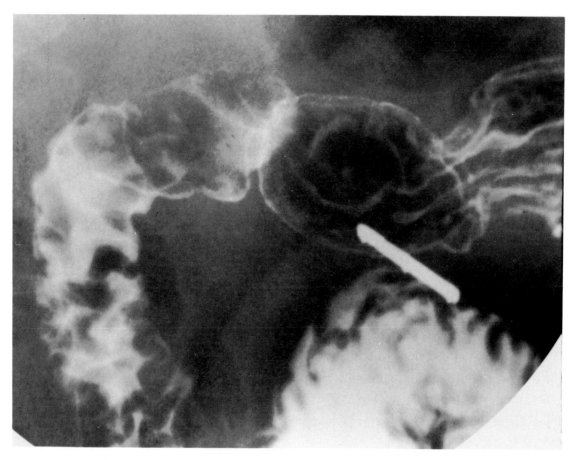

A 1.5-cm, round filling defect containing a central umbilication is present within the gastric antrum. This is the typical size, location, and appearance of ectopic (heterotopic) pancreas. The metallic marker is a measuring and compression device scored at 1-cm intervals.

Ectopic rests of pancreatic tissue have been identified in up to 14% of all autopsy specimens (Feldman and Weinberg, 1952). They are more commonly encountered than are gastric leiomyomas. Usually they are encountered incidentally, but any condition affecting the pancreas can also affect ectopic tissue. Diseases including pancreatitis, pseudocyst formation, carcinoma, and adenoma have been reported (Thoeni and Gedgaudas, 1980).

Although the distal stomach is usually involved, other locations including the duodenum, ileum, and within a Meckel diverticulum are possible (Dolan et al., 1974). Radiographically, they appear as umbilicated submucosal nodules, although nearly half may not contain the characteristic central depression (Kilman and Berk, 1977). The umbilication is not an ulceration; it is covered by normal epithelium. Rudimentary ducts may empty into this depression. These masses are often indistinguishable from a leiomyoma (Case 119) or other submucosal tumor (Case 123).

## Case 125

## EARLY GASTRIC CANCER

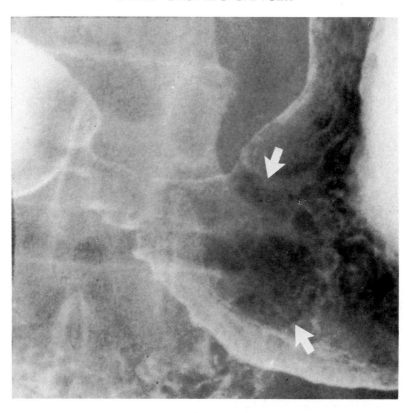

The antrum is deformed and irregular in contour. The mucosal pattern within the antrum is distorted with loss of the normal gastric folds and areae gastricae pattern. The margins *(arrows)* of the lesion are indistinct. Endoscopic biopsy and operation revealed a superficial spreading carcinoma without invasion beyond the muscularis mucosae.

The Japanese Endoscopic Society developed a classification for early gastric cancers. "Early" cancers refer to those tumors in which invasion is limited to the mucosa and submucosa (regardless of nodal or distant metastases). The three major types include:

Type I—protruded type, >5 mm

Type II—superficial growth which may be elevated (<5 mm) (IIa), flat (IIb), or depressed (IIc)

Type III—excavated type; this is usually seen in combination with type I or II tumors.

Early cancers are more frequently encountered in Japan, accounting for 30% of gastric tumors. The 5-year survival with these tumors approaches 90%. Nearly 10% may be synchronous (Marshak et al., 1983).

**Case 126**

## GASTRIC CARCINOMA: ABNORMAL FOLDS

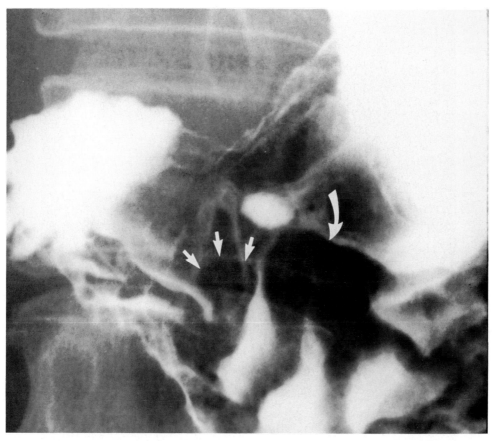

A small ulcer crater is present in the gastric antrum. Several abnormal folds are present adjacent to the ulcer crater, including fold clubbing *(arrows)* and fusion *(curved arrow).* The other surrounding folds are enlarged or effaced and not visible. At operation, a gastric adenocarcinoma was removed.

Early depressed cancers are often recognized by the characteristic changes of the converging folds about the cancer. Fold alteration usually includes clubbing, tapering, interruption (amputation), and fusion. When these findings are identified, a cancer should be suspected and an endoscopic biopsy should be performed.

## Case 127

# GASTRIC ADENOCARCINOMA: CARMAN'S MENISCUS SIGN

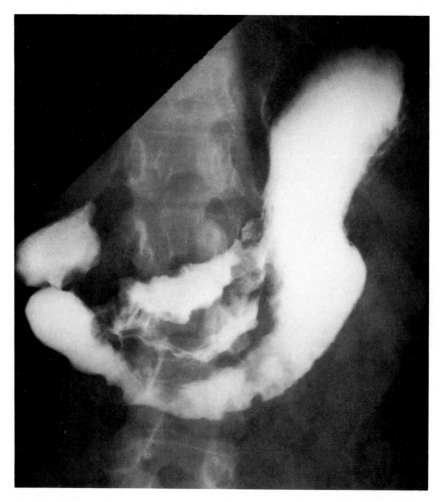

A large, ulcerated mass straddles the lesser curvature of the gastric body/antrum. The ulcer does not extend beyond the confines of the normal gastric lumen, and the surrounding mass has a lobulated contour. These findings are typical of a gastric carcinoma.

Gastric cancer remains a lethal disease. Most patients in this country have advanced-stage disease at diagnosis (65% with tumor, nodes, metastases stages III and IV) and a very low 5-year survival (<10% for these advanced-stage lesions) (Marshak et al., 1983).

Radiologic features of malignancy in lesions that are ulcerated include: (1) nodularity of the tissue surrounding the ulcer—often the orifice and floor of the crater are also nodular; (2) abrupt transition between the sur-

rounding tissue and the normal gastric wall; (3) the crater does not project beyond the normal confines of the gastric wall; (4) radiating folds stop at the edge of the surrounding tissue and do not reach the crater itself; (5) the crater is asymmetrically placed within the surrounding tissue; and (6) the crater is often wider than it is deep.

Carman's meniscus sign is demonstrated when the malignant ulcer straddles the lesser curvature and compression is applied apposing the margins of the surrounding tumor. The ulcer appears as a crescent (half moon) on the lesser curvature, with nodular tumor surrounding the periphery of the ulcer. This sign is reported to be pathognomonic of carcinoma.

## Case 128

## ULCERATING GASTRIC CARCINOMA

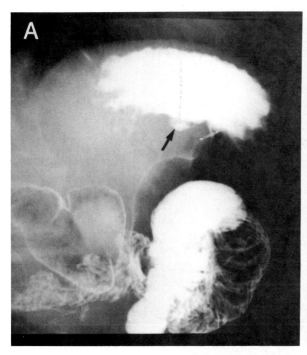

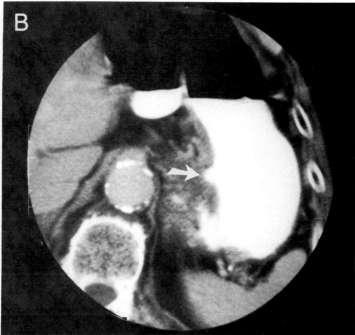

**A.** An ulcerated *(arrow)* mass is present along the lesser curvature of the gastric fundus. The benign or malignant nature of the surrounding mass is difficult to assess on this particular view. This is an unusual location for a benign peptic ulcer and endoscopy should probably be performed routinely to exclude malignancy in ulcers within the proximal stomach.

**B.** Marked gastric wall thickening is present along the lesser curvature of the gastric fundus. The medial margins (in the region of the gastrohepatic ligament) of the mass are poorly defined, suggesting possible extragastric extension. The ulceration *(arrow)* within the mass is seen clearly. Findings are characteristic of a gastric cancer.

There are several classification schemes that are recognized for gastric cancers. *Borrmann's classification* is generally used to stage advanced cancer (cancer that extends beyond the submucosa) and is based on the gross morphology of the tumor.

Type I—polypoid, nonulcerated (Cases 129, 130, and 131)

Type II—ulcerated, circumscribed margins; this may appear radiographically as infiltrating (Cases 127 and 128)

Type III—ulcerated, poorly circumscribed

Type IV—diffuse, infiltrating; linitis plastica (Cases 132, 133, and 134).

CT usually is not the primary imaging modality used for detecting mucosal-based disease of the stomach. It is valuable in assessing extraluminal disease extent. Normally the gastric wall is <5 mm thick (Komaki, 1982). Gastric wall thickening by itself is nonspecific and can be seen in various inflammatory and neoplastic disorders. Early gastric cancer cannot usually be detected at CT, but most advanced tumors are visible (approximately 80% sensitivity) (Komaki, 1986). The esophagogastric junction can appear thickened normally, and in questionable cases additional oral administration of contrast material or effervescent granules, or both, may be required to exclude a mass.

## Case 129

## POLYPOID GASTRIC CARCINOMA

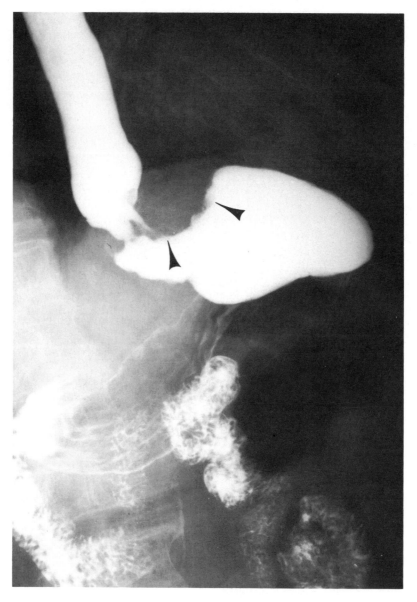

A polypoid filling defect *(arrowheads)* is present in the gastric fundus and cardia. Gastric adenocarcinoma was found at operation.

The incidence of gastric cancer has decreased in the United States. It now is the third most frequent gastrointestinal cancer after colorectal and pancreatic carcinoma (Boring et al., 1991). A few decades ago, gastric cancer was the most frequent gastrointestinal malignancy. There is considerable geographic variability throughout the world in the incidence of this disease.

High cancer rates are found in Japan, Finland, Iceland, and Chile. Several etiologic factors are likely to contribute to the development of this disease including high starch diets, polycyclic hydrocarbons (found in home-smoked foods), and nitrosamines (found in processed meats and vegetables). Patients with some gastric conditions—including atrophic gastritis, pernicious anemia, post-subtotal gastrectomy, and adenomatous polyps—are also considered to have a higher risk of gastric malignancy developing.

## Case 130

# POLYPOID GASTRIC CARCINOMA

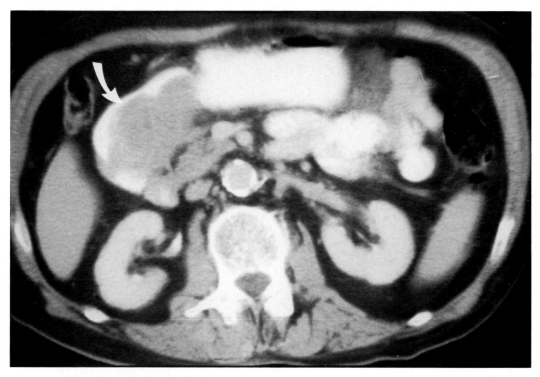

A large, polypoid, intraluminal, soft tissue mass *(arrow)* is present in the gastric antrum. Gastric adenocarcinoma was found at operation.

The use of routine preoperative CT for patients with known gastric cancer is controversial. Some investigators have found CT unreliable in determining the true extent of disease (Sussman et al., 1988). Nodal metastases can be particularly problematic, because normal-sized lymph nodes can contain metastases and enlarged lymph nodes may be hyperplastic. Solitary adenopathy was a common finding (62%) among false-positive examinations (Sussman et al., 1988). Some investigators observed that nonmalignant adenopathy will often (>80%) enhance with intravenously administered contrast material, whereas nodes replaced with tumor usually do not enhance (Komaki, 1986).

Despite these difficulties, no other examination except laparotomy can define disease extent better. At our institution, CT is utilized in selected preoperative cases to search for distant metastases to the liver and lungs and in the postoperative follow-up of these patients.

## Case 131

## POLYPOID, INFILTRATIVE GASTRIC CARCINOMA

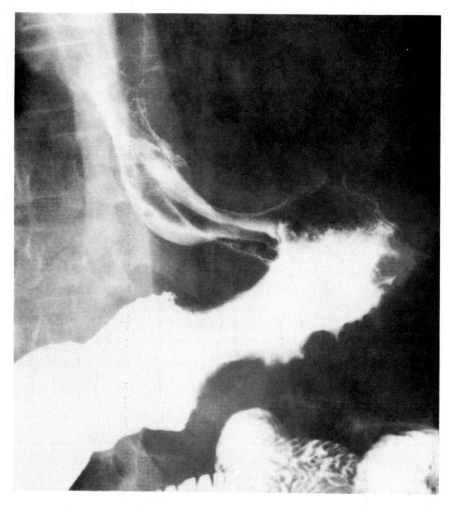

Several filling defects are seen within a nondistensible segment of the gastric body. The mass encases and narrows the stomach. Gastric folds can be seen at the level of the mass along the greater curvature. This is often found in patients with submucosal tumor extension. Gastric adenocarcinoma was found at surgical exploration.

Today, most patients with gastric cancers will have preoperative endoscopy for histologic confirmation. A correct diagnosis of gastric cancer can usually be made endoscopically; however, infiltrative tumors may be detected in only 70% of patients (Levine et al., 1990). The gastric cardia and the antrum beyond the incisura are the two most difficult regions from which to obtain adequate tissue samples.

Operation is the only treatment that can result in cure. Many authorities favor an extensive gastric and lymph node resection. Approximately 40% of patients with gastric cancer have advanced disease that precludes a curative resection. Many patients undergo a palliative bypass procedure to prevent obstruction or to relieve dysphagia.

**Case 132**

# SCIRRHOUS CARCINOMA OF THE STOMACH

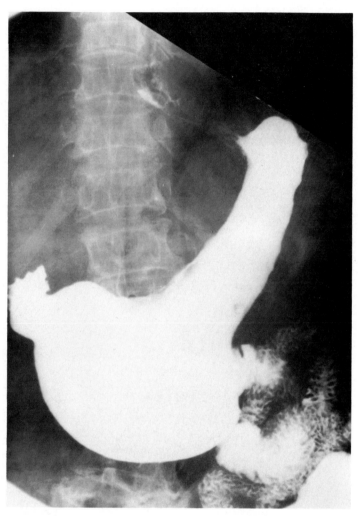

Marked narrowing is present within the gastric fundus and proximal body. This appearance of a markedly rigid and noncompliant gastric wall is typical of a scirrhous cancer.

Scirrhous carcinomas spread within the submucosa of the gastric wall, often inciting a desmoplastic reaction. Because of the narrowing and rigidity that often accompany these tumors, the radiographic appearance of the stomach has been likened to a leather bottle (linitis plastica). Gastric narrowing is not always detectable in all patients. In patients with these lesions, there may be mucosal nodularity, fold thickening, or ulceration.

Many conditions can present with similar radiographic findings. Breast cancer metastases can resemble scirrhous tumors and often narrow the gastric antrum. Omental metastases, often arising from a primary carcinoma in the transverse colon, can invade the stomach via the gastrocolic ligament and the stomach can resemble linitis plastica. Scarring from prior peptic ulcer disease, Crohn's disease, granulomatous infections, and antral gastritis can also cause antral narrowing. In elderly patients with atrophic gastritis, the antrum can be narrowed.

Histologic confirmation of scirrhous adenocarcinoma of the stomach may be difficult to obtain on the basis of an endoscopic biopsy. The disease is primarily located in the submucosal tissues and requires a deep biopsy specimen. In addition, the associated desmoplastic reaction may widely intersperse cancer cells between large areas of fibrosis.

**145**

**Case 133**

## SCIRRHOUS CARCINOMA

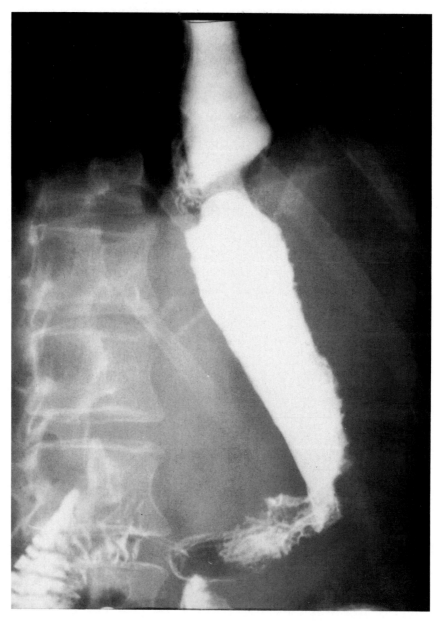

The entire stomach is nondistensible and tube-like as
a result of diffuse submucosal tumor—linitis plastica.

**Case 134**

## SCIRRHOUS CARCINOMA

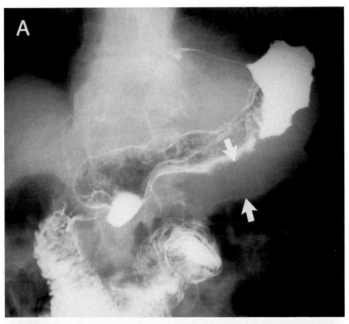

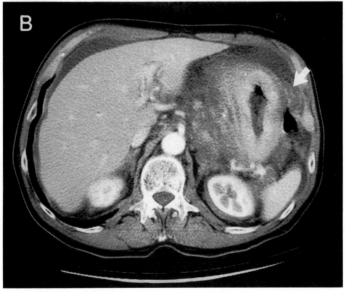

**A.** The wall of the stomach is markedly thickened *(arrows),* with narrowing and scalloping of the gastric contour.

**B.** The gastric wall is markedly thickened and enhances after the intravenous administration of contrast material. Extragastric extension *(arrow)* as well as ascites indicates tumor dissemination with intraperitoneal carcinomatosis.

Infiltrative tumors such as in this case are the type most frequently encountered today. Scirrhous tumors often enhance after intravenous administration of contrast material. These tumors often involve a large extent of the stomach and often spread to peritoneal surfaces. Polypoid and ulcerative tumors usually do not enhance.

Case 135

## METASTATIC GASTRIC CANCER

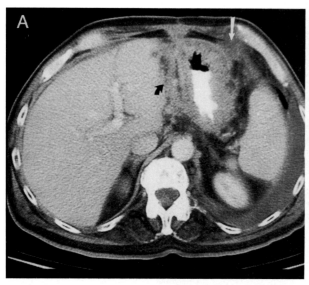 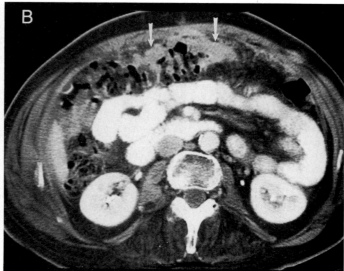

**A.** Circumferential thickening of the gastric fundus is due to a primary gastric carcinoma. The serosal contours are irregular and poorly defined. Abnormal soft-tissue masses are seen about the anterior peritoneal surface *(arrow)*. There is also soft-tissue thickening *(curved arrow)* within the gastrohepatic ligament, representing adenopathy. A left pleural effusion also is present.

**B.** Multiple soft-tissue masses *(arrows)* are seen within the omentum, anterior and adjacent to the transverse colon. The findings are typical of omental metastases.

The lesser and greater omentum represent tissues that are in direct contiguity with the gastric serosa. Once cancer extends to the serosa, extension to the omentum occurs in a majority of patients. More than 90% of patients have omental involvement if the tumor has reached the serosa, whereas only approximately a third of patients with tumor limited to the muscular layer will have omental tumor (Komaki, 1986).

Lymphatic metastases are common within nodes along the lesser curvature (within the gastrohepatic ligament) and greater curvature. Other commonly involved nodal groups include parapancreatic, para-aortic, and nodes around the middle colic artery.

After tumor spreads beyond the serosa, cells may seed the peritoneal cavity. Meyers eloquently described the usual routes of intraperitoneal tumor spread—often involving the pouch of Douglas, sigmoid mesocolon, right paracolic gutter, and small bowel mesentery (Meyers, 1988). Metastatic spread to the ovary is referred to as a Krukenberg tumor. Most liver and lung metastases occur as a result of hematogenous dissemination.

Direct invasion of gastric cancer to the pancreas or liver can be difficult to recognize at CT. Only if there are obvious findings of invasion should the diagnosis be made confidently.

## Case 136

## LYMPHOMA: POLYPOID

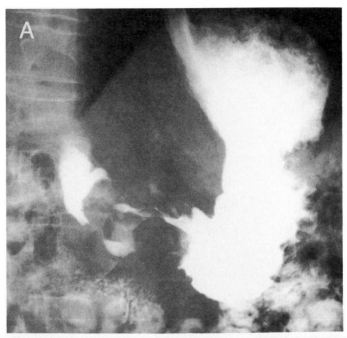

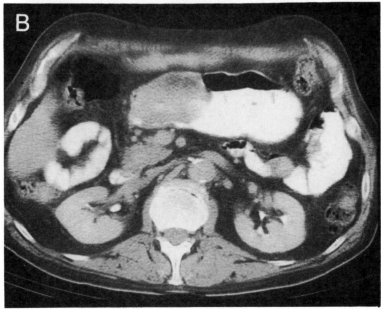

**A.** The gastric antrum is markedly narrowed by a large constricting mass.

**B.** A large polyploid mass arising from the anterior wall of the gastric antrum is present at CT. At operation, a large cell lymphoma was resected.

Solitary lymphomas, as in this case, can mimic gastric adenocarcinoma (Cases 129 and 130). The diagnosis may be difficult to make at endoscopic biopsy because the overlying mucosa may be intact and prevent adequate tumor sampling. For this reason, multiple biopsy specimens at sites of possible mucosal involvement are used.

Case 137

## LYMPHOMA: MULTIPLE SUBMUCOSAL MASSES

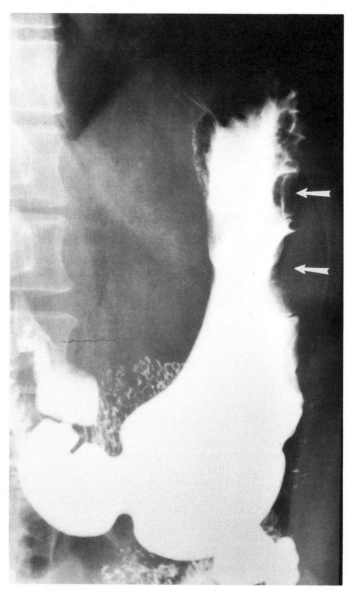

Multiple smooth-surfaced filling defects *(arrows)* are present in the gastric fundus along the greater curvature. Later, non-Hodgkin's lymphoma was proved.

The stomach is the most common extranododal site for non-Hodgkin's lymphoma. Disease confined to the stomach has a much better prognosis than does disseminated tumor, and it is often surgically resected rather than treated with chemotherapy. Radiation therapy also is used often.

Several radiographic forms of lymphoma have been identified: infiltrative (Cases 137, 139, and 140), ulcerative (Case 138), polypoid (Cases 136 and 138), and intraluminal-fungating (Case 136). There often is overlap among the radiographic forms that are seen. Radiographic features that are helpful in suggesting lymphoma include multiplicity of lesions, involvement of a large extent of the stomach, evidence for a submucosal origin of the tumor, extension of the tumor across the pylorus, and less luminal narrowing than expected compared to usual gastric adenocarcinoma.

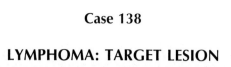

## Case 138

# LYMPHOMA: TARGET LESION

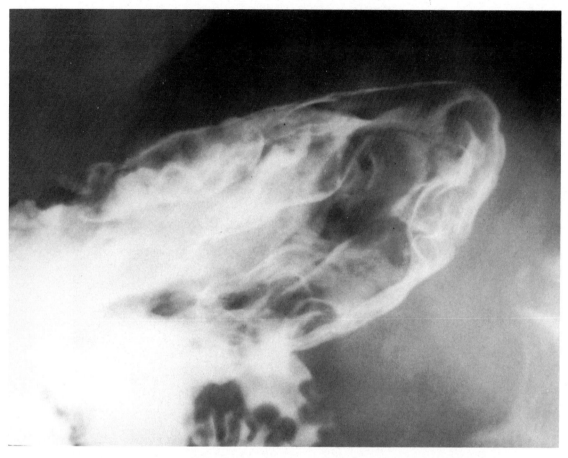

Multiple submucosal masses with central ulceration are present in the gastric fundus. Lymphoma was proved later.

Target lesions are an unusual presentation of lymphoma. Metastases should also be considered, especially melanoma (Case 145) and Kaposi's sarcoma.

## Case 139

## LYMPHOMA: DIFFUSE INFILTRATIVE

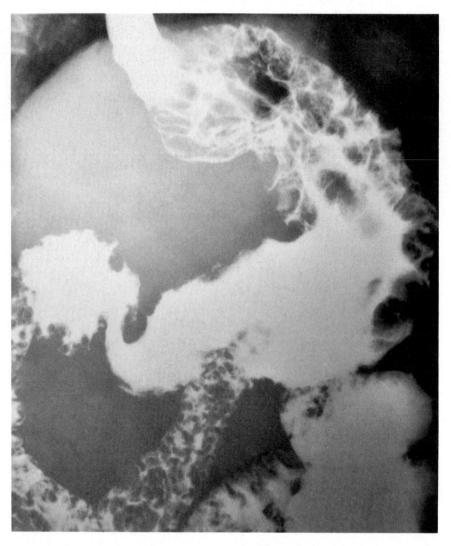

Marked rugal fold thickening is present throughout the stomach and in the duodenal bulb. Multiple nodules also are present in the duodenum.

Infiltrative lymphoma is often confined to the submucosal layers of the stomach. Ulcerations may be present. Despite extensive disease there is little restriction in gastric volume. Differential considerations include Ménétrier's disease (Case 110) and linitis plastica (gastric adenocarcinoma) (Cases 131, 133, and 134).

Ménétrier's disease usually affects the proximal stomach, and linitis plastica narrows the gastric lumen and produces a noncompliant affected segment. Lymphoma occasionally crosses the pylorus and affects the adjacent duodenum (as in this patient). Lymphomas can also occur within other regions of the alimentary tract. Because treatment and prognosis differ if the disease has spread beyond the stomach, it is often helpful to extend an upper gastrointestinal examination and study the small bowel as well.

Case 140

# LYMPHOMA: CT

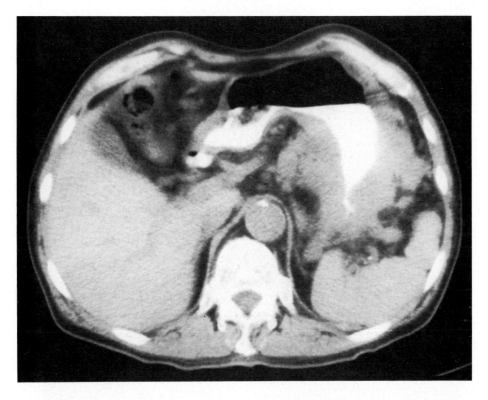

Marked wall thickening is seen within the gastric fundus and body. This amount of wall thickening is characteristic of lymphoma. Multiple enlarged perigastric lymph nodes are also present.

CT can be helpful in patients with known or suspected gastric lymphoma. The extent of extraluminal disease (usually adenopathy) can be documented and complications such as perforation and fistulization can be detected. Perigastric adenopathy is a common finding in patients with lymphoma, but it can also be found in patients with carcinoma (Case 135). Lymphadenopathy at or below the level of the renal pedicles is uncommon in patients with gastric carcinoma, but it has been reported in at least one-third of patients with lymphoma (Buy and Moss, 1982).

153

Case 141

## GASTRIC LEIOMYOSARCOMA

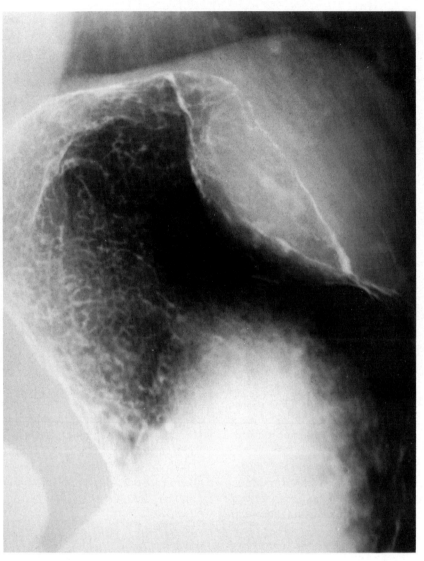

A large mass indents the gastric fundus. The surface of the mass is smooth and there appears to be a large extragastric component. The large size of the mass suggests malignancy, and a leiomyosarcoma was suggested. At operation, a leiomyosarcoma was removed.

Gastric leiomyosarcomas are unusual primary gastric tumors. Diagnosis of this tumor is important because it has a much better prognosis than does primary gastric adenocarcinoma. These tumors may present as primarily intramural masses; however, endogastric (Cases 120 and 121) or exogastric masses (Case 142) can also occur depending on the direction of growth. Surgical resection is the only curative treatment option. There are no definite radiographic criteria that differentiate leiomyomas from leiomyosarcomas. The larger the mass the more likely it is to be malignant. Most submucosal masses are surgically removed regardless of size, because even small tumors can harbor malignancy.

## Case 142

# LEIOMYOSARCOMA

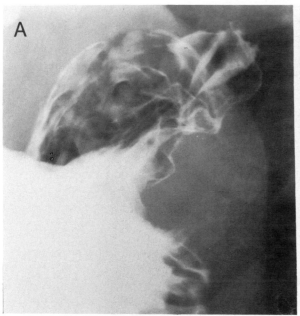

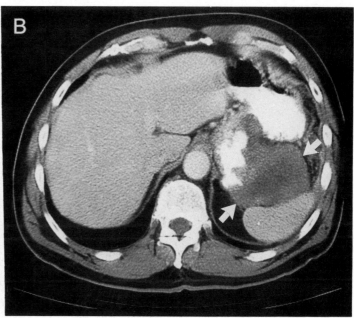

**A.** A smooth-surfaced mass is present in the posterior wall of the gastric fundus.

**B.** The mixed-density mass *(arrows)* is predominantly exophytic, lying between the posterior wall of the fundus and the spleen.

CT can be helpful in evaluating patients with smooth muscle tumors. These lesions can become large and often extend exophytically from the stomach. CT can assist in determining the origin and extent of these tumors. Large malignant tumors are often of heterogeneous density; because of necrosis, the central area is the density of water. In fact, one study stated that heterogeneity of the tumor was the most specific finding to suggest malignancy (Megibow et al., 1985). Metastases, when present, often spread to liver and peritoneal cavity. Metastases to local lymph nodes are unusual (Starr and Dockerty, 1955).

## Case 143

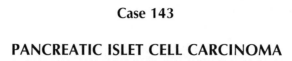

# PANCREATIC ISLET CELL CARCINOMA

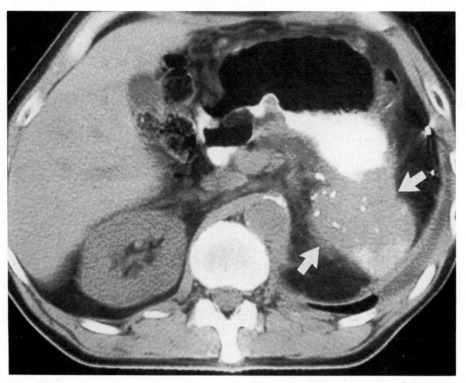

A mass *(arrows)* in the tail of the pancreas contains multiple coarse calcifications. Local direct invasion has occurred into the posterior wall of the gastric fundus and the spleen. An islet cell carcinoma was found surgically.

Pancreatic adenocarcinomas and islet cell carcinomas can invade locally into adjacent organs. Extrinsic mass effect, mural irregularity, and wall thickening of the stomach are common findings of locally invasive tumors arising from the pancreatic body and tail. Splenic vein thrombosis is a common associated finding in patients with pancreatic tumors in this location. As collaterals develop, gastric varices can often be identified on both CT (Case 162) and conventional barium studies (Case 160).

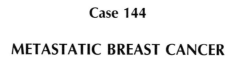

## Case 144

## METASTATIC BREAST CANCER

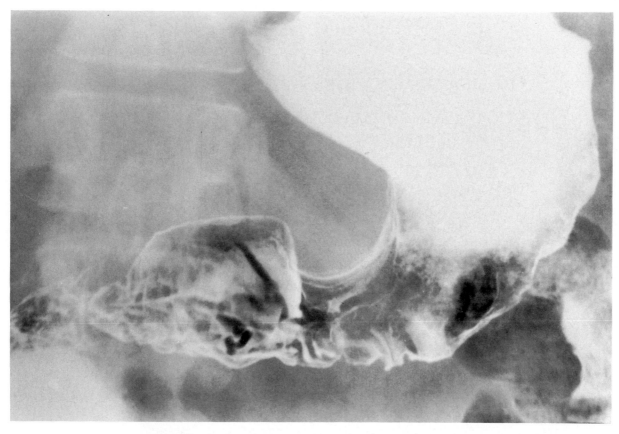

The greater curvature of the gastric body and antrum are deformed and nondistensible. This patient had known breast cancer, and the changes in the stomach were due to breast metastases.

Metastases from the breast to the stomach usually re-semble primary scirrhous carcinoma (Cases 132–134), with narrowing and rigidity of the lumen. Whenever a scirrhous carcinoma is identified in a woman, breast metastases should also be considered.

## Case 145

## METASTATIC MELANOMA

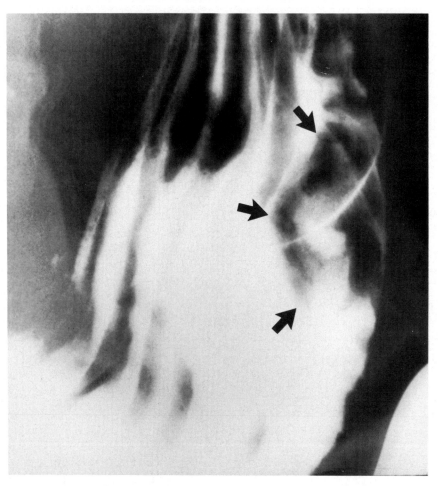

A mass *(arrows)* containing central ulceration is present in the stomach. This patient had a history of melanoma. Melanoma metastasis was proved later.

The radiographic appearance of melanoma metastasis is similar in the stomach and the small bowel. Usually a submucosal mass(es) containing a central ulceration is present. The appearance of these lesions has been described as a "target" or "bull's-eye" lesion. Although ulcerative metastases can cause gastrointestinal bleeding, other causes of bleeding should also be searched for in symptomatic cancer patients. Several studies have shown that in patients with gastroduode-nal bleeding and known cancer, a minority had malignant lesions causing the hemorrhage (Lightdale et al., 1973; Shivshanker et al., 1983). Severe gastritis and ulcers are most common in these patients.

Differential considerations of a solitary ulcerated lesion in the stomach include a smooth muscle tumor (Cases 119 and 121), primary gastric adenocarcinoma (Cases 126–128), lymphoma (Cases 136 and 138), or ectopic pancreatic rest (containing a central umbilication) (Case 124). Multiple lesions favor a diagnosis of metastases or lymphoma.

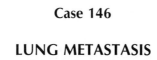

**Case 146**

## LUNG METASTASIS

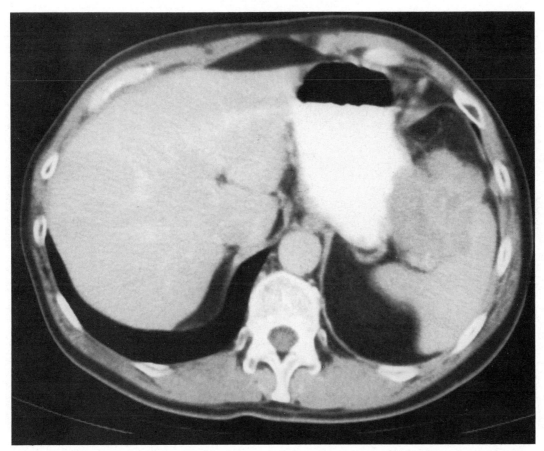

A lobulated soft tissue mass is present between the stomach and spleen. The mass indents the gastric fundus. Metastatic small cell carcinoma from a lung primary was later proved.

Metastases to the stomach from a primary lung lesion are relatively common, occurring in 3% to 26% of patients at autopsy (Libshitz et al., 1982). No characteristic appearance is associated with gastric metastases from lung cancer. Submucosal masses with a large extraluminal component can undergo central necrosis and ulceration. Most patients with metastases from breast cancer will appear to have linitis plastica (Case 144), whereas patients with melanoma often have bull's-eye lesions (Case 145).

## Case 147

## DIRECT INVASION

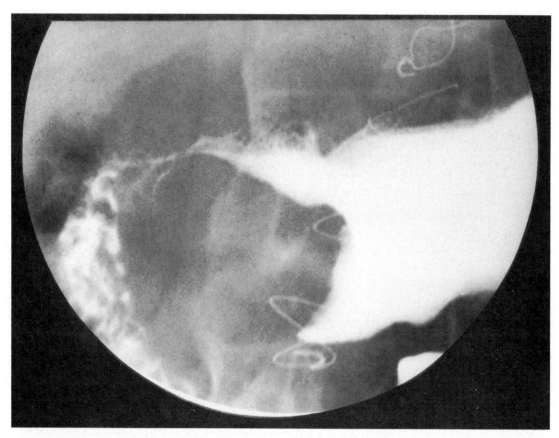

A large mass deforms the distal gastric antrum. A malignant process is suggested by the abrupt edge the mass makes with the normal gastric lumen, its lobulated surface, and its large size. This patient had a known islet cell carcinoma of the pancreas.

Direct invasion of the stomach usually occurs in patients with pancreatic or colonic malignancies. Mass effect, tethered and thickened folds, and occasionally ulceration can be identified radiographically.

## Case 148

## FUNDAL PSEUDOTUMOR: FUNDOPLICATION

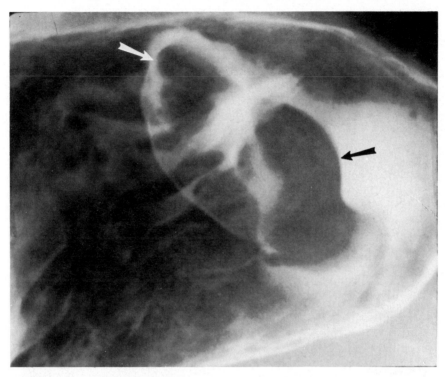

A symmetric, smooth filling defect *(arrows)* surrounds the esophagogastric junction. These findings are typical of a fundoplication filling defect.

There are different fundoplication procedures (Nissen 1, Nissen 2, Hill, Belsey) that are performed to correct gastroesophageal reflux. Any of these procedures may give the radiographic appearance of a pseudotumor. The Nissen 2 fundoplication generally is performed at our institution. This procedure involves wrapping a cuff of gastric fundus around the posterior esophagus and then suturing it together anteriorly. The cuff of fundus narrows the distal esophagus to prevent reflux. The main differential consideration is a neoplasm (Cases 128, 129, 131, and 142). A history of antireflux operation compatible with the typical radiographic findings (as in this case) usually makes the diagnosis straightforward.

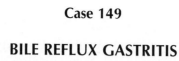

Case 149

# BILE REFLUX GASTRITIS

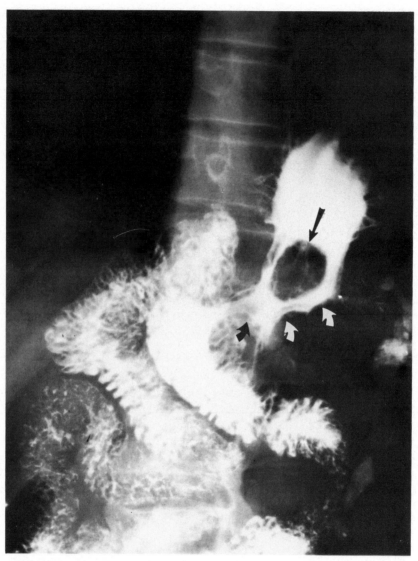

A Billroth II-type gastroenterostomy is present with a large filling defect *(long arrow)* within the gastric remnant. There is also narrowing and deformity *(curved short arrows)* of the remaining distal stomach and jejunum about the anastomosis. The filling defect was identified at endoscopy and found to be an inflammatory polyp. The markedly edematous folds were due to bile reflux gastritis. No tumor was present.

Gastritis after operation is common, but usually it resolves within a few weeks. Reflux of bile via the afferent loop in a patient with a Billroth II anastomosis can

also produce gastritis and can lead to considerable pain. Bile reflux gastritis rarely is diagnosed radiographically, but it may be suggested by identifying enlarged gastric folds (as seen in the distal portion of the gastric remnant in this patient). This patient's inflammatory polyp was probably secondary to chronic inflammatory changes from bile reflux. Other types of polyps (hyperplastic and adenomatous) can also develop in a gastric remnant. The filling defect in this case cannot be differentiated from a polypoid carcinoma. Endoscopic biopsy was necessary to make the distinction.

**Case 150**

## AFFERENT LOOP SYNDROME

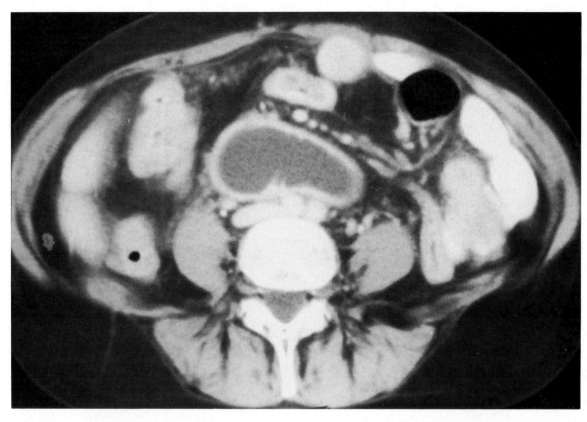

The duodenum is dilated and fluid-filled in this patient with a Billroth II-type gastroenterostomy. Findings are compatible with an afferent loop syndrome.

The afferent loop syndrome refers to dilatation of the afferent limb of a gastroenterostomy. The usual causes of this syndrome are obstruction of the loop from a recurrent ulcer, adhesions or internal herniation, or a nonphysiologic surgical anastomosis. The last cause often occurs when the afferent loop leads to the greater curvature of the stomach, and food preferentially emp-

ties into this limb. Fixed obstruction of the loop may lead to a blind loop syndrome with bacterial overgrowth, vitamin $B_{12}$ deficiency, and megaloblastic anemia. Perforation of the afferent limb with peritoneal spillage has been reported and may cause death.

Patients often have distension, pain, and nausea. Sudden bilious vomiting may be present if the afferent loop obstruction is relieved by uncoiling or unkinking of the small bowel loop. CT is helpful in directly imaging the fluid-filled and dilated afferent loop.

## Case 151

## AFFERENT LOOP SYNDROME

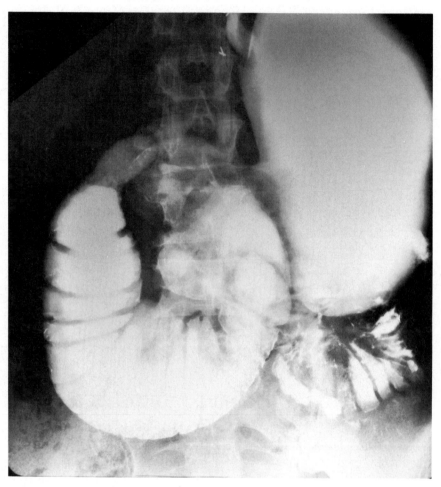

The afferent limb of a Billroth II anastomosis is markedly dilated. The cause of obstruction near the gastroenterostomy is not visible. At operation, the afferent limb was twisted and partially obstructed proximal to the anastomosis. The gastroenterostomy was surgically revised.

Conventional barium studies occasionally identify the site of distal obstruction and its cause (ulcer, adhesion). Often, however, only nonfilling of the afferent limb is detected. Preferential filling of the afferent loop and delayed emptying can often be appreciated fluoroscopically in patients with nonphysiologic anastomoses.

**Case 152**

## BLOWN DUODENAL STUMP

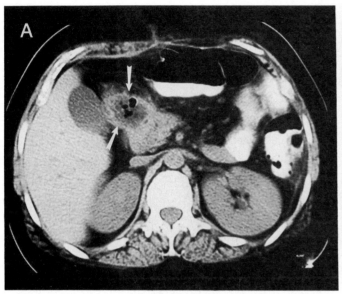 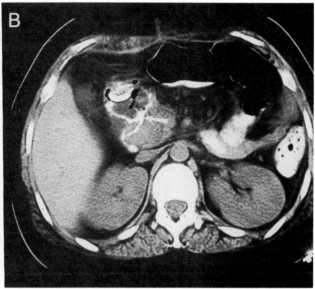

**A.** An abscess *(arrows)* containing fluid and air is adjacent to the duodenal stump in this patient with a recent Billroth II gastrojejunostomy.

**B.** A percutaneous drain was placed within the abscess. A sinogram demonstrates a communication *(arrow)* between the abscess and the duodenum. These findings are typical of a blown duodenal stump.

Breakdown or leakage of the duodenal stump is a serious complication after a Billroth II anastomosis. Recognition of this condition is important because it has a high mortality. Anastomotic breakdown can occur anytime between the first day and up to 3 weeks after op-

eration. Early intervention and drainage are important for proper management.

The diagnosis may be suggested by the findings on an abdominal plain film, by identifying extraluminal gas, or by abnormal soft tissue in the subhepatic space or about the duodenal stump. An upper gastrointestinal examination using water-soluble contrast material can help in confirming the diagnosis. Extravasated contrast material can be identified from the duodenal stump. CT is also an excellent modality to evaluate patients for this complication. The presence and location of abnormal fluid collections can be identified, and in some patients percutaneous drainage can be performed.

## Case 153

## GASTRIC REMNANT BEZOAR

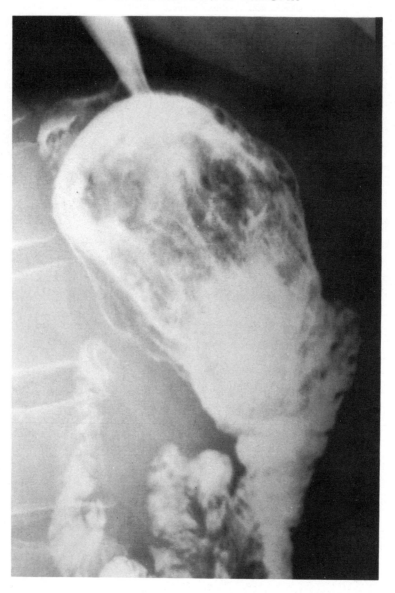

In this patient with a Billroth II-type gastroenterostomy with a persistent filling defect within the gastric remnant, contrast material could be seen to completely cover and surround the filling defect.

Bezoar formation, usually from retained vegetable matter (phytobezoar), is a relatively common complication in patients after a gastroenterostomy. Bezoar formation occurs as a result of surgical vagotomy that slows gastric transit and decreases acid production and of a narrowed gastroenterostomy stoma.

Radiologic diagnosis is based on finding a filling defect within the gastric remnant that is not attached to the gastric wall (Case 169). Often interstices within a phytobezoar fill with barium and give it a variegated appearance. Retained food can simulate a bezoar, and it is probably prudent to reexamine the fasting patient several hours later to see if the finding is still present. Yeast bezoars due to yeast overgrowth and blood-clot bezoars can occur and cause gastric-outlet obstruction.

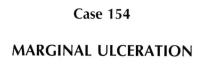

## Case 154

## MARGINAL ULCERATION

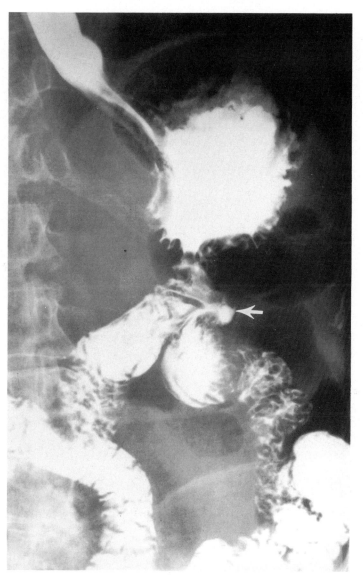

A Billroth II-type gastroenterostomy is shown with an ulcer crater *(arrow)* near the stoma within the efferent limb.

Marginal (or stomal) ulcer refers to a perianastomotic ulcer developing in patients after a gastroenterostomy. Most ulcers occur in the efferent limb of the jejunum, within 2 cm of the stoma. Marginal ulcers should raise suspicion of several possible conditions: incomplete vagotomy, retained gastric antrum, Zollinger-Ellison syndrome (Cases 106 and 155), hypercalcemia, smoking, or ulcerogenic drug abuse.

A spectrum of radiographic findings of peptic disease affecting the postanastomotic jejunum includes: typical ulcer craters, giant craters resembling large diverticula, thickened jejunal folds, and rigidity of the affected jejunal segment. Despite ideal radiographic techniques, some postoperative ulcers will not be detected (reports vary between 20% and 50%) (Ominsky and Moss, 1979). Endoscopy should be recommended for symptomatic patients with negative radiologic studies. Delayed diagnosis can lead to perforation bleeding or penetration—often into the colon, creating a jejunocolic fistula.

## Case 155

## MARGINAL ULCER

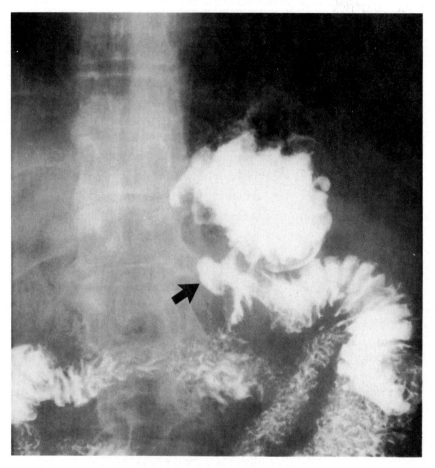

An ulcer crater *(arrow)* is present in the postanastomotic jejunum, involving the afferent limb of a Billroth II gastroenterostomy. A small gastric remnant remains.

This patient had multiple endocrine neoplasia syndrome, Type I with associated Zollinger-Ellison syndrome (a gastrin-secreting islet cell tumor).

## Case 156

# JEJUNOGASTRIC INTUSSUSCEPTION

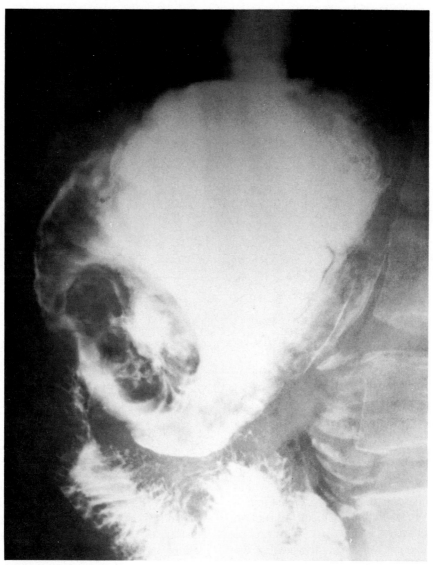

A filling defect is present within the gastric remnant. The defect is tubular and valvulae conniventes are seen within it. Findings are characteristic of a jejunogastric intussusception.

Clinically significant intussusception is an unusual complication after a gastroenterostomy. Intussusceptions can occur antegrade or retrograde, acutely or chronically, and early or late after operation. Patients with an acute intussusception develop clinical signs and symptoms of gastric-outlet obstruction, hematemesis, and an upper abdominal mass or fullness. Chronic intussusception is usually intermittent and self-reducing. Symptomatic patients should be regarded as surgical emergencies because of the high mortality associated with untreated patients in whom bowel perforation develops. The efferent limb is most commonly the intussuscipiens, but the afferent or both limbs can also intussuscept. A mass acting as a lead point should be searched for in patients with an antegrade intussusception, when the jejunum is the intussusceptum.

## Case 157

## POSTGASTRECTOMY CARCINOMA

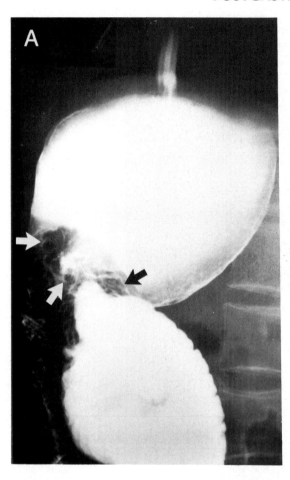

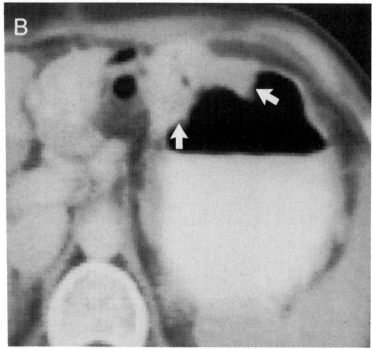

**A.** A lobulated filling defect *(arrows)* is present within the gastric remnant near the anastomosis. The stomach is distended because of partial mechanical obstruction from the mass.

**B.** Gastric wall thickening *(arrows)* at the level of the gastroenterostomy is confirmed at CT. Carcinoma was proved endoscopically.

Gastric carcinoma in a gastric remnant usually occurs either soon (several months) after surgical resection for gastric adenocarcinoma as a result of subtotal tumor removal or as a primary cancer developing 20 to 30 years after gastric surgery for ulcer disease. Some authors report a two- to sixfold increased risk of developing carcinoma within the gastric remnant in patients with a gastroenterostomy performed for managing gastric ulcer disease (Stalsberg and Taksdal, 1971). The increased risk is believed to be related to long-standing gastritis as a result of reflux of bile acids and pancreatic secretions into the stomach. Other investigators have not demonstrated an increased risk of cancer in these patients (Schafer et al., 1983).

Radiologic detection can be difficult. Filling defects, mucosal ulceration, and stomal or gastric pouch narrowing are the usual findings. Suspicious findings should be further evaluated by endoscopy. Examinations of the gastric remnant using the air-contrast technique are recommended, because the remaining pouch is rarely accessible for compression.

**Case 158**

## POSTGASTRECTOMY CARCINOMA

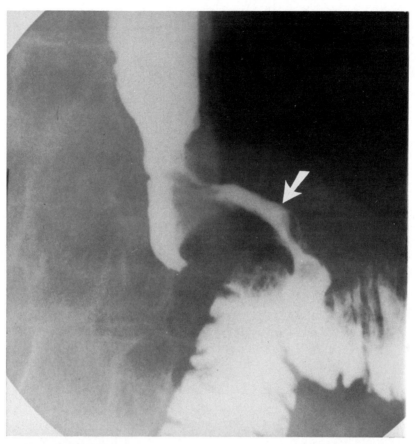

A Billroth II gastroenterostomy is present with a small and stenotic residual gastric remnant *(arrow)*. Mass effect deforms the distal esophagus eccentrically. This patient had an ulcerative and infiltrative adenocarcinoma of the gastric remnant.

Detection of gastric remnant cancers can be difficult. Baseline examinations can be helpful to assess for subtle changes in the gastric pouch. This examination illustrates an advanced case of remnant shrinkage due to carcinoma.

## Case 159

## POSTGASTRECTOMY CARCINOMA

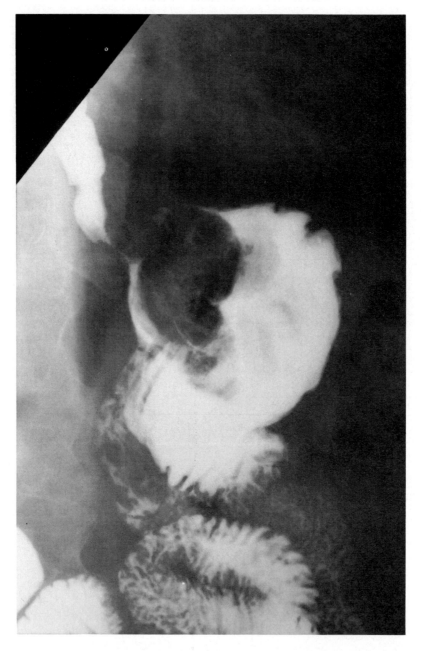

A polypoid intraluminal mass is present within the gastric remnant. A Billroth II gastroenterostomy had been performed 29 years before this examination. At operation, a polypoid adenocarcinoma was removed.

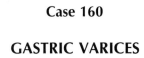

Case 160

## GASTRIC VARICES

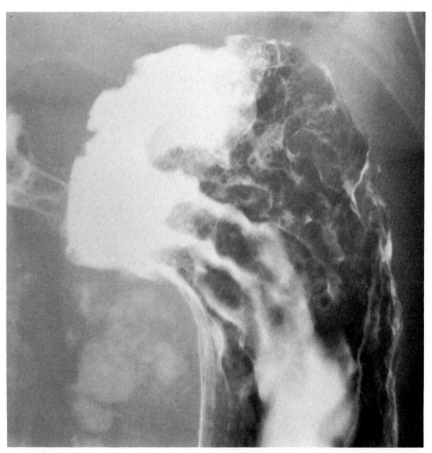

Multiple, serpentine filling defects are present in the gastric fundus. Findings are typical of gastric varices. A calcified mass is present in the region of the pancreas as a result of an islet cell carcinoma causing splenic vein occlusion.

Gastric varices can develop as a result of portal venous hypertension or splenic vein occlusion. Only one-third to one-half of patients with uphill esophageal varices from portal venous hypertension have gastric varices, but nearly all patients with gastric varices and portal venous hypertension have esophageal varices (Evans and Delany, 1953; Evans, 1959). This is probably the result of the subserosal location of gastric varices that in many patients cannot be detected by barium examination. Splenic vein occlusion usually is due to pancreatic disease (pancreatitis or pancreatic carcinoma), but it can be idiopathic in origin. Esophageal varices are absent in splenic vein occlusion because blood

flow travels from the short gastric veins to the gastric fundal plexus and returns to the portal circulation via the left gastric (coronary) vein.

Radiographic findings include serpentine filling defects; multiple, lobulated masses resembling a "bunch of grapes"; or even a single, polypoid fundal mass (Case 161). The double-contrast examination may be more sensitive in examining the fundus for varices, because this region is usually not accessible for adequate compression using the single-contrast technique. Examination of the esophagus for varices is important because both esophageal and gastric varices indicate portal venous hypertension. A normal esophagus suggests splenic vein occlusion.

Differential considerations for tortuous, thick fundal folds include Ménétrier's disease (Case 110), Zollinger-Ellison syndrome (Case 105), lymphoma (Case 139), and pancreatitis.

## Case 161

## GASTRIC VARICES

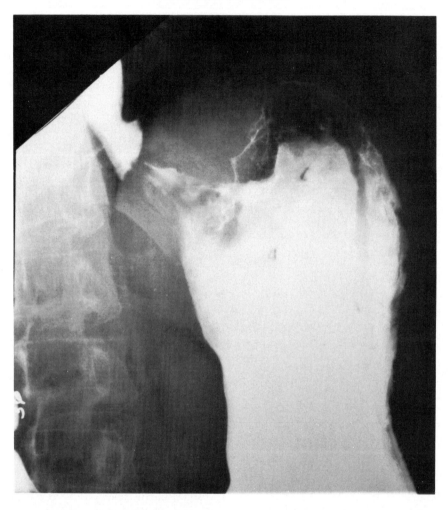

A lobulated mass is present within the gastric cardia and fundus. This mass resembles a carcinoma. Esophageal varices were present.

Gastric varices can, rarely, mimic a fundal tumor. The presence of esophageal varices in patients with portal venous hypertension should make the examiner consider a possible gastric pseudotumor. CT, MRI, sonography, or angiography may be helpful in determining the vascular nature of the mass (Case 162). These studies may also be able to determine the origin of the underlying disease causing the varices. Cirrhosis with portal venous hypertension and pancreatitis or pancreatic neoplasm with splenic vein thrombosis are common causes of gastric varices.

Case 162

# GASTRIC VARICES

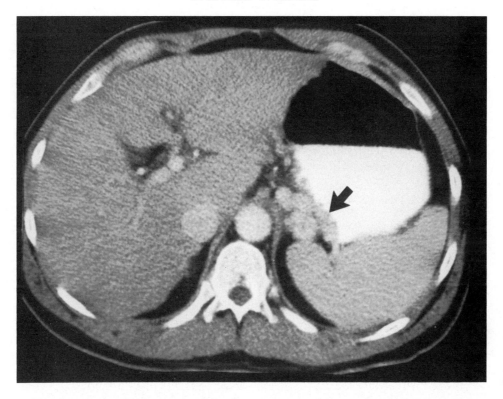

Enhancing, serpentine filling defects *(arrow)* are present within the gastric fundus medially. Short gastric varices are seen posteromedial to the stomach.

CT can be helpful in patients with known or suspected portal venous hypertension. Morphologic changes of cirrhosis can be identified in the liver. Splenomegaly is often present in patients with portal venous hypertension. Upper abdominal varices also can be directly visualized at CT. Common variceal locations include the peri-

esophageal tissues, gastric fundus, perigastric tissues, and left gastric (coronary vein) and retroperitoneal regions. Varices are tortuous, tubular structures that often cluster and appear masslike. It is common to identify varices around the stomach at CT that do not cause an impression on the gastric lumen. These varices would be missed on an upper gastrointestinal or endoscopic examination.

## Case 163

## VASCULAR IMPRESSIONS/AREAE GASTRICAE

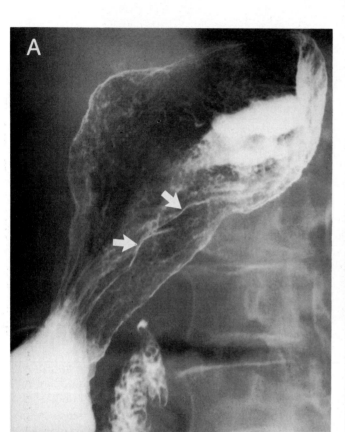

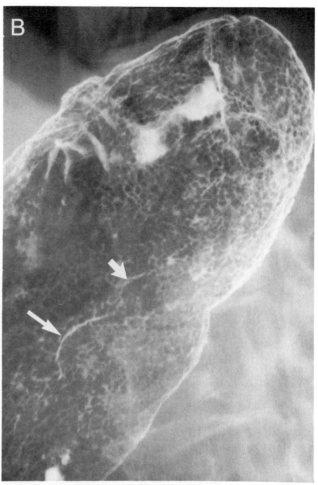

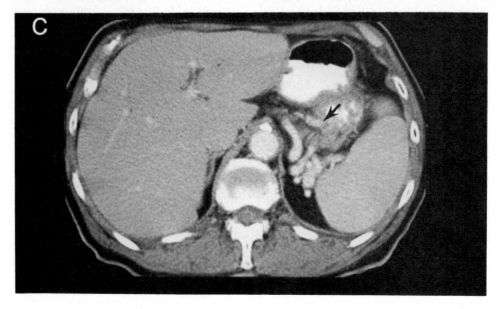

**A** and **B.** View of the gastric fundus and cardia with air distension shows a prominent areae gastricae pattern. Linear impressions *(arrows)* are also visible on the posterior wall as a result of vascular structures.

**C.** Multiple splenic vessels *(arrow)* are visible about the posterior gastric wall. Splenomegaly was present.

The normal surface pattern of the stomach on double-contrast examination is either a featureless or an areae gastricae pattern. Demonstration of the areae gastricae requires excellent mucosal coating with high density barium mixtures. This surface pattern is seen most frequently in the antrum. Prominence of this normal pattern has been reported in patients with nonspecific inflammation, intestinal metaplasia, and benign lymphoid hyperplasia. One study reported that a coarse areae gastricae pattern in the proximal stomach frequently was associated with increased gastric secretions and peptic ulcer disease (Watanabe et al., 1983).

Vascular impressions on the stomach are not normally identified. In this patient with splenomegaly the enlarged splenic vessels are visible.

## Case 164

## ANTRAL DIAPHRAGM

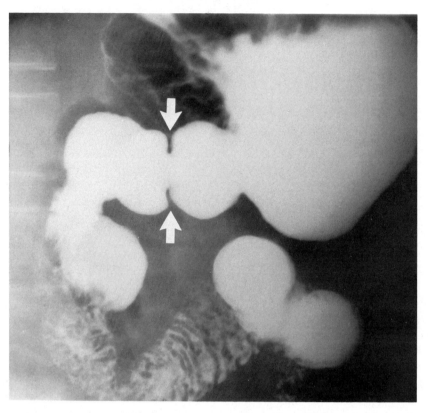

A region of bandlike narrowing *(arrows)* is present in the gastric antrum. This is the typical appearance of an antral diaphragm.

Antral diaphragms are thin mucosal membranes that usually encircle the antrum and narrow the gastric lumen. Most authorities believe they occur congenitally, but others believe they are acquired during adulthood as a result of scarring from peptic ulcer disease. Usually they are asymptomatic, unless the aperture through the diaphragm is less than 1 cm in diameter. Occasionally they are multiple and partial. Symptomatic diaphragms are usually treated by balloon dilatation over a guidewire.

Radiologic recognition depends on adequate distension of the stomach. A bandlike narrowing of the antrum is seen when the antrum is profiled correctly. The usual location is within a few centimeters of the pylorus.

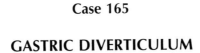

## Case 165

## GASTRIC DIVERTICULUM

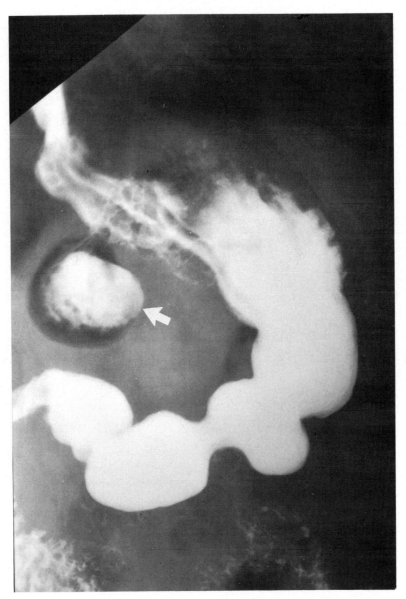

A moderate-sized diverticulum *(arrow)* arises from the gastric fundus posteriorly. Its narrow neck arises near the esophagogastric junction.

Diverticula of the stomach are unusual congenital entities. Most arise from the posterior surface of the gastric fundus near the esophagogastric junction. Symptoms are rarely associated with diverticula, but bleeding has been reported (Brown and Priestley, 1938).

Radiologic recognition of these entities depends on identifying mucosal folds within the diverticulum and observing its characteristic changing size and shape. A connecting neck is also a helpful finding.

## Case 166

## GASTRIC DIVERTICULUM

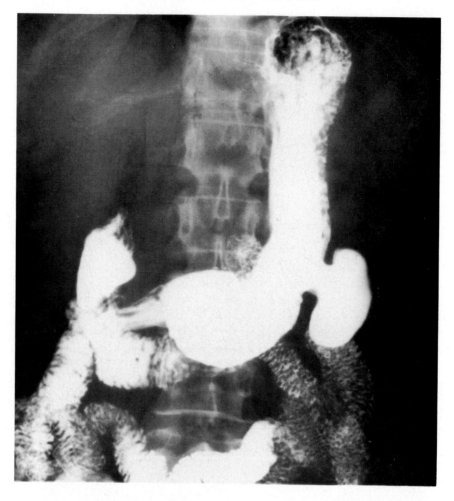

A diverticulum arises from the greater curvature of the gastric body. This is an unusual location for a diverticulum. Most true diverticula arise from the posterior fundal region.

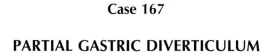

## Case 167

## PARTIAL GASTRIC DIVERTICULUM

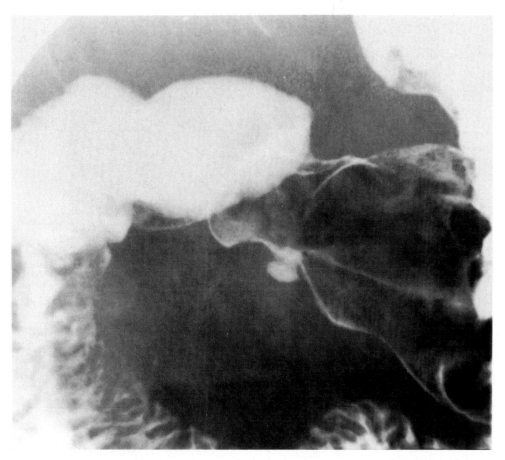

An intramural collection of barium is present along the greater curvature of the gastric antrum. This had the appearance of an ulcer crater but was observed fluoroscopically to change in size and shape. The location and its variable shape are typical of partial gastric diverticula.

A partial gastric diverticulum is a protrusion of mucosa into the muscular wall of the stomach without disturbing the serosa. These entities are rare (found in approximately 0.05% of the population) and asympto-

matic. Their importance lies in differentiating them from a peptic ulcer. Most partial diverticula are located along the greater curvature of the antrum. They often have a narrow neck and change in shape during fluoroscopic visualization. Ectopic pancreatic tissue (Case 124) in the distal stomach is reported to be a frequent finding in these patients. The exact role this aberrant tissue plays in the development of these diverticula is unclear.

## Case 168

# GASTRIC VOLVULUS

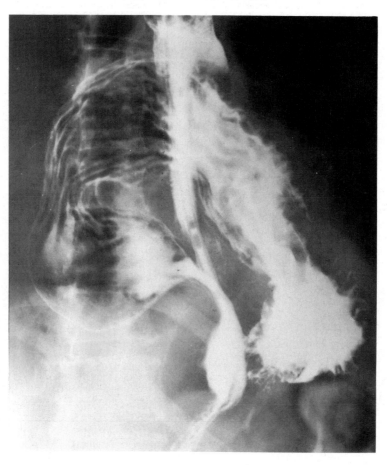

An intrathoracic stomach is present and has rotated 180° around the longitudinal axis of the stomach, with the greater curvature cephalad to the lesser curvature. This "upside-down stomach" is characteristic of organoaxial volvulus. No obstruction is present, but a nasogastric tube could not be passed into the stomach.

Gastric volvulus is a rare occurrence defined as 180° torsion along either the longitudinal axis of the stomach (organoaxial) or about the gastric mesentery (mesenteroaxial). Ischemia and gangrene can develop in either type, requiring emergency surgical repair.

Organoaxial volvulus is the more common type, and it is often associated with a long-standing hiatal hernia, paraesophageal hernia, or eventration of the diaphragm. The intrathoracic stomach rotates so that the greater curvature is located superiorly, with the gastric body cranial to the fundus (as seen in this case). This type of volvulus often presents as an upside-down stomach. Acute symptoms are those of epigastric pain, retching without vomitus, and an inability to pass a nasogastric tube. Mesenteroaxial volvulus presents with the pylorus and antrum folded anteriorly and superiorly. This type often causes either partial or complete obstruction in the pyloroantral region.

Radiologic examination usually demonstrates an intrathoracic location of the stomach and the anatomic alterations described above. It may not be possible to demonstrate filling or emptying of the stomach if obstruction is present.

## Case 169

## BEZOAR

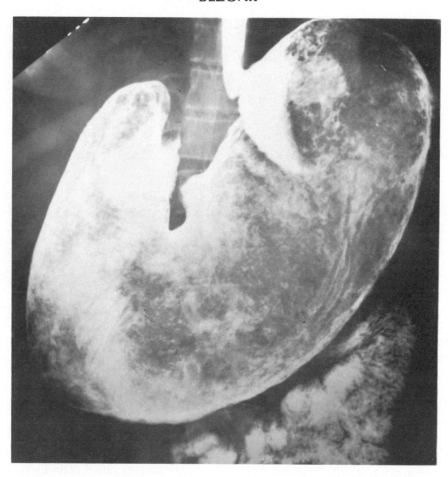

A huge filling defect occupies the entire gastric lumen. A trichobezoar was removed surgically.

Bezoars are concretions of ingested material. They are most commonly composed of vegetable material (phytobezoar), hair (trichobezoar), or other substances. Various foods (persimmons, berries, other fruits, vegetables, milk), mucus, pitch, tar, antacids, shellac, and furniture polish have been reported to form bezoars. Delayed gastric emptying, diminished gastric acid and pepsin production, excess or abnormal mucus production, dietary content, and improper mastication are factors that can contribute to bezoar formation. Patients

*From Bender CE. In: Marshak RH, Lindner AE, Maklansky D, eds.* Radiology of the stomach. *Philadelphia: WB Saunders,* **1983:**542–555. *By permission of the publisher.*

with prior gastric surgery are particularly prone to bezoar development (Case 153).

Radiographic features of a bezoar include a mottled soft tissue mass on abdominal plain films. A filling defect is present within the stomach on barium studies. The defect is not attached to the wall and contrast material often collects within the interstices of the bezoar. Complications are rare but include obstruction, ulceration, hemorrhage, and perforation. Gastric tumors (carcinoma [Case 130], lymphoma [Case 136], smooth muscle tumors [Cases 120–122]) are the most important differential consideration. Free movement of the mass within the stomach and the lack of attachment of the mass to the stomach can usually distinguish it from a true neoplasm.

## Case 170

# EMPHYSEMATOUS GASTRITIS

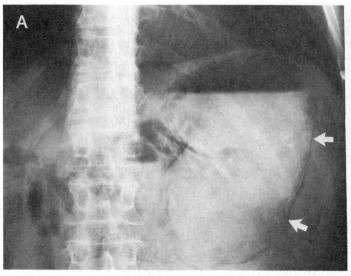 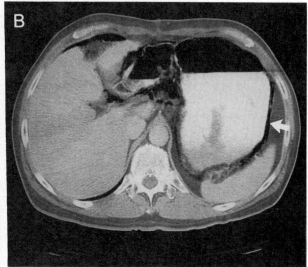

**A.** Intramural gas *(arrows)* is present throughout the fluid- and gas-filled stomach.

**B.** Intramural gastric air *(arrow)* is confirmed at CT. In addition, retroperitoneal gas is seen in the region of the lesser sac. This patient was on steroid medication and recovered uneventfully without operation. Benign pneumatosis was diagnosed clinically because of the absence of abdominal symptoms or signs.

Emphysematous gastritis refers to gas within the stomach wall. Infection with a gas-forming organism— i.e., *Escherichia coli* or *Clostridium perfringens*—is a common cause. These patients are usually severely ill and often die. Other causes of intramural gastric gas include gastric obstruction (due to a pyloric or prepyloric ulcer or tumor) with associated increased intragastric pressure, severe vomiting, and mucosal disruption due to ischemia, infection, or corrosive ingestion. Clinical evaluation of the patient and a brief history are often helpful in excluding many of these causes. Patients receiving steroids are particularly prone to develop intramural pneumatosis that has no clinical sequelae. Benign pneumatosis usually is encountered in either the small bowel or colon (Cases 342 and 466–468).

Radiologically, a gas-like lucency is identified within the gastric wall. The diagnosis can often be made successfully on abdominal plain films, upper gastrointestinal barium studies, or CT. It is impossible to differentiate infectious from noninfectious pneumatosis on the radiograph.

## Case 171

# GASTRIC-OUTLET OBSTRUCTION

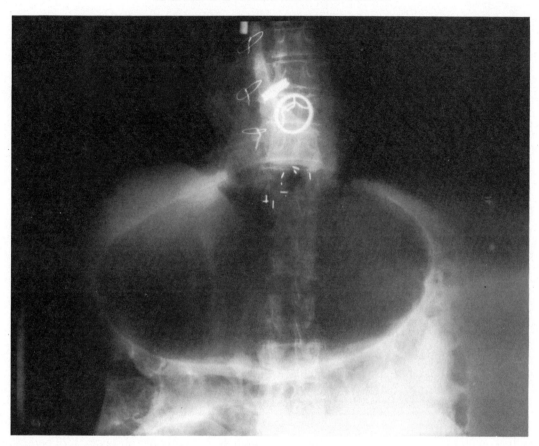

The stomach is dilated and distended with air. Findings are consistent with mechanical obstruction of the gastric outlet or gastric atony. This patient had an adynamic ileus that resolved with conservative therapy.

In a fasting patient, gastric dilatation with retained food and fluid can be secondary to either mechanical obstruction or gastric atony (adynamic ileus). Many diseases can cause mechanical obstruction, including peptic ulcer disease, neoplasms (usually malignant), inflammatory stenosis (Crohn's disease, pancreatitis), and other less common conditions. An even longer list of conditions can cause nonobstructive gastric dilatation (atony), including postoperative ileus, peritonitis, diabetes mellitus, various neuromuscular disorders, numerous medications, electrolyte abnormalities, and others. Radiologic assessment can be helpful to separate mechanical from nonobstructive gastric dilatation. It may be necessary to empty the stomach with nasogastric suction in order to adequately examine it. In high-grade mechanical gastric-outlet obstruction, the cause of obstruction may not be evident on the barium examination. Endoscopy can be helpful in some patients, particularly those with neoplastic obstruction in whom tissue confirmation of the diagnosis can be obtained. No obstruction will be encountered in patients with gastric ileus. Peristalsis often will be weak or absent in these patients.

**185**

## Case 172

# GASTRIC-OUTLET OBSTRUCTION

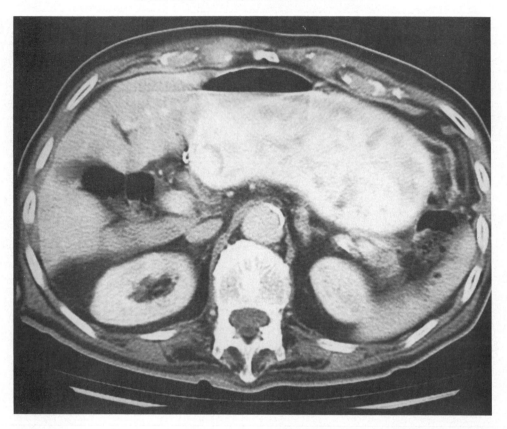

The stomach is abnormally distended with contrast material and residual food. This amount of retained food is abnormal if the patient has fasted for at least 4 hours prior to the examination. Gastric-outlet obstruction can be suggested by this examination, but the cause is not visible. A surgical clip is visible near the gastroduodenal anastomosis in this patient with a known Billroth I anastomosis. An anastomotic stricture was identified at endoscopy.

Postoperative obstruction at a stoma (either Billroth I or II anastomoses) can be secondary to several causes. Postoperative ileus can mimic a mechanical obstruction, but it usually resolves within 2 to 3 days after op-

eration. Fluoroscopic observation of peristaltic contractions can be most helpful in excluding paralytic ileus. Mechanical obstruction at the stoma can be due to postoperative submucosal edema or hematoma (which usually resolves in 2 to 3 weeks after operation), mechanical problems due to the surgical design of the anastomosis, stricture (secondary to postoperative fibrosis, stomal ulceration, recurrent constricting tumor), bezoar, internal hernia, or jejunogastric intussusception.

A conventional upper gastrointestinal examination can be helpful in confirming the presence of significant obstruction, and often the cause may be identified.

| DIFFERENTIAL DIAGNOSES | CASE NUMBER |
|---|---|
| ***FILLING DEFECTS*** | |
| Malignant | |
|    Carcinoma | 126–131, 157, 159 |
|    Leiomyosarcoma | 141, 142 |
|    Metastases | 145, 146 |
|    Lymphoma | 136–139 |
| Benign | |
|    Polyp(s) | 114–118 |
|    Leiomyoma | 119–122 |
|    Lipoma | 123 |
|    Erosions (edema) | 95, 108 |
|    Varices | 160–162 |
|    Folds | 91 |
|    Fundoplication defect | 148 |
|    Food | 169, 172 |
| ***NARROWING*** | |
| Common | |
|    Peptic scarring | 105, 190 |
|    Carcinoma | 132–134 |
|    Metastases | 144, 147 |
|    Lymphoma | 136, 140 |
| Uncommon | |
|    Corrosive ingestion | 107 |
|    Crohn's disease | 109 |
|    Other granulomatous diseases (sarcoid, tuberculosis, syphilis) | 112 |
|    Eosinophilic gastroenteritis | |
| ***THICKENED FOLDS*** | |
| Normal variant | 91 |
| Varices | 160–162 |
| Lymphoma | 139 |
| Ménétrier's disease | 110 |
| Zollinger-Ellison syndrome | 105 |
| Peptic ulcer disease | 96, 98 |
| Gastritis | 149 |
| Carcinoma | 126 |
| ***ULCERATIVE LESIONS*** | |
| Peptic or stress ulcer | 95–102 |
| Superficial gastric erosions | 95, 108 |
| Zollinger-Ellison syndrome | 105, 106 |
| Smooth muscle tumor | 119, 121 |
| Carcinoma | 126–128 |
| Metastases | 145 |
| Lymphoma | 138 |

## SELECTED READINGS

### Normal Stomach

Cimmino CV. Sign of the burnous in the stomach. *Radiology* **1960**;75:722–724

*Komaki S. Normal or benign gastric wall thickening demonstrated by computed tomography. *J Comput Assist Tomogr* **1982**;6:1103–1107

Laufer I. Stomach. In: Laufer I, ed. *Double contrast gastrointestinal radiology with endoscopic correlation.* Philadelphia: WB Saunders, **1979**:155–239

MacKintosh CE, Kreel L. Anatomy and radiology of the areae gastricae. *Gut* **1977**;18:855–864

Marks WM, Callen PW, Moss AA. Gastroesophageal region: source of confusion on CT. *AJR* **1981**;136:359–362

Megibow AJ. Stomach. In: Megibow AJ, Balthazar EJ, eds. *Computed tomography of the gastrointestinal tract.* St. Louis, CV Mosby, **1986**:99–174

Tim LO, Bank S, Marks IN, et al. Benign lymphoid hyperplasia of the gastric antrum—another cause of "etat mammelonne." *Br J Radiol* **1977**;50:29–31

### Peptic Ulcer Disease

Allison JE. Gastrocolic fistula as a complication of gastric lymphoma. *Am J Gastroenterol* **1973**;59:499–504

*Amberg JR, Zboralske FF. Gastric ulcers after 70. *Am J Roentgenol* **1966**;96:393–399

*Boyle JD. Multiple gastric ulcers. *Gastroenterology* **1971**;61:628–631

Burhenne HJ. Postoperative radiology. In: Margulis AR, Burhenne HJ, eds. *Alimentary tract radiology,* 4th ed, vol 1. St. Louis: CV Mosby, **1989**:1551–1633

*Cronan J, Burrell M, Trepeta R. Aphthoid ulcerations in gastric candidiasis. *Radiology* **1980**;134:607–611

Fraser GM. The double contrast barium meal in patients with acute upper gastrointestinal bleeding. *Clin Radiol* **1978**;29:625–634

*Gelfand DW, Dale WJ, Ott DJ. The location and size of gastric ulcers: radiologic and endoscopic evaluation. *AJR* **1984**;143:755–758

Golstein H, Jamin M, Schapiro M, Boyle JD. Gastric retention associated with gastroduodenal disease. *Am J Dig Dis* **1966**;11:887–897

*Jensen RT, Gardner JD, Raufman J-P, Pandol SJ, Doppman JL, Collen MJ. Zollinger-Ellison syndrome: current concepts and management. *Ann Intern Med* **1983**;98:59–75

Kirsh IE. Benign and malignant gastric ulcers: roentgen differentiation. An analysis of 142 cases proved histologically. *Radiology* **1955**;64:357–365

*Kottler RE, Tuft RJ. Benign greater curve gastric ulcer: the "sump-ulcer." *Br J Radiol* **1981**;54:651–654

Laufer I. Stomach. In: Laufer I, ed. *Double contrast gastrointestinal radiology with endoscopic correlation.* Philadelphia: WB Saunders, **1979**:166–173

Laufer I, Hamilton J, Mullens JE. Demonstration of superficial gastric erosions by double contrast radiography. *Gastroenterology* **1975**;68:387–391

Laufer I, Thornley GD, Stolberg H. Gastrocolic fistula as a complication of benign gastric ulcer. *Radiology* **1976**;119:7–11

*Levine MS, Creteur V, Kressel HY, Laufer I, Herlinger H. Benign gastric ulcers: diagnosis and follow-up with double-contrast radiography. *Radiology* **1987**;164:9–13

Levine MS, Verstandig A, Laufer I. Serpiginous gastric erosions caused by aspirin and other nonsteroidal antiinflammatory drugs. *AJR* **1986**;146:31–34

Madrazo BL, Halpert RD, Sandler MA, Pearlberg JL. Computed tomographic findings in penetrating peptic ulcer. *Radiology* **1984**;153:751–754

Nelson SW. The discovery of gastric ulcers and the differential diagnosis between benignancy and malignancy. *Radiol Clin North Am* **1969** April;7:5–25

Nolan DJ. *The double-contrast barium meal: a radiologic atlas.* Aylesbury, Buckinghamshire: HM + M Publishers, **1980**:81–91

Norris JR, Haubrick WS. The incidence and clinical features of penetration in peptic ulceration. *JAMA* **1961**;178:386–389

*Pulvertaft CN. Comments on the incidence and natural history of gastric and duodenal ulcer. *Postgrad Med J* **1968**;44:597–602

Rimer DG. Gastric retention without mechanical obstruction. *Arch Intern Med* **1966**;117:287–299

Scott-Harden WG. Radiology of acute upper digestive tract bleeding. *J R Coll Physicians Lond* **1974**;8:365–374

Thompson G, Somers S, Stevenson GW. Benign gastric ulcer: a reliable radiologic diagnosis? *AJR* **1983**;141:331–333

Thompson WM. Unusual manifestations and compli-

*Cited in text.

cations of peptic ulcer disease. *Contemp Diagn Radiol* 1983;6:1–5

Thompson WM, Kelvin FM, Gedgaudas RK, Rice RP. Radiologic investigation of peptic ulcer disease. *Radiol Clin North Am* 1982 Dec;20:701–720

Thompson WM, Norton G, KeWin FM, Rice RP. Unusual manifestations of peptic ulcer disease. *Radiographics* 1981;1:1–16

Zboralske FF, Stargartder FL, Harell GS. Profile of roentgenographic features of benign greater curvature ulcers. *Radiology* 1978;127:63–67

### Other Inflammatory Disorders

Ariyama J, Wehlin L, Lindstrom CG, Wenkert A, Roberts GM. Gastroduodenal erosions in Crohn's disease. *Gastrointest Radiol* 1980;5:121–125

Burkhart CR, Wilkinson RH Jr. Inflammatory pseudotumors of the stomach. *Cancer* 1965;18:1310–1316

Chazan BI, Aitchison JD. Gastric tuberculosis. *Br Med J* 1960;2:1288–1290

Cohen WN. Gastric involvement in Crohn's disease. *Am J Roentgenol* 1967;101:425–430

Cooley RN, Childers JH. Acquired syphilis of the stomach: report of two cases. *Gastroenterology* 1960;39:201–207

Fahimi HD, Deren JJ, Gottlieb LS, Zamcheck N. Isolated granulomatous gastritis: its relationship to disseminated sarcoidosis and regional enteritis. *Gastroenterology* 1963;45:161–175

*Farman J, Faegenburg D, Dallemand S, Chen C-K. Crohn's disease of the stomach: the "ram's horn" sign. *Am J Roentgenol* 1975;123:242–251

*Fieber SS, Rickert RR. Hyperplastic gastropathy: analysis of 50 selected cases from 1955–1980. *Am J Gastroenterol* 1981;76:321–329

Gonzalez G, Kennedy T. Crohn's disease of the stomach. *Radiology* 1974;113:27–29

Laufer I, Costopoulos L. Early lesions of Crohn's disease. *AJR* 1978;130:307–311

*Martel W, Abell MR, Allan TNK. Lymphoreticular hyperplasia of the stomach (pseudolymphoma). *Am J Roentgenol* 1976;127:261–265

Muhletaler CA. Caustic lesions of the stomach and duodenum. In: Marshak RE, Lindner AE, Maklansky D, eds. *Radiology of the stomach.* Philadelphia: WB Saunders, 1983:527–541

Nevin IN, Turner WW, Gardner HT. Early and late roentgenologic findings in corrosive gastritis. *Am J Roentgenol* 1959;81:603–608

Olmsted WW, Cooper PH, Madewell JE. Involvement of the gastric antrum in Ménétrier's disease. *Am J Roentgenol* 1976;126:524–529

Perez CA, Sturim HS, Kouchoukos NT, Kamberg S. Some clinical and radiographic features of gastrointestinal histoplasmosis. *Radiology* 1966;86:482–487

Reese DF, Hodgson JR, Dockerty MB. Giant hypertrophy of gastric mucosa (Ménétrier's disease): a correlation of the roentgenographic, pathologic, and clinical findings. *Am J Roentgenol* 1962;88:619–626

### Benign Neoplasms

Bose B, Candy J. Gastric leiomyoblastoma. *Gut* 1970;11:875–880

*Dolan RV, ReMine WH, Dockerty MD. The fate of heterotopic pancreatic tissue: a study of 212 cases. *Arch Surg* 1974;109:762–765

*Feczko PJ. Incidental filling defects (polyps) in the stomach. In: Thompson WM, ed. *Common problems in gastrointestinal radiology.* Chicago: Year Book, 1989:183–190

*Feczko PJ, Halpert RD, Ackerman LV. Gastric polyps: radiological evaluation and clinical significance. *Radiology* 1985;155:581–584

*Feldman M, Weinberg T. Aberrant pancreas: a cause of duodenal syndrome. *JAMA* 1952 March;148:893–898

Fernandez MJ, Davis RP, Nora PF. Gastrointestinal lipomas. *Arch Surg* 1983;118:1081–1083

*Kilman WJ, Berk RN. The spectrum of radiographic features of aberrant pancreatic rests involving the stomach. *Radiology* 1977;123:291–296

Marshak RH, Lindner AE, Maklansky D. Submucosal tumors, benign and malignant. In: Marshak RH, Lindner AE, Maklansky D, eds. *Radiology of the stomach.* Philadelphia: WB Saunders, 1983;216–234

Megibow AJ, Balthazar EJ, Hulnick DH, Naidich DP, Bosniak MA. CT evaluation of gastrointestinal leiomyomas and leiomyosarcomas. *AJR* 1985;144:727–731

Palmer ED. Benign intramural tumors of the stomach: a review with special reference to gross pathology. *Medicine* 1951;30:81–179

ReMine SG, Hughes RW Jr, Weiland LH. Endoscopic gastric polypectomies. *Mayo Clin Proc* 1981;56:371–375

Seifert E, Elster K. Gastric polypectomy. *Am J Gastroenterol* 1975;63:451–456

*Smith HJ, Lee EL. Large hyperplastic polyps of the stomach. *Gastrointest Radiol* 1983;8:19–23

*Thoeni RF, Gedgaudas RK. Ectopic pancreas: usual and unusual features. *Gastrointest Radiol* **1980**;5:37–42

Ushio K, Sasagawa M, Doi H, et al. Lesions associated with familial polyposis coli: studies of lesions of the stomach, duodenum, bones and teeth. *Gastrointest Radiol* **1976**;1:67—80

### Malignant Neoplasms

Balfe DM, Koehler RE, Karstaedt N, Stanley RJ, Sagel SS. Computed tomography of gastric neoplasms. *Radiology* **1981**;140:431–436

Balfe DM, Mauro MA, Koehler RE, et al. Gastrohepatic ligament: normal and pathologic CT anatomy. *Radiology* **1984**;150:485–490

Bolondi L, Casanova P, Caletti GC, Grigioni W, Zani L, Barbara L. Primary gastric lymphoma versus gastric carcinoma: endoscopic US evaluation. *Radiology* **1987**;165:821–826

*Boring CC, Squires TS, Tong T. Cancer Statistics, 1991. *CA* **1991** Jan/Feb;41:19–36.

Brandt D, Muramatsu Y, Ushio K, et al. Synchronous early gastric cancer. *Radiology* **1989**;173: 649–652

Brooks JJ, Enterline HT. Primary gastric lymphomas: a clinicopathologic study of 58 cases with long-term follow-up and literature review. *Cancer* **1983**;51:701–711

Bryk D, Elguezabal A. Roentgen problems in evaluating the atrophic stomach of the elderly. *Am J Roentgenol* **1975**;123:236–241

*Buy J-N, Moss AA. Computed tomography of gastric lymphoma. *AJR* **1982**;138:859–865

Carman RD. A new roentgen-ray sign of ulcerating gastric cancer. *JAMA* **1921**;77:990–992

Coller FA, Kay EB, McIntyre RS. Regional lymphatic metastases of carcinoma of the stomach. *Arch Surg* **1941**;43:748–761

Derchi LE, Banderali A, Bossi C, et al. The sonographic appearances of gastric lymphoma. *J Ultrasound Med* **1984**;3:251–256

Henke F, Lubarsch O. *Handbuch der speziellen pathologischen Anatomie und Histologie*, vol 4. Berlin: Springer, **1926**:865

Joffe N. Metastatic involvement of the stomach secondary to breast carcinoma. *Am J Roentgenol* **1975**;123:512–521

*Komaki S. Normal or benign gastric wall thickening demonstrated by computed tomography. *J Comp Assist Tomogr* **1982**;6:1103–1107

*Komaki S. Gastric carcinoma. In: Meyers MA, ed. *Computed tomography of the gastrointestinal*

*tract: including the peritoneal cavity and mesentery*. New York: Springer-Verlag, **1986**:23–54

Komaki S, Toyoshima S. CT's capability in detecting advanced gastric cancer. *Gastrointest Radiol* **1983**;8:307–313

Kurtz RC, Sherlock P. Carcinoma of the stomach. In: Berk JE, Haubrich WS, Kalser MH, Roth JLA, Schaffner F, eds. *Bockus gastroenterology*, 4th ed, vol 2. Philadelphia: WB Saunders, **1985**: 1278–1304

*Levine MS, Kong V, Rubesin SE, Laufer I, Herlinger H. Scirrhous carcinoma of the stomach: radiologic and endoscopic diagnosis. *Radiology* **1990**;175:151–154

*Libshitz HI, Lindell MM, Dodd GD. Metastases to the hollow viscera. *Radiol Clin North Am* **1982** Sept;20:487–499

*Lightdale CJ, Kurtz RC, Boyle CC, Sherlock P, Winawer SJ. Cancer and upper gastrointestinal tract hemorrhage. Benign causes of bleeding demonstrated by endoscopy. *JAMA* **1973**; 226:139–141

*Marshak RH, Lindner AE, Maklansky D. Carcinoma of the stomach. In: Marshak RH, Lindner AE, Maklansky D, eds. *Radiology of the stomach*. Philadelphia: WB Saunders, **1983**:108–146

Marshak RH, Lindner AE, Maklansky D. Lymphoma of the stomach. In: Marshak RH, Lindner AE, Maklansky D, eds. *Radiology of the stomach*. Philadelphia: WB Saunders, **1983**;235–262

*Megibow AJ, Balthazar EJ, Hulnick DH, Naidich DP, Bosniak MA. CT evaluation of gastrointestinal leiomyomas and leiomyosarcomas. *AJR* **1985**;144:727–731

Megibow AJ, Balthazar EJ, Naidich DP, Bosniak MA. Computed tomography of gastrointestinal lymphoma. *AJR* **1983**;141:541–547

Menuck LS, Amberg JR. Metastatic disease involving the stomach. *Am J Dig Dis* **1975**;20:903–913

*Meyers MA. *Dynamic radiology of the abdomen: normal and pathologic anatomy*, 3rd ed. New York: Springer-Verlag, **1988**:198

Nelson SW. The discovery of gastric ulcers and the differential diagnosis between benignancy and malignancy. *Radiol Clin North Am* **1969** April:7:5-15

Rubesin SE, Levine MS, Glick SN. Gastric involvement by omental cakes: radiographic findings. *Gastrointest Radiol* **1986**;11:223–228

Sherrick DW, Hodgson JR, Dockerty MB. The roentgenologic diagnosis of primary gastric lymphoma. *Radiology* **1965**;84:925–932

*Shivshanker K, Chu DZJ, Stroehlein JR, Nelson

RS. Gastrointestinal hemorrhage in the cancer patient. *Gastrointest Endosc* **1983**;29:273–275

*Starr GF, Dockerty MB. Leiomyomas and leiomyosarcomas of the small intestine. *Cancer* **1955**;8: 101–111

*Sussman SK, Halvorsen RA Jr, Illescas FF, et al. Gastric adenocarcinoma: CT versus surgical staging. *Radiology* **1988**;167:335–340

Wolf BS. Observations on roentgen features of benign and malignant gastric ulcers. *Semin Roentgenol* **1971**;6:140–150

Zornoza J, Dodd GD. Lymphoma of the gastrointestinal tract. *Semin Roentgenol* **1980**;15:272–287

### Postoperative Conditions

Bachman AL, Parmer EA. Radiographic diagnosis of recurrence following resection for gastric cancer. *Radiology* **1965**;84:913–924

Berkowitz D, Cooney P, Bralow SP. Carcinoma of the stomach appearing after previous gastric surgery for benign ulcer disease. *Gastroenterology* **1959**;36:691–697

Brown CD, Kraus JW. Afferent loop syndrome revisited: new emphasis on ultrasound and computerized tomography. *South Med J* **1981**;74:599–601

Burhenne HJ. The iatrogenic afferent-loop syndrome. *Radiology* **1968**;91:942–947; 928.

Burrell M, Curtis AM. Sequelae of stomach surgery. *CRC Crit Rev Diagn Imaging* **1977**;10:17–97

Burrell M, Touloukian JS, Curtis AM. Roentgen manifestations of carcinoma in the gastric remnant. *Gastrointest Radiol* **1980**;5:331–341

Caudell WS, Lee CM Jr. Acute and chronic jejunogastric intussusception. *N Engl J Med* **1955**;253: 635–640

Devor D, Passaro E Jr. Jejunogastric intussusception: review of 4 cases—diagnosis and management. *Ann Surg* **1966**;163:93–96

Feldman F, Seaman WB. Primary gastric stump cancer. *Am J Roentgenol* **1972**;115:257–267

Gale ME, Gerzof SG, Kiser LC, et al. CT appearance of afferent loop obstruction. *AJR* **1982**; 138:1085–1088

Madsen P. The afferent-loop syndrome: a roentgen and cineroentgenographic study. *Acta Chir Scand* **1965**;129:417–424

McBurney RP, Farrar T, Sanders RL. Gastrojejunal ulcer and gastrojejunocolic fistula. *Am Surg* **1958**;24:709–713

Moseley RV. Pyloric obstruction by phytobezoar following pyloroplasty and vagotomy. *Arch Surg* **1967**;94:290–291

*Ominsky SH, Moss AA. The postoperative stomach: a comparative study of double-contrast barium examinations and endoscopy. *Gastrointest Radiol* **1979**;4:17–21

Palmer ED. Further observations on postoperative gastritis: histopathologic aspects, with a note on jejunitis. *Gastroenterology* **1953**;25:405–415.

Perttala Y, Peltokallio P, Leiviskä T, Sipponen J. Yeast bezoar formation following gastric surgery. *Am J Roentgenol* **1975**;125:365–373

Poppel MH. Gastric intussusceptions. *Radiology* **1962**;78:602–608

*Schafer LW, Larson DE, Melton LJ III, Higgins JA, Ilstrup DM. The risk of gastric carcinoma after surgical treatment for benign ulcer disease. A population-based study in Olmsted County, Minnesota. *N Engl J Med* **1983**;309:1210–1213

Schatzki R. The significance of rigidity of the jejunum in the diagnosis of postoperative jejunal ulcers. *Am J Roentgenol* **1968**;103:330–338

Schulman A. Anastomotic, gastrojejunal ulcer: accuracy of radiological diagnosis in surgically proven cases. *Br J Radiol* **1971**;44:422–433

Segal AW, Bank S, Marks IN, Rubinstein Z. Bezoars occurring in the gastric remnant after gastrectomy. *S Afr Med J* **1970**;44:1176–1180

*Stalsberg H, Taksdal S. Stomach cancer following gastric surgery for benign conditions. *Lancet* **1971**;2:1175–1177

Szemes G, Amberg JR. Gastric bezoars after partial gastrectomy: report of five cases. *Radiology* **1968**;90:765–768

Thorfinnson PC, Brow JR. Reflux bile gastritis. *J Can Assoc Radiol* **1974**;25:263–268

Wychulis AR, Priestley JT, Foulk WT. A study of 360 patients with gastrojejunal ulceration. *Surg Gynecol Obstet* **1966**;122:89–99

### Miscellaneous Conditions

Balthazar EJ, Megibow A, Naidich D, LeFleur RS. Computed tomographic recognition of gastric varices. *AJR* **1984**;142:1121–1125

Belgrad R, Carlson HC, Payne WS, Cain JC. Pseudotumoral gastric varices. *Am J Roentgenol* **1964**;91:751–756

Bender CE. Gastric bezoars. In: Marshak RH, Lindner AE, Maklansky D, eds. *Radiology of the stomach*. Philadelphia: WB Saunders, **1983**:542–555

*Brown PW, Priestley JT. Massive and recurrent gastro-intestinal hemorrhage from diverticulum of the stomach. *Proc Staff Meet Mayo Clin* **1938**;13:270–272

Campbell JB, Rappaport LN, Skerker LB. Acute mesentero-axial volvulus of the stomach. *Radiology* **1972**;103:153–156

Carter R, Brewer LA III, Hinshaw DB. Acute gastric volvulus. A study of 25 cases. *Am J Surg* **1980**;140:99–105

Clements JL Jr, Jinkins JR, Torres WE, et al. Antral mucosal diaphragms in adults. *AJR* **1979**; **133:1105–1111**

*Evans JA, Delany F. Gastric varices. *Radiology* **1953**;60:46–51

*Evans KT. Oesophageal and gastric varices. *Br J Radiol* **1959**;32:233–240

Feliciano DV, van Heerden JA. Pyloric antral mucosal webs. *Mayo Clin Proc* **1977**;52:650–653

Flachs K, Stelman HH, Matsumoto PJH. Partial gastric diverticula. *Am J Roentgenol* **1965**; 94:339–342

Gerson DE, Lewicki AM. Intrathoracic stomach: when does it obstruct? *Radiology* **1976**; 119:257–264

McCain AH, Bernardino ME, Sones PJ Jr, Berkman WA, Casarella WJ. Varices from portal hypertension: correlation of CT and angiography. *Radiology* **1985**;154:63–69

Muhletaler C, Gerlock AJ Jr, Goncharenko V, Avant GR, Flexner JM. Gastric varices secondary to splenic vein occlusion: radiographic diagnosis and clinical significance. *Radiology* **1979**;132:593–598

Rice RP, Thompson WM, Kelvin FM, Kriner AF, Garbutt JT. Gastric varices without esophageal varices. An important preendoscopic diagnosis. *JAMA* **1977**;237:1976–1979

Samuel E. Gastric diverticula. *Br J Radiol* **1955**;28: 574–578

Seaman WB, Fleming RJ. Intramural gastric emphysema. *Am J Roentgenol* **1967**;101:431–436

Sos T, Meyers MA, Baltaxe HA. Nonfundic gastric varices. *Radiology* **1972**;105:579–580

Treichel J, Gerstenberg E, Palme G, Klemm T. Diagnosis of partial gastric diverticula. *Radiology* **1976**;119:13–18

Turnbull AR, Michell RC. Interstitial emphysema of the stomach. *Br J Surg* **1979**;66:350–351

*Watanabe H, Magota S, Shiiba S, Ebata K, Yoshiya K. Coarse areae gastricae in the proximal body and fundus: a sign of gastric hypersecretion. *Radiology* **1983**;146:303–306

# Duodenum

## Case 173

## NORMAL DUODENAL BULB

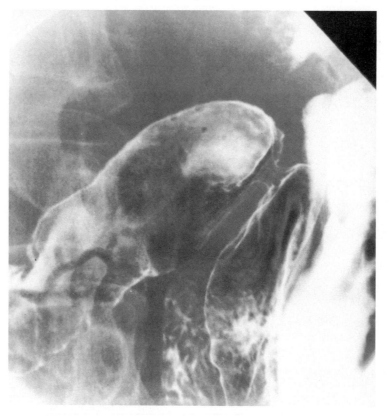

A normal double-contrast view of the duodenal bulb is illustrated. The normal duodenal bulb has been likened to a "cap" with the open end of the cap nearest the pylorus and the top of the cap near the junction of the first and second portions of the duodenum. The square corners of the proximal duodenum are important landmarks because they often become blunted and deformed as a result of scarring from peptic ulcer disease. A pattern of tiny interlacing spheres can often be appreciated on normal double-contrast examinations.

## Case 174

## NORMAL DUODENAL BULB

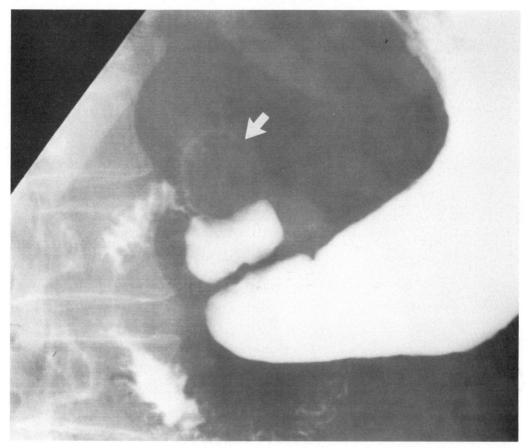

A faint peripheral rim of calcification is seen within a gallstone *(arrow)*. The gallbladder indents the superior aspect of the duodenal bulb.

The normal gallbladder frequently causes an indentation on the duodenal bulb. Occasionally, the distended gallbladder may also cause an impression on the lateral aspect of the descending duodenum. Diseases affecting the gallbladder or common bile duct can secondarily involve the duodenum because of their proximity.

## Case 175

## NORMAL DUODENAL BULB

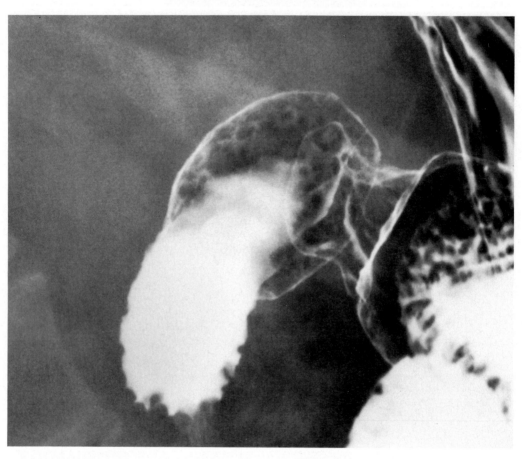

Small, nodular filling defects are present within the duodenal bulb. The small uniform size and shape of these filling defects are consistent with a normal duodenal lymphoid pattern.

The normal duodenal bulb can have a variable surface pattern on double-contrast examinations. Most often the mucosa is featureless and smooth. Occasionally a fine reticular pattern is seen that is less coarse than the areae gastricae within the stomach. Small, rounded filling defects (Case 176) and discrete punctate collections (without a halo of edema) can be seen normally (Case 177).

Normal filling defects should be distinguished from Brunner's gland hyperplasia. The filling defects of Brunner's gland hyperplasia are larger and less numerous than in this case (Case 182). Mounds of edema surround superficial erosions (Case 95) that can also present as filling defects. Filling defects due to lymphoid nodules are usually only 1 to 2 mm in diameter, numerous, and uniform size (Case 278). Duodenal mucosal changes that resemble a coarse areae gastricae pattern in the stomach are usually abnormal and have been associated with peptic ulcer disease, Crohn's disease, and celiac disease (Glick et al., 1984).

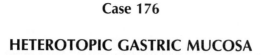

## Case 176

## HETEROTOPIC GASTRIC MUCOSA

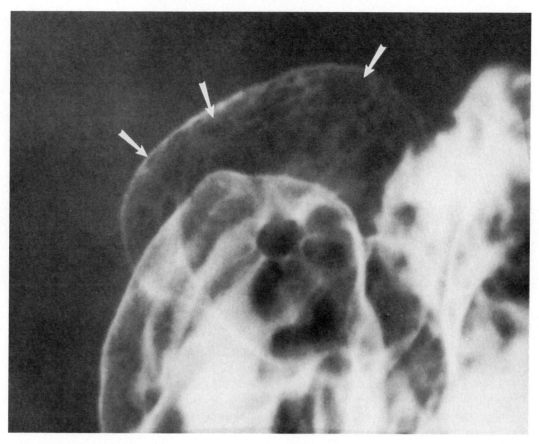

Multiple tiny filling defects of variable size *(arrows)* are present within the duodenal bulb. This appearance is consistent with heterotopic gastric mucosa within the duodenum.

The normal duodenal mucosa can vary in appearance, but it is often either featureless or a fine nodular pattern. Heterotopic gastric mucosa is a congenital, benign, and asymptomatic condition consisting of islands of gastric mucosa within the duodenal bulb. It has been suggested that this type of mucosa may have a protective effect against peptic ulcer disease (Smithuis and Vos, 1989). Radiographically, raised nodules, often with an angular configuration, that measure one to several millimeters in diameter can be seen about the py-

lorus either diffusely or in clusters. Differential considerations include effervescent granules, Brunner's gland hyperplasia, and lymphoid nodular hyperplasia. Brunner's glands are usually larger, less numerous, and more uniform size (Case 182). Lymphoid nodules (Case 278) are small and uniform size, usually evenly distributed throughout the duodenum. Effervescent granules change size and shape on different views as they dissolve. Gastric metaplasia of duodenal epithelium can also occur, analogous to Barrett's metaplasia in the esophagus (Shousha et al., 1983). This condition is commonly associated with peptic ulcer disease. The mucosal changes in metaplasia cannot be appreciated radiologically because the lesions are flat.

## Case 177

## NORMAL DUODENAL BULB

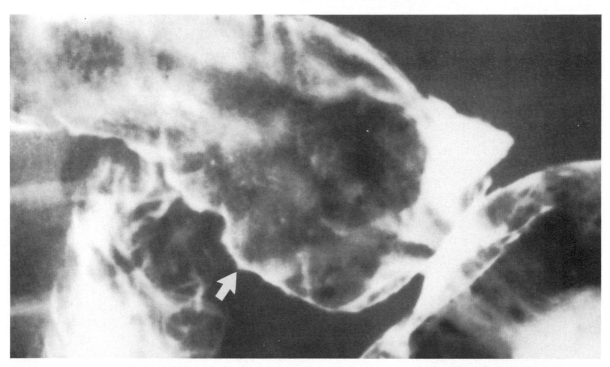

Multiple, tiny speckled collections of barium are present in the duodenal bulb.

This is a relatively uncommon normal variant. They are usually numerous and may extend to the duodenal apex. Seen tangentially, they may appear as tiny triangular irregularities *(arrow)*. Although the exact cause of these findings is unknown, it has been suggested that they may represent barium caught at the intersection of mucosal sulci (Glick et al., 1984). Differential considerations include erosions (Cases 95 and 276) and barium precipitates. Erosions are usually fewer in number and surrounded by a halo of edema. Barium precipitates are dense, discrete, and appear as clumps of high-density material without irregularity (on the mucosal surface) when viewed tangentially.

**Case 178**

## NORMAL DUODENUM: CT

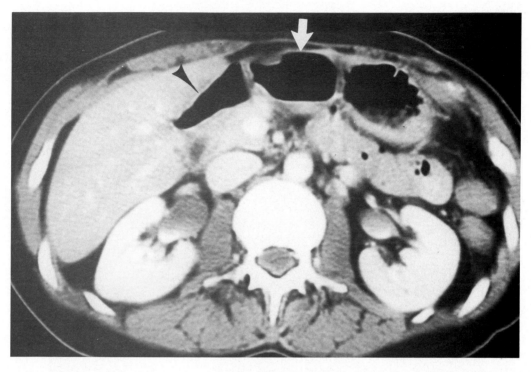

The body and antrum *(arrow)* of the stomach as well as the duodenal bulb *(arrowhead)* are distended with air. The normal cap-like shape of the duodenal bulb is seen. The duodenum distal to the bulb was visible on lower CT sections.

## Case 179

## FLEXURAL PSEUDOPOLYP

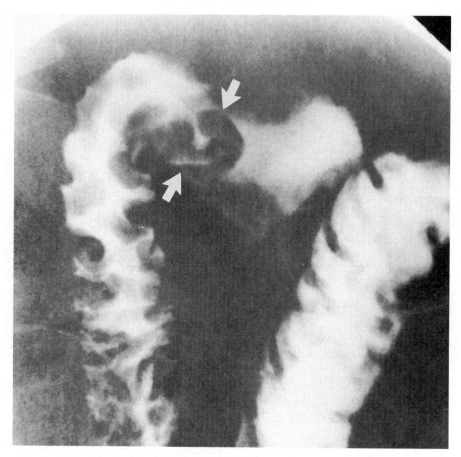

A polypoid filling defect *(arrows)* is present near the junction of the first and second portions of the duodenum. This is the typical appearance of a flexural pseudopolyp. Redundant mucosa is often present at the junction of the first and second portions of the duodenum. This extra mucosa combined with some buckling medially as the duodenum curves can resemble a polyp (Case 183), a small ulcer (Case 185), or ectopic pancreatic tissue (Case 124). The changing size and configuration of a pseudopolyp can be visualized at fluoroscopy during duodenal filling and emptying.

## Case 180

## NORMAL DUODENUM

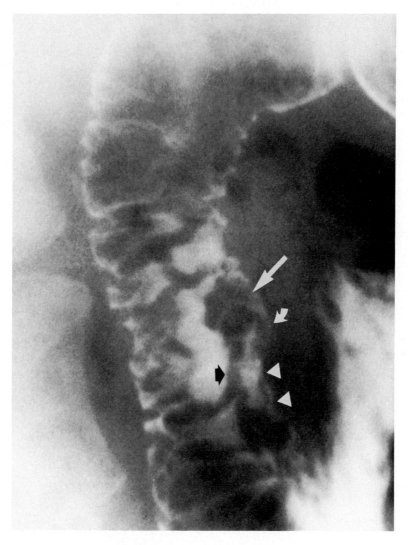

The normal circular valvulae conniventes are seen within the second portion of the duodenum. The papilla of Vater *(white straight arrow)* is seen along the medial wall of the duodenum as a rounded filling defect. A longitudinal fold *(black short arrow)* extends inferiorly from the papilla.

The papilla of Vater normally varies in diameter between 5 and 15 mm. It usually appears as a filling defect within the medial aspect of the second portion of the duodenum. The typical arrangement of folds about the papilla can be helpful in identifying its location. The promontory *(white curved arrow)* is a fixed projection along the medial wall of the duodenum. The major papilla is always on or just below the promontory. The medial duodenal wall just distal to the promontory is referred to as the straight segment *(white arrowheads)*. Often a vertical fold *(black short arrow)* can be identified extending from the papilla of Vater downward, parallel to the straight segment. The accessory papilla (not seen) is located about 1 cm proximal to the papilla. The duct of Santorini empties into the duodenum via this duct. The accessory papilla varies considerably in size and may not always be visible. These structures are important because they should not be confused with abnormal masses.

## Case 181

# NORMAL DUODENUM

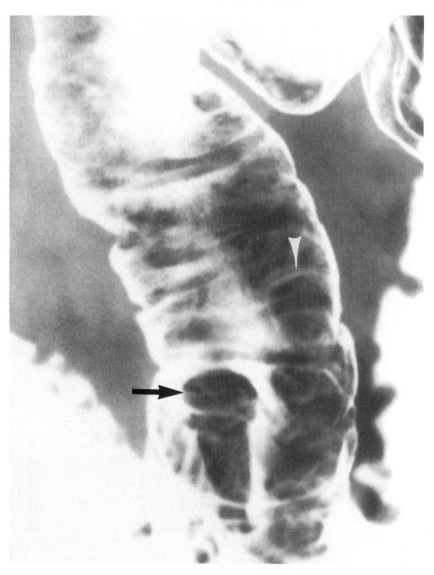

The normal major papilla *(arrow)* and minor papilla *(arrowhead)* are visible in the descending duodenum.

The radiographic appearance of the major papilla varies considerably. The most dramatic appearance occurs when a prominent longitudinal fold encircles the papilla and extends approximately 2 cm distally, as in this case. It is important not to mistake the papilla for a tumor. The minor papilla, 1 to 2 cm proximal to the major papilla, rarely exceeds 4 mm in diameter (Ferrucci et al., 1970).

## Case 182

## BRUNNER'S GLAND HYPERPLASIA

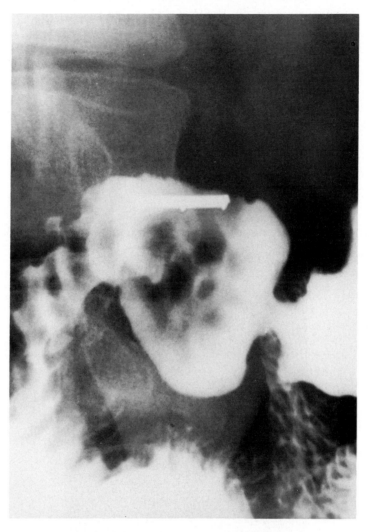

Multiple filling defects of various size are present within the duodenal bulb. These findings are typical of Brunner's gland hyperplasia. A metallic marker embedded on a radiolucent compression paddle is projected over the bulb.

Brunner's glands are normal glandular elements located predominantly in the proximal portion of the duodenum. Glandular secretions are rich in mucus and bicarbonate, substances that protect the duodenum against acid. Hyperplasia of these glands occurs mainly in response to peptic ulcer disease. Radiographically, nodular filling defects can be seen in the duodenal bulb and the second portion of the duodenum.

Differential considerations include thickened folds from duodenitis (Case 184), which can often be obliterated with compression. Crohn's disease often involves a more extensive portion of the duodenum and is often associated with changes in the distal stomach and small bowel (Cases 208 and 209). Nodular lymphoid hyperplasia usually presents with smaller, uniform-size, and diffusely and evenly distributed nodular filling defects (Case 278). Heterotopic gastric mucosa is usually smaller and confined to the duodenal bulb (Case 176).

## Case 183

## BRUNNER'S GLAND ADENOMA

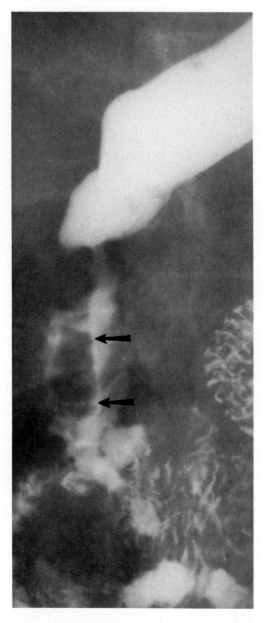

A sausage-shaped, well-demarcated filling defect *(arrows)* is present within the second portion of the duodenum. A Brunner gland adenoma was removed.

Brunner's gland adenoma is an unusual manifestation of Brunner's gland hyperplasia. Histologically, both hyperplasia and hypertrophy are seen. No neoplastic elements are present. Radiologically, this entity is indistinguishable from other polypoid lesions, including adenomas (Case 224) and lipomas (Case 225).

Case 184

# DUODENITIS: ZOLLINGER-ELLISON SYNDROME

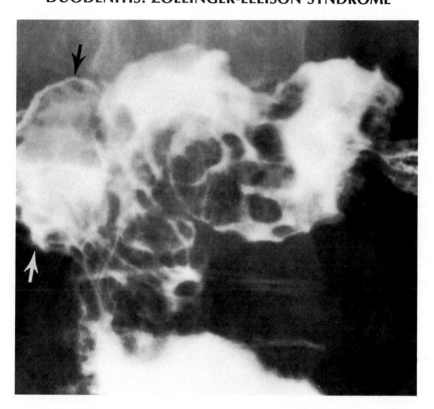

Multiple thick and nodular folds are present in the first and second portions of the duodenum. This patient had known Zollinger-Ellison syndrome and secondary duodenitis. A diverticulum *(arrows)* is seen lateral to the descending duodenum.

The most frequent cause of thickened duodenal folds is peptic ulcer disease. The folds may be enlarged secondary to edema, or Brunner's gland hyperplasia (Case 182) may simulate fold thickening. Usually, multiple, enlarged discrete nodules that form a cobblestone appearance are present in patients with Brunner's gland hyperplasia. Patients with pancreatitis (Case 201), uremia (undergoing chronic dialysis), Crohn's disease (Case 209), giardiasis (Case 270), sprue (Case 210), Whipple's disease (Case 272), and lymphoma (Case 271) can present with thickened duodenal folds. Other less common causes include duodenal varices and cystic fibrosis (Case 238).

## Case 185

## DUODENAL ULCER: TINY NICHE

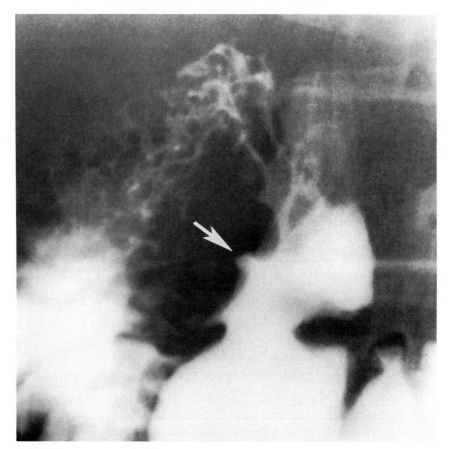

The duodenum is deformed along its inferior margin. A small ulcer niche *(arrow)* with a surrounding mound of edema is present.

Duodenal ulcers are common problems and are encountered 2 to 3 times more often than gastric ulcers. More males are affected than females. Correlation between clinical symptoms and radiographic findings is often imprecise. Some patients with relatively large duodenal ulcers remain asymptomatic, whereas other patients have typical symptoms and normal radiologic findings.

The key radiologic finding is a persistent collection of barium in the duodenal bulb that does not change shape with compression or peristalsis. Ulcers can vary in shape from pinpoint erosions to linear niches to the commonest round crater. Duodenal deformity is often associated with ulcers but is not present in many cases. Folds usually can be seen to radiate up to an ulcer crater.

## Case 186

## LINEAR DUODENAL ULCER

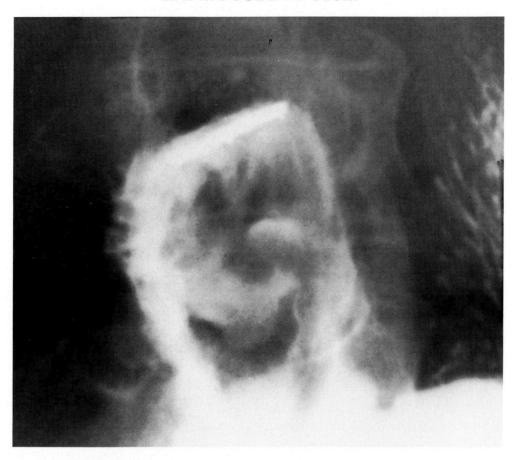

A linear ulcer crater is present in the (deformed) duodenal bulb. A poorly defined filling defect surrounds the ulcer crater and represents a mound of edema. A metallic measuring device (2 cm in length) is attached to the compression paddle.

Linear ulcers of the duodenum and stomach are common (representing about 6% of all visible craters) but may be overlooked because they resemble lines of barium caught between rugal folds (Braver et al., 1979). The duodenal bulb may not be deformed in the presence of a circular ulcer crater; however, moderate to severe deformity is present in at least 50% of linear ulcerations (Braver et al., 1979). It has been suggested that the likelihood of a linear ulcer increases as the deformity becomes more severe. Linear ulcer craters often have fuzzy, blurred margins whereas the lines between folds are sharp and well defined. Linear ulcers can develop de novo or can be seen during the healing phase of a common circular ulcer. Folds can be seen to radiate to the base of the ulcer crater, a finding analogous to usual round craters. If radiating folds are visible but no barium collection is seen, then the ulcer has healed and only a residual scar persists.

## Case 187

# DUODENAL BULB CRATER

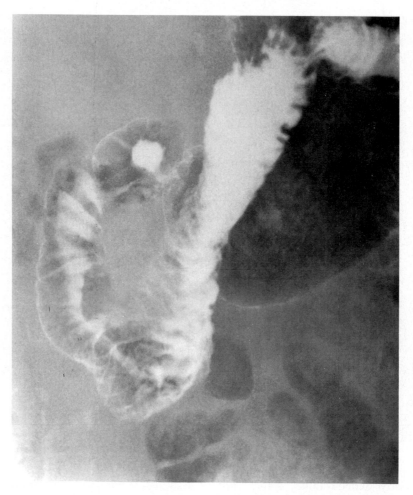

A persistent, round ulcer crater is present in the duodenal bulb. Folds radiate up to the crater. This is the classic appearance of a duodenal ulcer.

This radiograph was obtained with the patient in the supine position. Because barium collected within the crater, its location is within the posterior duodenal wall. An anteriorly located ulcer crater would appear as a ring shadow in this position, because barium would empty from the crater, leaving the ulcer edges barium-coated. Anteriorly located ulcers can be difficult to detect using only the double-contrast technique. Compression of the duodenal bulb is an important part of every upper gastrointestinal examination. Using compression, most anterior wall ulcers can be identified.

Duodenal ulcers are identifed less frequently than in the past because of improved medical therapy. Duode-nal ulcers alone are rarely malignant. These ulcers tend to follow the same morphologic patterns as benign gastric ulcers. Most are located along the anterior surface of the duodenum within the bulb. Acute ulcers without fibrosis can heal without scarring. Chronic ulcers with submucosal fibrosis usually result in residual duodenal deformity. Complications of duodenal ulcers are similar to those of peptic gastric ulcers: bleeding, perforation, obstruction, and penetration. Perforation is more common among duodenal ulcers (Cases 191–196). Penetration of the ulcer into adjacent structures can occur—e.g., pancreas, omentum, biliary tract, colon, liver, and mesocolon. Multiple duodenal ulcers can be identified in 10% to 15% of patients (Classen, 1973). The presence of multiple, postbulbar ulcerations should suggest the possibility of Zollinger-Ellison syndrome (Case 200).

### Case 188

## DUODENAL ULCER: GIANT

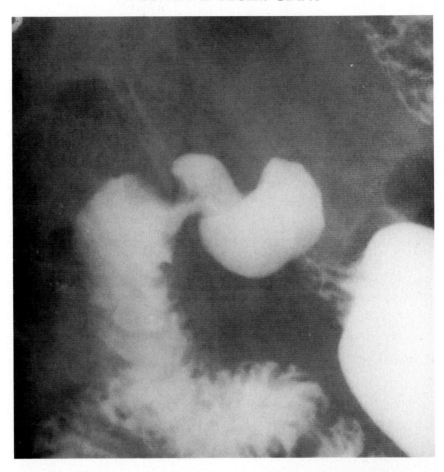

A large ulcer crater resides at the junction of the first and second portions of the duodenum. A symmetric mound of edema causes a filling defect around the ulcer base. An ulcer this size is sometimes referred to as a giant ulcer crater.

Giant ulcers have been described as ulcers larger than 2 to 2.5 cm in diameter or as those replacing most of the duodenal bulb. These ulcers may be so large as to mimic a normal duodenal configuration. Recognition is dependent on observing the fixed shape and size of the ulcer, which contains no normal duodenal folds. Narrowing of the duodenum proximal and distal to the ulcer is common. The complication rate and mortality are higher with this type than with usual duodenal ulcers (Lumsden et al., 1970).

## Case 189

## DUODENAL SCARRING

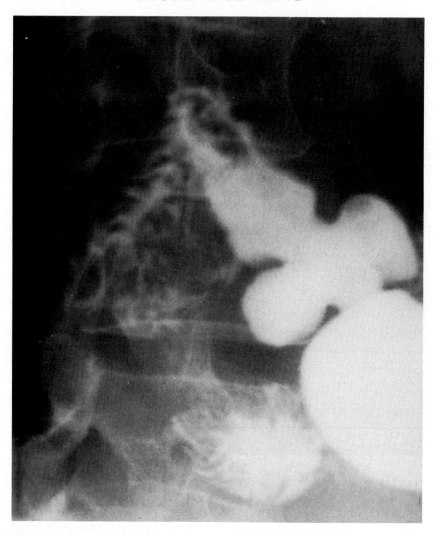

The duodenal bulb is deformed and resembles a cloverleaf. This is the classic appearance of duodenal bulb scarring from a peptic ulcer.

Scarring of the duodenal bulb from previous peptic ulcer disease is a common finding. A centrally located duodenal bulb ulcer characteristically produces this cloverleaf deformity. The challenge to the radiologist is to exclude an active ulcer in the scarred bulb. Some-times this is impossible and endoscopy should be recommended to directly examine the mucosa. Active ulcers are fixed abnormalities within the duodenum that do not change shape with peristalsis. Scarred duodenal bulbs will change shape as the duodenum fills and empties. Compression should be routinely performed to exclude concomitant ulcers within the deformed bulb.

**Case 190**

## PEPTIC ULCER DISEASE: SCARRING

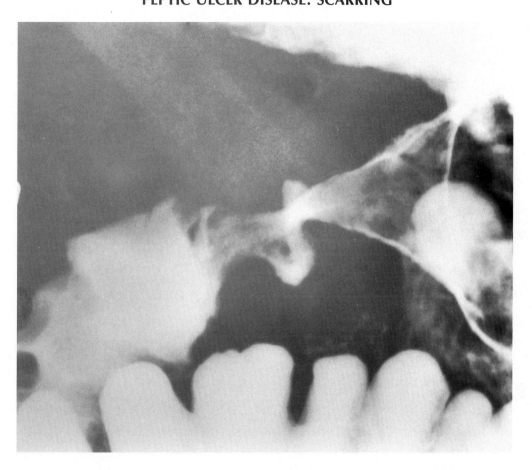

Two collections of barium protrude from the pyloric channel. Deformity of the distal gastric antrum and duodenal bulb is present as a result of previous peptic ulcer disease.

On a single radiograph it is impossible to determine if the changes in the pyloric canal are due to ulcerations or are the result of scarring from previous ulcer disease. This distinction is not always possible, and in equivocal examinations endoscopy should be performed. Generally, deformed regions as a result of prior inflammation and scarring will change shape during fluoroscopic observation, whereas ulcers are fixed collections that maintain their shape with filling and emptying. In this patient, changes were seen in the configuration of the pyloric collections. At endoscopy, no active ulcer crater was found. The typical changes of scarring from peptic ulcer disease are also present in the gastric antrum and duodenal bulb. The normal square shoulders of these structures are replaced by smooth-tapered narrowing.

Less severe ulcer disease will result in less deformity. As a small ulcer heals, a tiny linear excavation often remains (Case 186). The typical changes from a round crater to a small linear collection, combined with disappearance of the patient's symptoms, are excellent evidence for healing. Endoscopy is necessary to differentiate a reepithelialized scar from an active linear ulcer.

## Case 191

## PNEUMOPERITONEUM: UPRIGHT

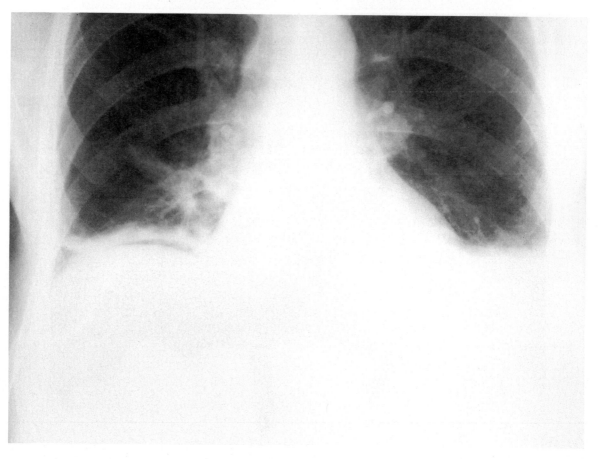

Free air is present beneath the right diaphragm. This patient was found to have a perforated peptic ulcer.

Spontaneous pneumoperitoneum is nearly always due to a perforated viscus. It has been estimated that nearly three-quarters of these patients have a perforated peptic ulcer (Edwards and Foster, 1962). Other causes of pneumoperitoneum include perforation of the colon or small bowel secondary to mechanical obstruction or adynamic ileus, toxic megacolon from inflammatory bowel disease, perforation of a diverticulum, pneumatosis intestinalis, or introduction of air via the female genital tract.

An upright view of the abdomen with the x-ray beam centered on the diaphragm is useful for diagnosing free air. Pneumoperitoneum is seen as a crescent of gas positioned between the diaphragm and liver on the right or the diaphragm and spleen/stomach on the left. Overpenetration of the abdomen may make identification of free air difficult. In some patients, the x-ray technique used for examining the chest will best demonstrate the finding.

**Case 192**

## PNEUMOPERITONEUM: UPRIGHT, DECUBITUS

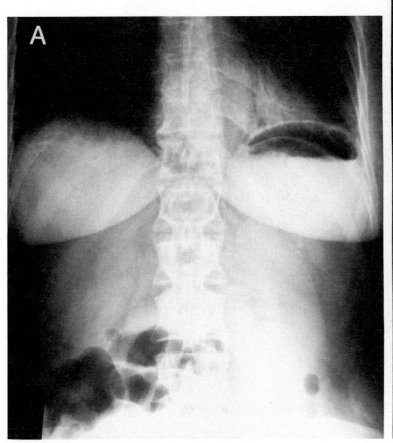

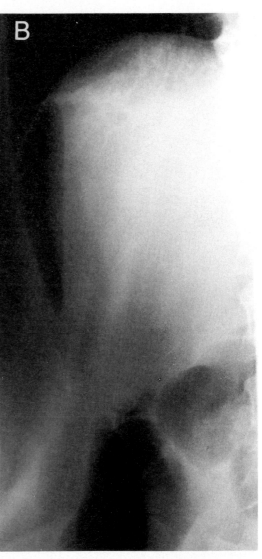

**A.** Free intraperitoneal air is present beneath the left diaphragm. Gas is seen on both sides of the stomach (fundus) wall. This finding is known as Rigler's sign (Case 193). A perforated peptic ulcer was found at operation.

**B.** Left lateral decubitus view demonstrates free intraperitoneal air between the liver and the right abdominal body wall.

The left lateral decubitus view can be helpful in ex-

amining patients who are too ill to sit or stand for an upright view or in patients with equivocal findings of pneumoperitoneum. If only small quantities of free air are present, it is helpful to have patients remain on their left side for approximately 10 min before taking the radiograph. This enables small quantities of gas to collect in the nondependent portion of the peritoneal cavity.

## Case 193

# PNEUMOPERITONEUM: RIGLER'S SIGN

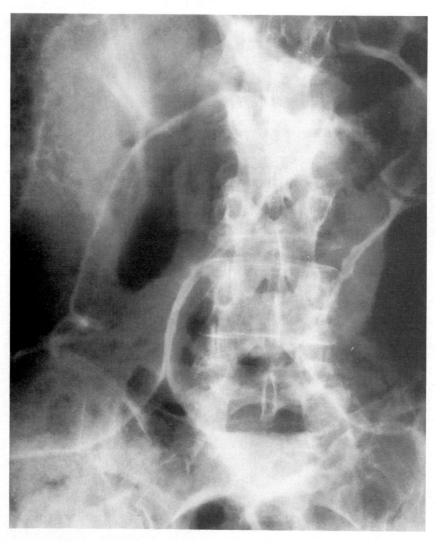

Both sides of the small bowel wall are identified. This finding is referred to as "Rigler's sign." Only in the presence of pneumoperitoneum can both the mucosal and serosal surfaces of the bowel be identified. Normally, the serosal surface is not visible as it blends imperceptibly with other contiguous soft-tissue structures. Moderate to large quantities of free intraperitoneal air are usually present when this finding is detected on radiographs taken with the patient in the supine position.

Case 194

# PNEUMOPERITONEUM

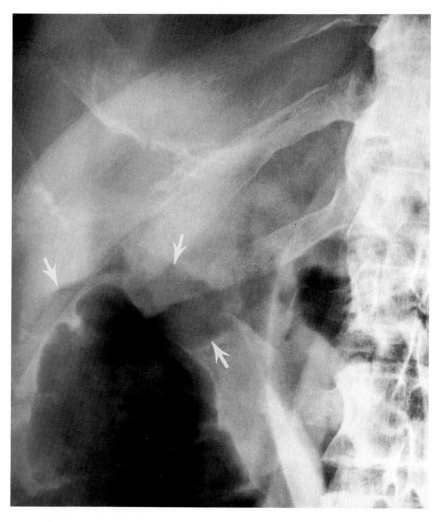

A lucent collection of gas *(arrows)* is present beneath the liver's edge, positioned just superior to the hepatic flexure of the colon. This is a characteristic appearance for free intraperitoneal air on an abdominal radiograph taken with the patient supine.

There are several radiographic signs of pneumoperitoneum on supine abdominal radiographs. The "football sign" refers to a large central lucency over the abdomen due to a large quantity of free air. "Rigler's sign" refers to visualizing both sides of the bowel wall (Case 193). Occasionally, the falciform ligament (Case 196) or urachus will be outlined by air and visible on a flat abdominal film. This case demonstrates a common finding of pneumoperitoneum: gas collecting beneath the liver edge. In addition, free air can also collect anterior to the liver and appear as a poorly defined homogeneous lucency projected over the liver (Case 195).

## Case 195

## PNEUMOPERITONEUM: SUPINE

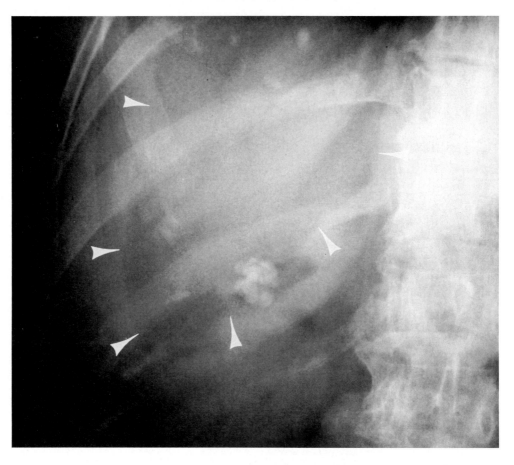

A lucent collection of air *(arrowheads)* is visible over the anterior surface of the liver on this abdominal radiograph taken with the patient in the supine position. This is an important finding of pneumoperitoneum. Free air can be demonstrated on abdominal plain films in up to three-fourths of patients with perforated ulcers (Edwards and Foster, 1962). When a perforated viscus is suspected, an emergent examination using water-soluble contrast material can be helpful to localize the site of the leak. Depending on the clinical status of the patient, urgent surgical exploration without additional imaging studies may be necessary. Postoperative pneumoperitoneum is also a common cause of free air. The time required for free air to resolve depends in part on body habitus. Obese individuals will reabsorb intraperitoneal air faster than will asthenic individuals (Bryant et al., 1963). The amount of air left within the abdomen at operation also is an important factor. Large amounts of intraperitoneal air will take longer to resolve than will small quantities.

## Case 196

## PNEUMOPERITONEUM: CT

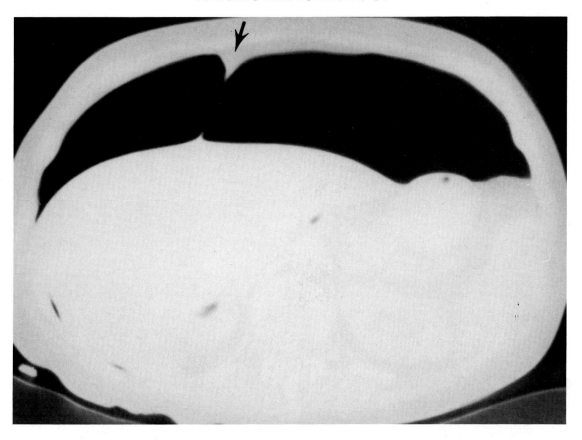

A large amount of free air is present in the peritoneal cavity. The falciform ligament *(arrow)* is seen in the right anterior part of the abdomen.

CT is a sensitive technique for detecting pneumoperitoneum but is rarely necessary as the primary examination for making the diagnosis. Extraluminal air is seen anteriorly in the nondependent portion of the peritoneal cavity.

**217**

## Case 197

## DOUBLE PYLORUS

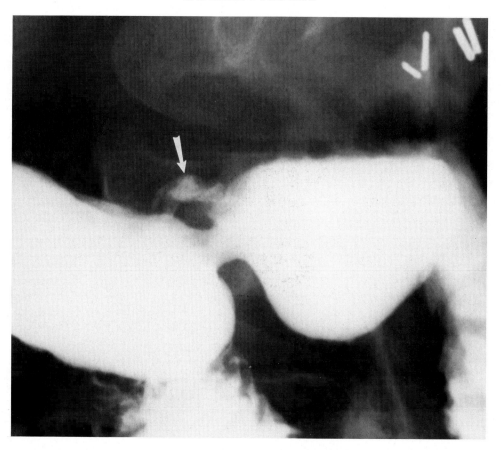

Two pyloric channels are present on this radiograph taken with the patient in the prone position. The most superior channel *(arrow)* connects the lesser curvature of the gastric antrum with the apex of the duodenal bulb.

The majority of cases of multichannel pylorus are secondary to a persistent fistula from peptic ulcer disease or Crohn's disease. Rarely, this finding may represent a congenital abnormality. No treatment may be necessary if no active ulcer is present.

# POSTBULBAR ULCER

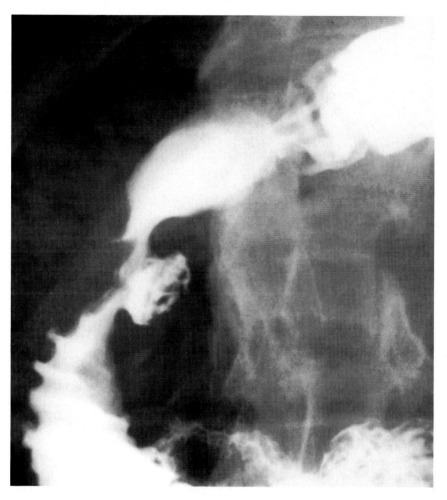

A round ulcer crater lies along the medial aspect of the second portion of the duodenum. There is associated duodenal narrowing, concentric edema about the crater, and fold thickening.

Duodenal ulcers most commonly occur in the duodenal bulb. Postbulbar ulcers are unusual, but when they develop they are usually located proximal to the ampulla and often along the medial wall of the descending duodenum. It has been estimated that 1 in 20 peptic ulcers is located beyond the duodenal bulb (Rodriguez et al., 1973). Ulcerations should be considered malignant or evidence for a gastrin-secreting tu-

mor (Zollinger-Ellison syndrome) should be looked for if an ulcer is identified distal to the ampulla of Vater (Case 200). Healing of these ulcers can result in a ring stricture of the duodenum. Ring strictures can be difficult to diagnose, often requiring distension of the duodenum with either barium or effervescent gas. Associated ulcer niches can also be easily overlooked and should be suspected if a focal area of narrowing is encountered in the postbulbar duodenum. CT may be useful in assessing for the complications of peptic ulcer disease: abscess, fistula, and pancreatitis. CT has no primary role in the diagnosis of peptic ulcers.

## Case 199

## POSTBULBAR ULCER

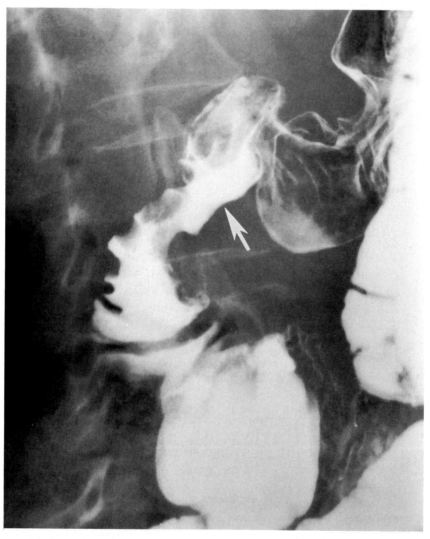

A large ulcer crater lies in the proximal and medial aspect of the descending duodenum *(arrow)*. Thickened folds are seen to radiate up to the crater. Duodenal narrowing is present at the level of the ulceration. A postbulbar ulceration was confirmed endoscopically.

**Case 200**

# POSTBULBAR ULCER: ZOLLINGER-ELLISON SYNDROME

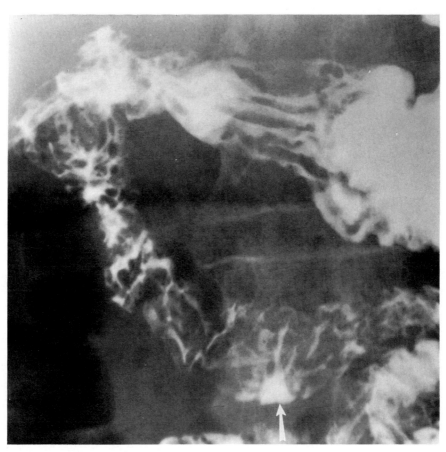

An ulceration *(arrow)* is present within the fourth portion of the duodenum. The ulcer has benign features radiographically, with no associated mass and folds that radiate to the edge of the crater. This patient was found to have Zollinger-Ellison syndrome.

Peptic ulcers in patients with Zollinger-Ellison syndrome most commonly occur in the pylorus and proximal duodenal region (Ellison and Wilson, 1964). Ulcers occurring distal to the ampulla are usually malignant, except in patients with Zollinger-Ellison syndrome. Normally, acidic gastric secretions will be neutralized by the alkaline pancreatic secretions in the postampullary duodenum. Multiple ulcers occur in about 10% of patients with Zollinger-Ellison syndrome (Ellison and Wilson, 1964). The stomach and duodenum may appear hypotonic with dilatation of the duodenum ("megaduodenum"). Thickened duodenal folds and Brunner's gland hyperplasia may also be present (Case 184).

## Case 201

## ACUTE PANCREATITIS

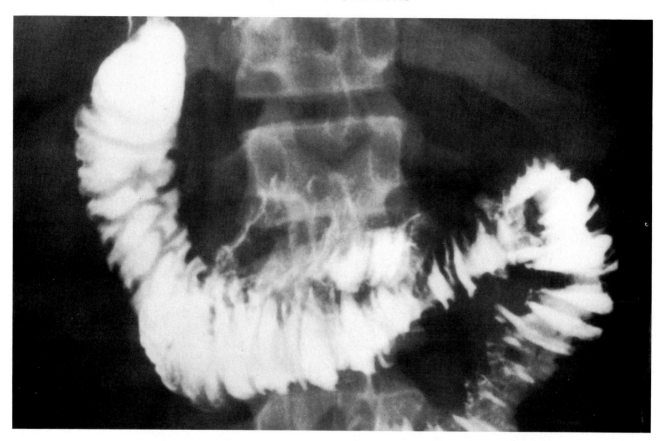

Thickened folds are present in the distal duodenum and proximal jejunum. These findings are nonspecific but were secondary to acute pancreatitis.

Inflammatory exudate from acute pancreatitis most commonly pools in the left anterior pararenal space. The duodenal-jejunal flexure (as seen in this case) and proximal descending colon are often secondarily affected by these inflammatory fluids. Pancreatitis can also be associated with inflammatory changes affecting the entire duodenal sweep (Cases 202 and 203) and small bowel (as fluid tracts into the small bowel mesentery). Other common causes of thickened, proximal small bowel folds include Whipple's disease (Case 272), giardiasis (Case 270), cryptosporidiosis, and *Mycobacterium avium-intracellulare*. The last two are usually found in immunocompromised hosts.

**Case 202**

## PANCREATITIS

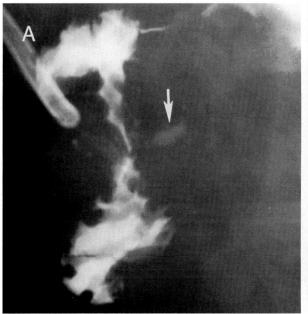

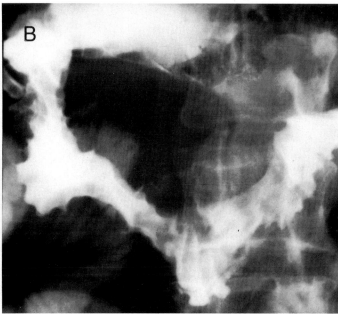

**A.** The folds of the descending duodenum are thickened and the lumen is narrowed. A calculus *(arrow)* is present in the distal main pancreatic duct.

**B.** The duodenal loop has markedly thickened folds, and the second and third portions are narrowed. These findings were secondary to a relapsing attack of acute pancreatitis in a patient with chronic pancreatitis.

Evaluation of patients with known or suspected pancreatitis is usually performed at CT. CT can directly image the pancreas and the surrounding organs and tissues. The role of intraluminal contrast studies in these patients is limited. Evaluation for complications of pancreatitis—including obstruction, leak, and fistula—is the most frequent indication for intraluminal contrast studies today. Changes of pancreatitis involving the duodenum include thickened folds (due to edema), spasm, and mass effect (from the enlarged pancreas or peripancreatic effusion). Thickened folds may be rela-

tively localized or can involve the entire duodenal sweep. Enlargement of the pancreatic head causes a reverse-three appearance of the duodenum and has been described as the epsilon or Frostberg sign (Case 220). This sign can also be seen in carcinoma of the pancreas. A pancreatic mass may displace the stomach anteriorly or depress the duodenojejunal flexure. Deformity of the duodenal bulb may simulate a duodenal ulcer. A significant amount of gas throughout the duodenum due to duodenal ileus can be seen on plain-film examinations and is a helpful finding when present.

The presence of pancreatic calculi is diagnostic of chronic pancreatitis. These calculi lie within the main pancreatic duct or its lateral side branches. Small calculi are more readily detected at CT than on abdominal radiographs.

## Case 203

## PANCREATITIS: FOCAL STENOSIS

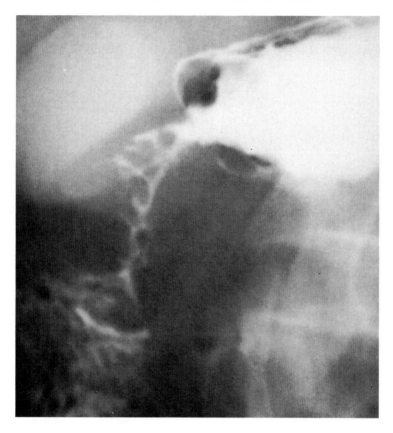

The proximal duodenum is markedly narrowed. The mucosa through this region is intact, and the narrowing ends abruptly. The findings are secondary to pancreatitis.

Occasionally, patients with pancreatitis will have a region of focal stenosis in the proximal duodenum. This narrowing is believed to be due to pancreatitis-induced edema and spasm. A persistent stricture can develop. The stenosis may mimic a carcinoma because of the abrupt edges and focal nature of the narrowing. Identifying intact mucosa through the stenosis is a key finding in distinguishing it from a tumor. A history of pancreatitis is also helpful information.

**Case 204**

## PANCREATITIS

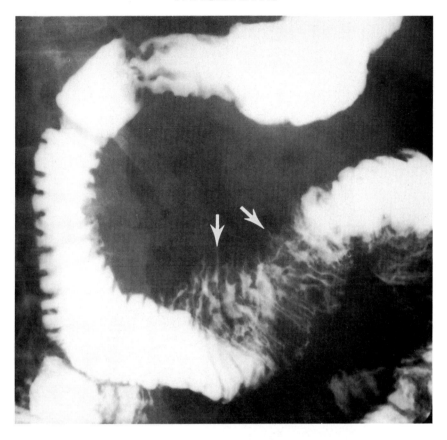

The duodenal C-loop is mildly widened. Tethered folds *(arrows)* are present along the cranial aspect of the transverse duodenum. This patient had acute pancreatitis clinically.

Tethered folds of the bowel usually develop secondary to either an extraluminal inflammatory or a neoplastic process. Normally the folds of the bowel are oriented perpendicular to the lumen and meet the edge of the bowel wall with a square, flat appearance. Tethered folds usually appear to be pulled from the normal bowel wall toward a central area extrinsic to the bowel. The folds are usually pointed and elongated.

## Case 205

## PANCREATIC PSEUDOCYST

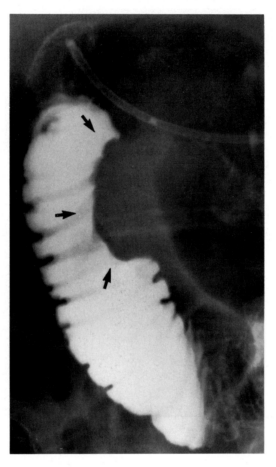

A lobulated filling defect *(arrows)* deforms the medial wall of the descending duodenum. This mass appears to arise from an intramural location. This patient had a recent history of pancreatitis, and a pseudocyst was found later and drained surgically.

Pancreatic pseudocysts are a complication of acute pancreatitis. An extrapancreatic fluid collection may develop as a result of the inflammatory process. If the fluid persists, it may become organized into a well-defined, encapsulated, surgically drainable collection. Depending on the location and size of the pseudocyst, deformity of the duodenum or the stomach may occur. Pseudocysts may occasionally penetrate the serosa and occasionally the muscularis of an intestinal segment.

The duodenum is most commonly involved. These pseudocysts resemble an intramural mass (as in this case). Pancreatic pseudocysts have been reported in locations distant from the pancreas—including mediastinal and pelvic collections. Some pseudocysts undergo spontaneous fistulization into the gastrointestinal tract and require no treatment. Others may require surgical drainage because of persistent pain and intestinal or biliary obstruction and to prevent potential cyst rupture. The most important differential considerations include pancreatic neoplasms. Usually a history of pancreatitis and typical findings at CT make this distinction relatively easy.

**Case 206**

## ACUTE PANCREATITIS WITH PANCREATIC ABSCESS

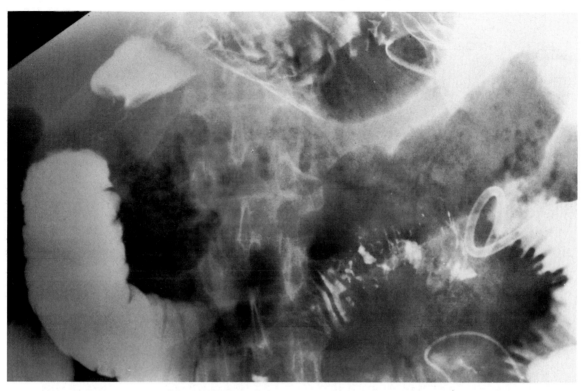

A mottled collection of gas is present within the pancreatic bed. There is a region of focal narrowing in the proximal duodenum. A drainage catheter is seen in the left upper quadrant. The location and appearance of the extraluminal gas are pathognomonic of a pancreatic abscess.

Pancreatic abscess is a dreaded complication of severe acute pancreatitis. High morbidity and mortality are associated with this disease. Pancreatic necrosis is present in many patients with abscess; however, infection of a peripancreatic fluid collection(s) is possible without pancreatic parenchymal necrosis. If a pancreatic abscess is suspected, a CT scan is the best initial examination. Diagnosis of this condition from plain films often occurs for patients with nonspecific abdominal complaints or incidentally when radiographs are obtained for documenting tube position. The key radiographic finding of a pancreatic abscess is a variable amount of extraluminal gas within the pancreatic bed. The gas collection may appear either mottled or homogeneous.

Case 207

## CROHN'S DISEASE

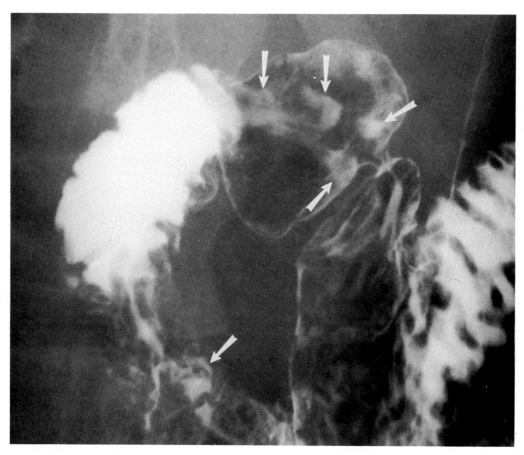

Multiple flat ulcerations *(arrows)* are present within the duodenal bulb and descending duodenum in this patient with known Crohn's disease. These ulcers were confirmed endoscopically.

Crohn's disease affecting the upper gastrointestinal tract is most common within the proximal duodenum. Aphthous ulcers are probably the earliest radiologic lesion detectable. The ulcers in Crohn's disease can vary in appearance from pinpoint ulcers with surrounding halos of edema (aphthous ulcers) to small shallow ulcerations (as seen in this case).

Duodenal erosions are nonspecific lesions. They can be caused by various medications (aspirin and nonsteroidal anti-inflammatory agents), drugs (alcohol), and infectious agents (herpesvirus and cytomegalovirus). The erosions found in patients with Crohn's disease are often identical to those due to other conditions. The clinical setting is an important consideration in these patients. Usually patients with duodenal Crohn's disease will also have radiologic findings in the more distal small bowel.

## Case 208

## CROHN'S DISEASE

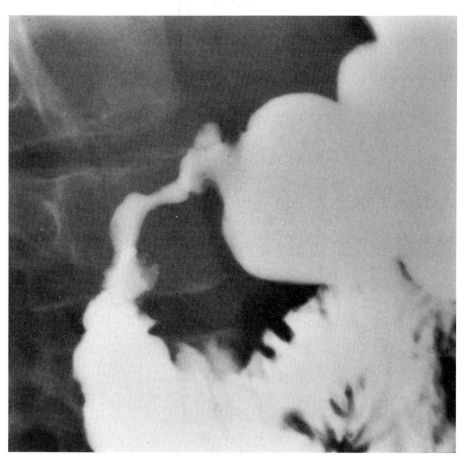

Marked deformity of the pylorus and proximal duodenum is present in this patient with known Crohn's disease.

Chronic changes of Crohn's disease involving the duodenum mimic the findings of Crohn's disease found elsewhere in the small bowel. These changes vary from slight luminal narrowing and mucosal thickening to marked narrowing and irregularity causing gastric ob-struction. Similar changes can affect the gastric antrum. A differential consideration in this case is scarring from previous peptic ulcer disease. If the diagnosis of Crohn's disease is not definite, it is often worthwhile extending the examination to include the remainder of the small bowel, because often other characteristic lesion(s) will be found (Cases 292–298).

## Case 209

## CROHN'S DISEASE

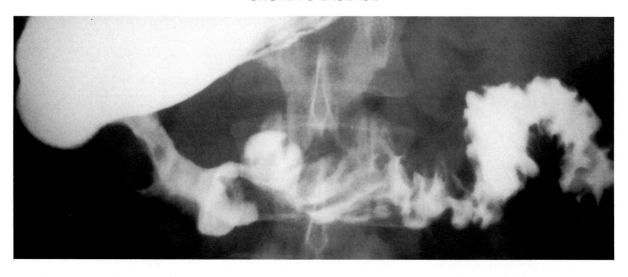

Duodenal narrowing, luminal irregularity, and sacculations (secondary to asymmetric bowel wall involvement) are visible throughout most of the transverse duodenum. This patient had known Crohn's disease.

## Case 210

# ADULT CELIAC DISEASE

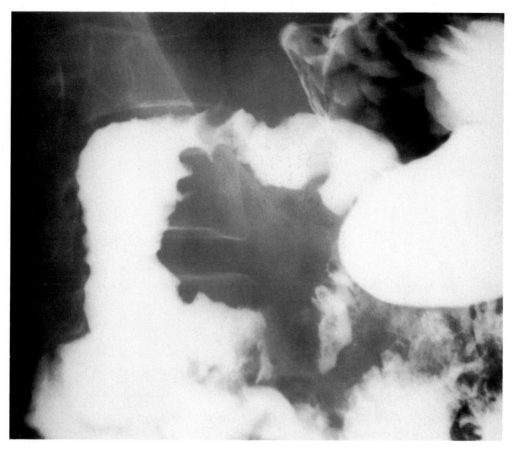

The duodenum is mildly dilated and thickened folds are present in its first and second portions. This patient had known adult celiac disease (nontropical sprue).

Changes of sprue are usually most marked in the jejunum and ileum (Cases 286–289), but changes in the duodenal mucosa can also be identified both radiographically and endoscopically in a majority of patients. Both villous atrophy and inflammatory changes are usually found histologically. Celiac disease probably impairs the protective effects of the duodenal mucosa against peptic damage.

The radiographic findings of sprue in the duodenum include thickened and often nodular duodenal folds. Duodenal erosions and luminal dilatation may be seen. Brunner's gland hyperplasia is often present. Small (1–4 mm), angular filling defects have been reported, resulting in a mosaic or "bubbly" appearance of the duodenal bulb (Jones et al., 1984). Patients with longstanding disease may have an atrophic, featureless, duodenal mucosal pattern.

## Case 211

## ADENOCARCINOMA

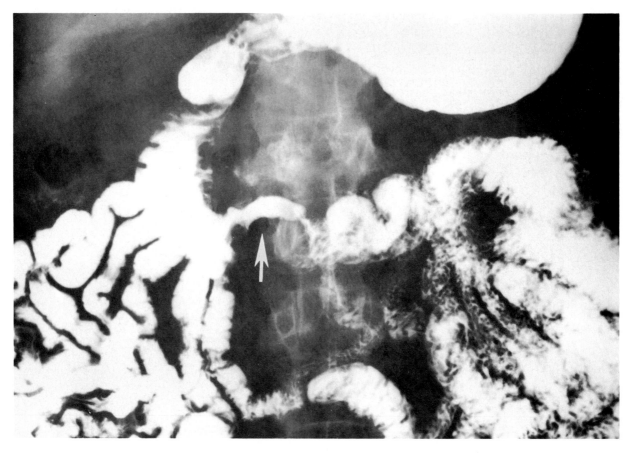

Focal, eccentric narrowing *(arrow)* is present within the third portion of the duodenum. The intraluminal characteristics of the lesion are featureless and devoid of any normal mucosal markings because of the ulcerated surface. Adenocarcinoma was removed surgically.

Adenocarcinoma is the primary malignant tumor that most frequently affects the duodenum. These tumors are most commonly found distal to the ampulla. Short segmental regions of narrowing ("apple core") with abrupt edges or polypoid masses are most commonly encountered (Cases 328 and 329).

## Case 212

# ADENOCARCINOMA

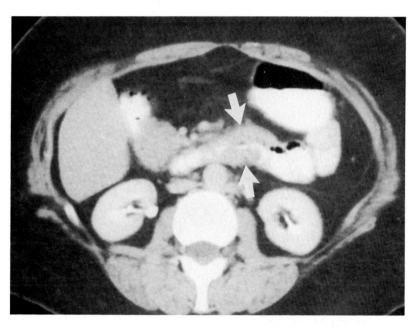

Short, segmental bowel-wall thickening *(arrows)* is present within the fourth portion of the duodenum. Primary adenocarcinoma of the duodenum was removed surgically.

*From Dudiak KM, Johnson CD, Stephens DH. AJR* ***1989;****152:995–998. By permission of the American Roentgen Ray Society.*

CT is rarely the primary imaging test to evaluate for a duodenal tumor. Occasionally, a mass will be discovered incidentally. Adenocarcinomas characteristically cause short, segmental wall thickening of the duodenum. Luminal narrowing is often present. CT is particularly helpful in assessing extraluminal tumor extent, including invasion of adjacent organs, regional adenopathy, and liver metastases.

## Case 213

## AMPULLARY ADENOCARCINOMA

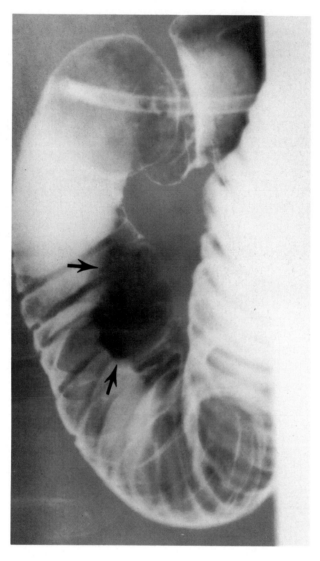

A lobulated filling defect *(arrows)* occupies the medial wall of the second portion of the duodenum. Adenocarcinoma of the ampulla was removed at operation.

Carcinomas involving the ampulla of Vater are nearly always adenocarcinomas arising from the duodenum, distal common bile duct, or distal pancreatic duct. They may present as a polypoid mass or as an annular constricting lesion. Obstruction of the biliary tree is common. Malignant lesions usually have an irregular surface contour. Duodenal adenomas and adenocarcinomas may present as a manifestation of Gardner's syndrome (Case 374).

Differential considerations include a normal ampullary filling defect (Cases 180 and 181) and an edematous papilla, usually due to an impacted distal common bile stone. Edematous changes nearly always present with the enlarged papilla having a smooth surface.

Endoscopic retrograde cholangiopancreatography is usually indicated in any patient with a suspected ampullary lesion. The tumor is often directly visible and a biopsy specimen can be obtained. Surgical treatment is usually pancreatoduodenectomy (Whipple's procedure).

## Case 214

## LYMPHOMA

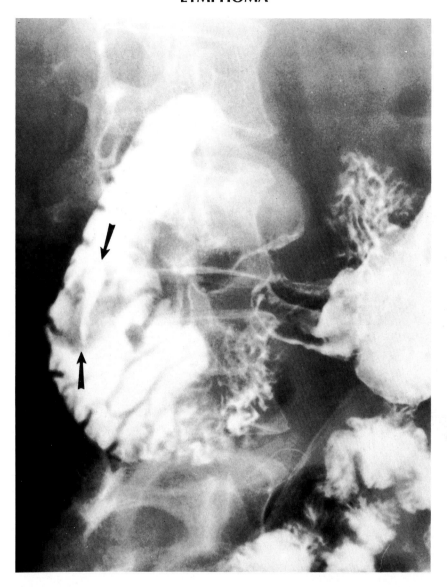

A well-defined mass *(arrows)* with smooth borders is present within the second portion of the duodenum. The mass contains a linear ulcer crater. Any of the primary duodenal tumors could have this appearance, including adenocarcinoma (Case 211), leiomyoma, leiomyosarcoma (Case 216), and lymphoma. Lymphoma was removed surgically. Notice the well-defined minor and major papillae located medial to the tumor.

## Case 215

## LYMPHOMA

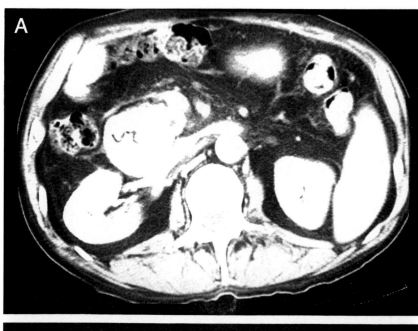

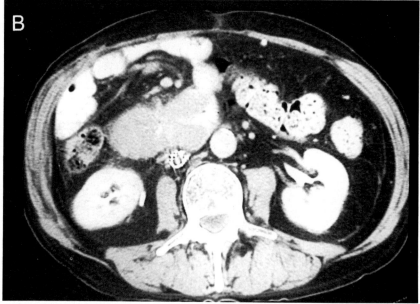

**A** and **B.** A long segment of circumferential bowel-wall thickening involves the second portion of the duodenum. A large ulceration is present within the lesion (best seen in **A**). Primary duodenal lymphoma was removed surgically.

Lymphoma involving the duodenum is unusual. It may present as a solitary mass, as one of many lesions within the alimentary tract, or as an ulcerated mass. Occasionally, the ulcer crater is larger than the associated unaffected bowel lumen (aneurysmal ulceration). Characteristic findings of lymphoma on CT include a long segment of marked bowel-wall thickening (as seen in this case). Regional or diffuse adenopathy may be associated with the mass.

## Case 216

# LEIOMYOSARCOMA

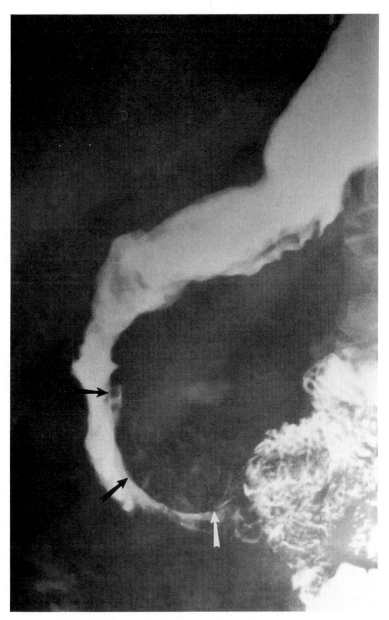

An extramucosal mass *(arrows)* narrows and deforms the duodenum at the junction of its second and third portions. The smooth surface of the lesion indicates its extramucosal location. Calcification is present within the mass. At operation, a leiomyosarcoma was removed.

Leiomyosarcomas are often impossible to differentiate radiologically from leiomyomas. They are intramu-

ral tumors with a smooth surface. Tumoral calcification (as seen in this case) is usually specific for smooth muscle tumors. Large lesions and ulcerative lesions are more likely sarcomatous. Bulky lesions with areas of central necrosis are typically encountered at CT. Often the tumor appears larger at CT than anticipated from the barium study.

## Case 217

## METASTASES

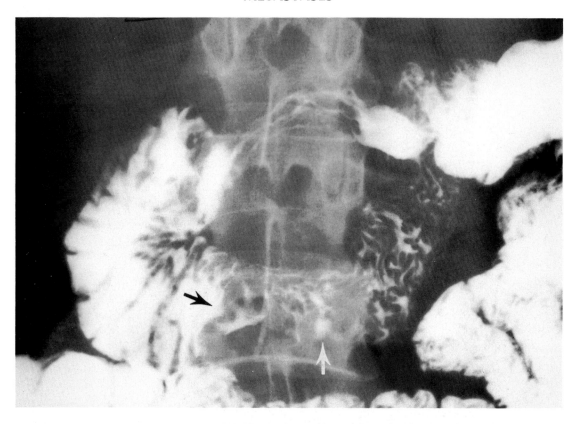

Two ulcerated and lobulated filling defects *(arrows)* are present in the third portion of the duodenum. This patient had a known squamous cell carcinoma of the lung that had metastasized to the duodenum.

Metastasis to the duodenum can occur from either direct invasion or by lymphatic or hematogenous dissemination. Direct invasion occurs most commonly in patients with pancreatic carcinoma (mass effect and ulceration usually along the medial aspect of duodenum), gallbladder carcinoma, gastric or colonic carcinoma, or renal adenocarcinoma. Retroperitoneal adenopathy from distant tumors can compress and narrow the duodenum. Hematogenous metastases most commonly arise from lung cancer and melanoma. Multiple lesions in the gastrointestinal tract are commonly encountered with both hematogenous metastases and lymphoma.

## Case 218

## METASTASIS

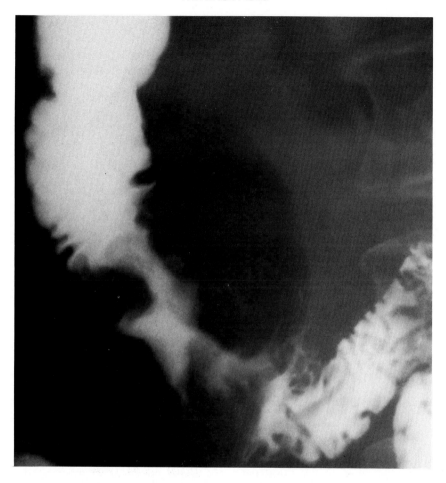

An ulcerated, annular constricting mass is present within the second portion of the duodenum. This mass was a metastatic large cell carcinoma from a primary lesion in the lung.

This tumor is radiographically indistinguishable from a primary duodenal adenocarcinoma (Case 211). Statistically, a metastasis to the duodenum is more likely than is a primary adenocarcinoma.

## Case 219

## METASTASIS

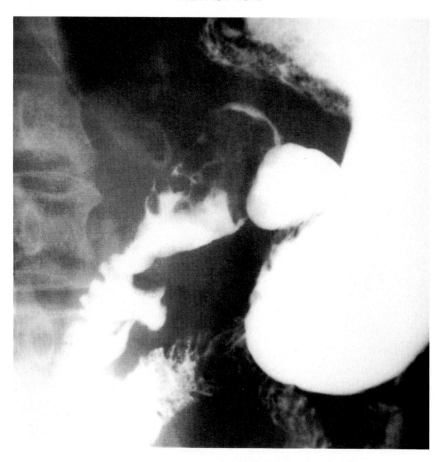

A large polypoid mass fills most of the duodenal bulb. This mass was due to metastatic renal adenocarcinoma. A diverticulum is present along the medial aspect of the second portion of the duodenum.

Renal adenocarcinomas can directly invade or metastasize hematogenously to the alimentary tract. Either route of spread can lead to bulky, polypoid filling defects, as seen in this case.

## Case 220

## PANCREATIC ADENOCARCINOMA

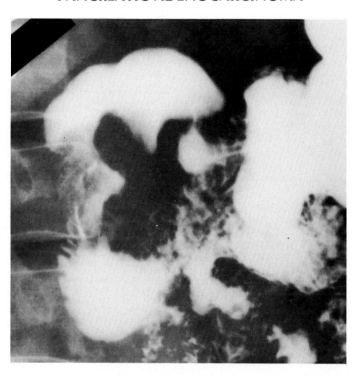

The second portion of the duodenum is narrowed and distorted, with ulceration along its medial border. This is a typical example of the reverse three or epsilon sign described by Frostberg.

Barium examinations are no longer the modality of choice for examination of the pancreas. Direct pancreatic imaging with CT or sonography is preferable. Many intraluminal contrast examinations in patients

*From Stephens DH. In: Margules AR, Burhenne HJ, eds. Alimentary tract radiology, 4th ed, vol 2. St. Louis: Mosby—Year Book, 1989:1167—1194. By permission of the publisher.*

with pancreatic cancer will be negative. Radiographic findings vary depending on the size of the tumor and its location within the pancreas. Tumors in the pancreatic head can compress, invade, and ulcerate the medial border of the duodenal sweep and inferior aspect of the gastric antrum. Masses in the pancreatic body and tail usually cause mass effect and tethering of the gastric body and fundus. Extension of tumor can also occur along the normal tissue planes and ligaments of the transverse colon and duodenojejunal flexure.

## Case 221

# PANCREATIC ISLET CELL CARCINOMA

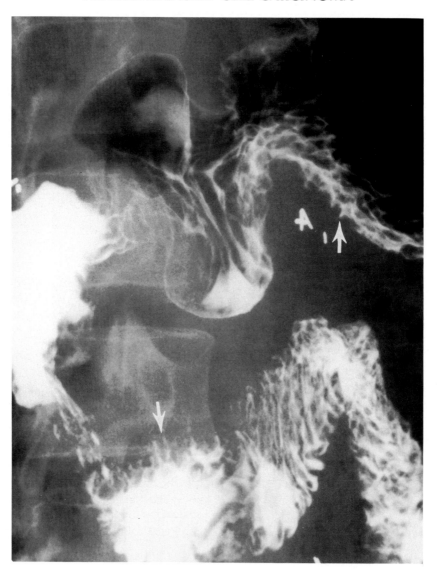

Fixed narrowing of the distal portion of the stomach and duodenum is present. Both antral and duodenal folds are tethered *(arrows)* from serosal invasion by this patient's known islet cell carcinoma. Surgical clips are present from a prior unsuccessful attempt at tumor resection.

The classic changes on the duodenum produced by a mass in the pancreatic head include mass effect or displacement on the medial wall of the duodenum, mucosal tethering, the epsilon sign of Frostberg, and a tubular impression on the duodenum from the obstructed and dilated common bile duct. Many of these changes are absent or difficult to detect unless the tumor is quite large. Today, CT has replaced conventional barium studies for evaluating patients with suspected pancreatic disease.

## Case 222

## PROLAPSING GASTRIC POLYPS

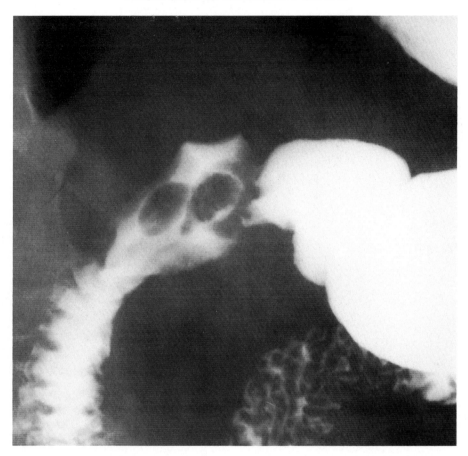

Two polypoid filling defects are present within the duodenal bulb. At fluoroscopy, these could be observed to traverse the pylorus and return to the stomach. These were found to be hyperplastic gastric polyps and were removed by endoscopic polypectomy.

Gastric polyps are more common than duodenal pol-

yps. In fact, most duodenal bulb polyps are actually gastric polyps that have prolapsed through the pylorus into the duodenum. Fluoroscopic observation can be helpful in watching the polyps move between stomach and duodenum and in identifying the pedicle.

## Case 223

## POLYPOSIS

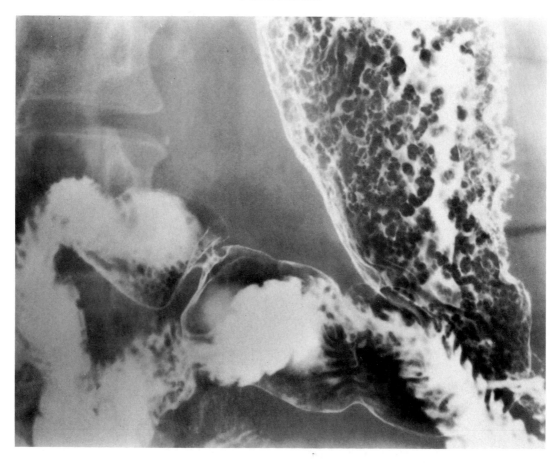

Multiple tiny filling defects are present within the duodenal bulb. Larger and more numerous polyps are also present in the stomach in this patient with Gardner's syndrome.

Duodenal polyps are rare; when present, they are usually adenomas, leiomyomas, or lipomas. Multiple polyps in the duodenum can be present in patients with a polyposis syndrome. Although little is known about the incidence and distribution of extracolonic polyps in familial polyposis, they are recognized more frequently today. Gastric polyps in familial polyposis (and Gardner's syndrome) are most commonly hyperplastic, although adenoma also can be found (Feczko, 1989). Duodenal polyps are usually adenomatous. Because patients with Gardner's syndrome (a variant of familial polyposis) have an increased incidence of ampullary carcinoma, the duodenum should be carefully assessed in all patients with familial polyposis. Hamartomas are usually present in Peutz-Jeghers syndrome.

Other causes of multiple filling defects in the duodenal bulb include heterotopic gastric mucosa (Case 176), benign lymphoid hyperplasia, and Brunner's gland hyperplasia (Case 182). Heterotopic gastric mucosa usually appears as multiple, tiny, angular filling defects. Lymphoid nodular hyperplasia consists of tiny, round, uniform filling defects that usually diffusely involve the entire small bowel (Case 278). Brunner's gland hyperplasia is often larger and involves fewer filling defects that vary in size.

## Case 224

## VILLOUS ADENOMA

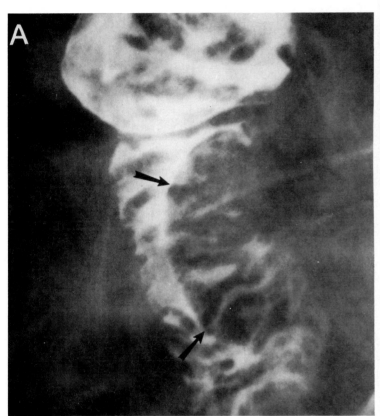

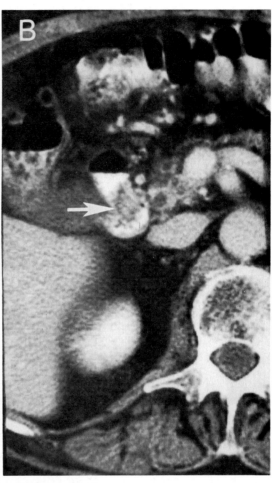

**A.** A well-defined mass *(arrows)* is located in the region of the ampulla.

**B.** A soft-tissue mass causes focal wall thickening *(arrow)* of the medial wall of the second portion of the duodenum. A villous adenoma was removed at operation.

Benign tumors of the duodenum are unusual. Villous adenomas often have a raspberry or cauliflowerlike surface, although the surface of the tumor in this case does not appear villous. These tumors can be suggested radiographically when barium fills the many tiny surface interstices. There is a higher incidence of malignant transformation within villous adenomas than is found in usual tubular adenomatous polyps.

CT is never a primary diagnostic tool in polyp detection. Occasionally, however, polyps will be incidentally discovered. CT is most helpful in determining the extraluminal extent of disease. Local tumor invasion, regional lymphadenopathy, and liver and lung metastases can be assessed preoperatively at CT.

## Case 225

## LIPOMA

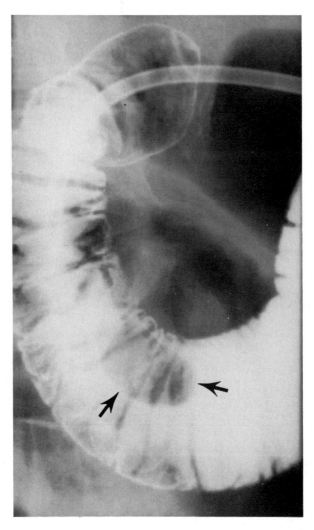

A well-circumscribed mass *(arrows)* is located at the junction of the second and third portions of the duodenum. Its smooth surface suggests a submucosal origin of the tumor. The sausage shape of the mass suggests it is soft and pliable. A lipoma was removed surgically.

Lipomas are submucosal tumors that nearly always have a smooth surface and are compressible at fluoroscopy. These tumors may change shape during a peristaltic contraction. They may grow to a large size.

## Case 226

## LIPOMA

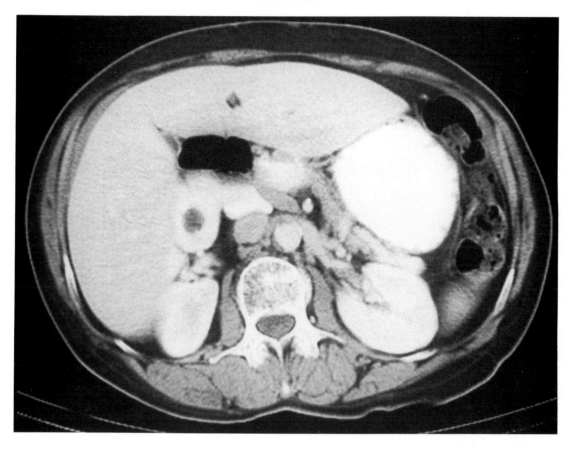

A mass the density of fat is present within the duodenum. The mass is well circumscribed. This radiographic appearance is typical and pathognomonic for a lipoma. No further diagnostic tests should be necessary.

Case 227

## PROLAPSED GASTRIC MUCOSA

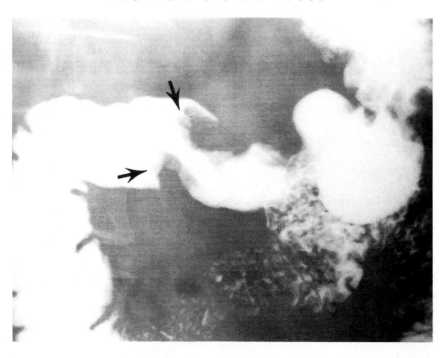

A symmetric filling defect *(arrows)* is seen within the base of the duodenal bulb. At fluoroscopy this was an inconstant finding; it was most noticeable as a gastric peristaltic wave passed through the antrum.

Gastric mucosal prolapse is an incidental finding without any known clinical significance in nearly 20% of the population (Levin and Felson, 1951). The radiologic appearance varies depending on the amount of mucosal redundancy and duodenal protrusion.

**Case 228**

## PROLAPSED GASTRIC MUCOSA

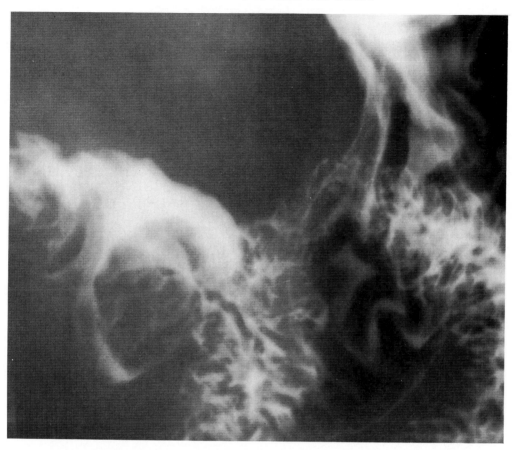

A polypoid filling defect is present in the duodenal bulb. At fluoroscopy this was seen to partially reduce.

Considerable redundancy of the gastric mucosa can mimic a prolapsing gastric polyp. Polyps can slip back and forth through the pylorus, but they can always be identified in either the stomach or the duodenum. Redundant gastric mucosa will only be identifiable as an inconstant filling defect in the duodenum. It usually disappears in the absence of antral peristalsis and with full distension of the stomach.

## Case 229

## DIVERTICULA

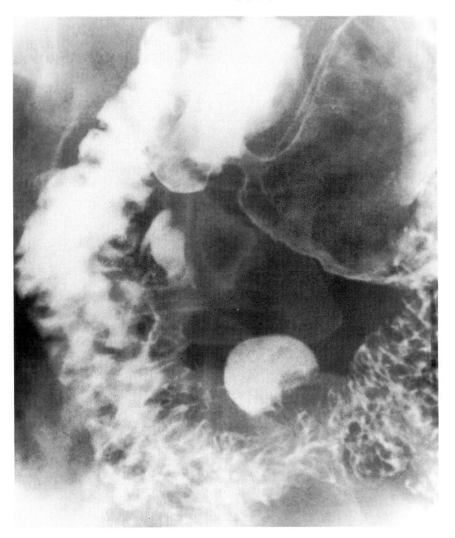

Two diverticula arise from the second and third portions of the duodenum.

Diverticula can occur at any location in the duodenum, but they most commonly arise from the medial wall of its second portion. Usually these are of little clinical significance; however, rarely hemorrhage and perforation have been reported. Differentiation of diverticula from ulcers can often be made by observing duodenal folds entering the diverticula and the diverticulum changing shape and size.

Case 230

# INTRALUMINAL DUODENAL DIVERTICULUM

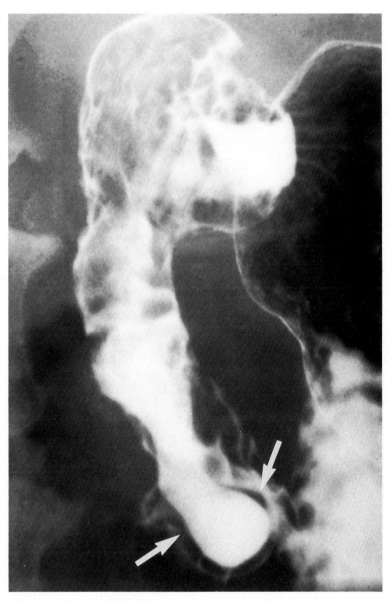

A barium-filled, polypoid, intraluminal mass *(arrows)* is present within the descending duodenum. This is the typical appearance of an intraluminal duodenal diverticulum.

An intraluminal duodenal diverticulum is believed to develop secondary to an intraluminal duodenal diaphragm. The diaphragm usually arises at or near the papilla of Vater. The diaphragm balloons within the duodenum, eventually developing into a sac. Most patients present with intermittent obstructive symptoms and abdominal pain. An obstructive diverticulum near the papilla of Vater may be associated with pancreatitis (Nosher and Seaman, 1975).

The radiologic appearance of these diverticula has been likened to a wind sock. Usually a radiolucent band, representing the diverticular wall, surrounds the diverticulum. If the diverticulum is not filled with barium it will resemble a pedunculated polyp (Case 183).

## Case 231

## INFANTILE HYPERTROPHIC PYLORIC STENOSIS

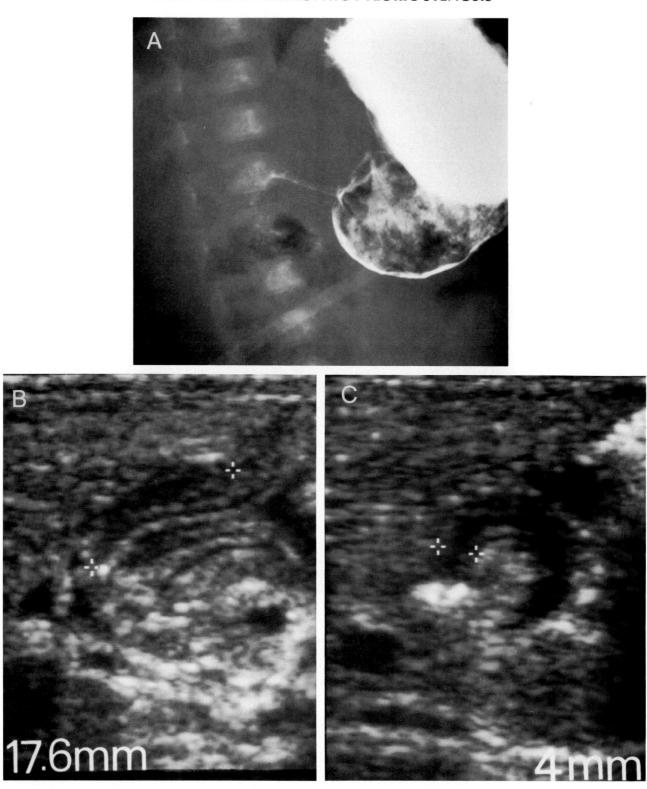

**A.** The pyloric canal is elongated. Very little barium passes into the duodenum with subsequent fluoroscopic observation.

**B.** The pyloric canal is elongated (17.6 mm) on this transverse sonogram.

**C.** The pylorus is seen in cross section on this longitudinal sonogram. The pyloric muscle is abnormally thickened (4 mm).

Hypertrophic pyloric stenosis is a disease that usually affects males; they present after the second week of life with symptoms of gastric outlet obstruction. Pathologically, there is thickening and hypertrophy of the gastric antral musculature. The exact cause of this developmental problem is unknown.

Ultrasound examination of patients with a suspected diagnosis of hypertrophic pyloric stenosis has now become the initial imaging modality in many centers. Ultrasound can be used to directly visualize and measure the hypertrophic muscular mass and elongated pyloric canal. Generally, an abnormally thick pyloric muscle, ≥4 mm (as seen in **C**), is the most helpful sonographic criterion. Overlap exists in the measurements of muscle and canal length in patients with and without the disease (Blumhagen et al., 1988). If the conventional upper gastrointestinal examination is performed, a spectrum of narrowed and elongated pyloric canals exists. Complete opacification of the pyloric canal is not necessary if the typical appearance of a "pyloric beak" or "shoulder sign" is identified. Occasionally, more than one pyloric canal can be identified.

Case 232

# PYLORIC TORUS DEFECT WITH HYPERTROPHIC PYLORIC STENOSIS

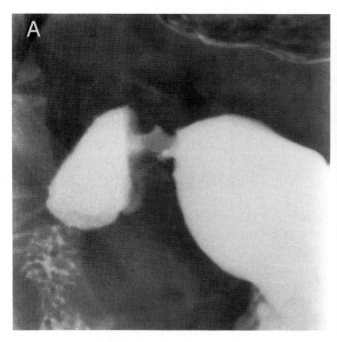 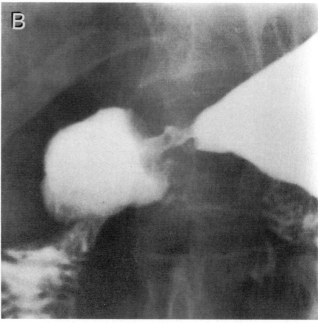

**A** and **B.** An angular-shaped collection of barium is seen in an elongated pyloric canal. The triangular collection was observed at fluoroscopy to change shape. The findings are consistent with adult hypertrophic pyloric stenosis.

The normal pylorus is composed of two prominent muscle bundles that converge toward the lesser curvature known as the torus. In some patients these muscular bundles may diverge far enough to allow mucosa to prolapse between them. This prolapse creates an angular-shaped niche within the pyloric canal that can simulate a pyloric channel crater. A pyloric torus niche is transient and will change shape and possibly disappear with fluoroscopic observation or serial films. It has been reported in 14% of normal patients (Bremner,

1968) and is also prominent in patients with hypertrophic pyloric stenosis.

Adult hypertrophic stenosis is a rare condition. Patients frequently complain of nausea, postprandial upset, intermittent vomiting, and heartburn. Radiologically, the pyloric canal is narrowed and elongated. The torus defect is often identified and the pyloric muscle mass indents the base of the duodenal bulb. Nearly half of all patients will have concomitant gastric ulceration.

Differential considerations include a pyloric ulcer, carcinoma, and antral gastritis. A fixed pyloric channel should be viewed with suspicion, and endoscopy with biopsy should be recommended to exclude neoplasm.

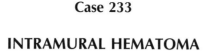

# Case 233

# INTRAMURAL HEMATOMA

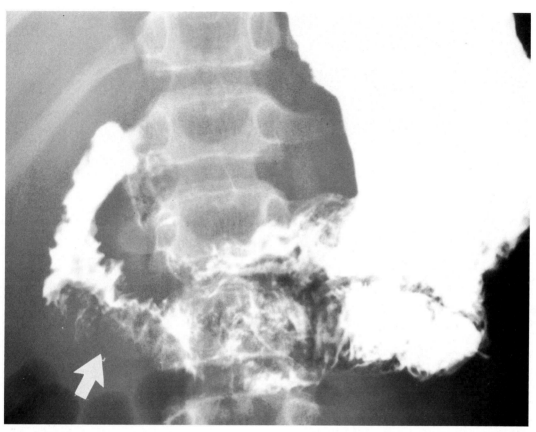

A localized mass *(arrow)* indents and narrows the duodenum at the junction of its second and third portions. This child was brought to the emergency room after falling from playground equipment onto the abdomen. A duodenal hematoma is most likely, considering the history of trauma.

Hemorrhage can affect any portion of the gastrointestinal tract, but the small bowel is most frequently affected. Anticoagulants, trauma, and bleeding diatheses are the usual causes. Patients suffering blunt abdominal trauma usually have masslike changes involving the duodenum because of its lack of mobility and retroperitoneal fixation. Spontaneous hematomas can occur anywhere in the small or large bowel and involve the bowel more diffusely. Usually the condition is self-limited and the hematoma is gradually resorbed. Clearing of the hematoma can usually be appreciated within

1 week, with complete resolution in 2 to 3 weeks (Balthazar and Einhorn, 1976).

Radiographic findings include a segmental region of fold thickening where the folds are straight and have been likened to a "stack of coins." Smooth or scalloped narrowing of the duodenum with effacement of the folds can also be seen, as in this case. It is important to assess for a duodenal leak (extravasated contrast material or extraluminal gas), an important complication of a severe injury (Case 234).

Differential considerations include any process causing localized fold thickening, including an adjacent abscess (Case 206), pancreatitis (Case 201), or infarction. Infiltration of the bowel wall with tumor could also have a similar appearance (Case 271). Generally, the diagnosis is obvious if recent trauma has occurred.

## Case 234

## TRAUMATIC PERFORATION

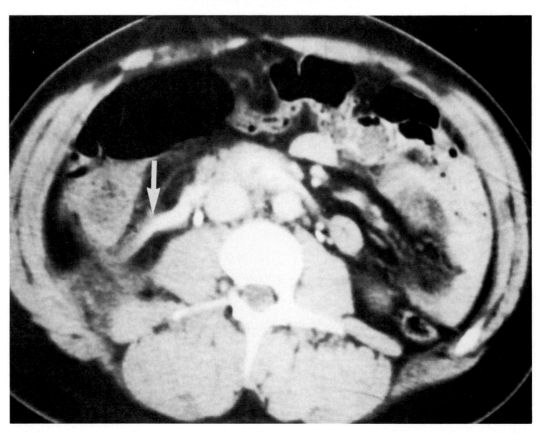

Extravasated orally administered contrast material *(arrow)* is tracking from the region of the retroperitoneal duodenum into the right anterior pararenal space. Hazy soft-tissue stranding is also present in the right flank. This patient was in a motor vehicle accident and suffered a blow to the abdomen. The location of the extraluminal contrast material and history of abdominal trauma are consistent with duodenal perforation, which was surgically confirmed and repaired.

The diagnosis of duodenal perforation is often not apparent clinically. If the diagnosis is delayed beyond 24 hours, reports suggest that mortality may reach 65%. Repair within 24 hours has only a 5% mortality (Roman et al., 1971). For traumatic duodenal perforation, the most important finding on plain films is retro-

peritoneal air. Other nonspecific findings include psoas obliteration, segmental ileus near the duodenum, and scoliosis. Plain-film findings of duodenal perforation are present in only one-third of patients (Toxopeus et al., 1972). Free intraperitoneal air is unusual in traumatic duodenal perforations, and it is more commonly encountered in patients with a perforated peptic ulcer. CT can directly visualize the duodenum and adjacent tissues. CT findings of a traumatic duodenal perforation include extravasated gas or orally administered contrast material, fluid collection in the anterior pararenal space, and considerable soft-tissue stranding in the retroperitoneum. Retroperitoneal gas and fluid can also occur from traumatic injuries to the thorax, bladder, or pancreas.

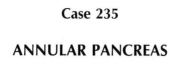

Case 235

# ANNULAR PANCREAS

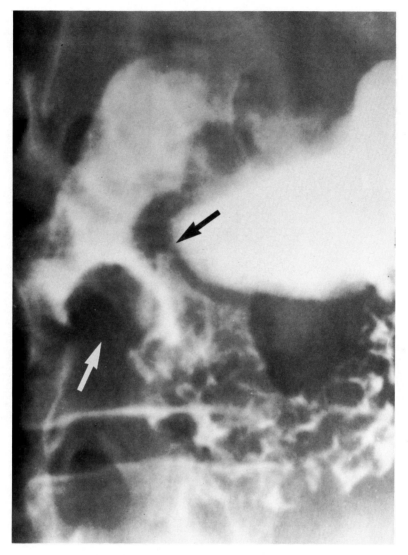

A well-defined filling defect *(arrows)* with associated narrowing of the descending duodenum is present. At operation, an annular pancreas was removed.

Annular pancreas is a congenital abnormality in which the dorsal and ventral pancreatic tissues encircle and narrow the duodenum at or above the level of the ampulla. Complete duodenal obstruction often occurs in the neonatal period. In these patients, the classic "double bubble" is present with gas in the distended stomach and proximal duodenum. Less-severe narrowing may be asymptomatic or lead to symptoms that are delayed until adulthood (Kiernan et al., 1980). Endoscopic retrograde cholangiopancreatography is diagnostic of this condition when the ventral pancreatic duct is seen to encircle the duodenum.

## Case 236

# SUPERIOR MESENTERIC ARTERY SYNDROME

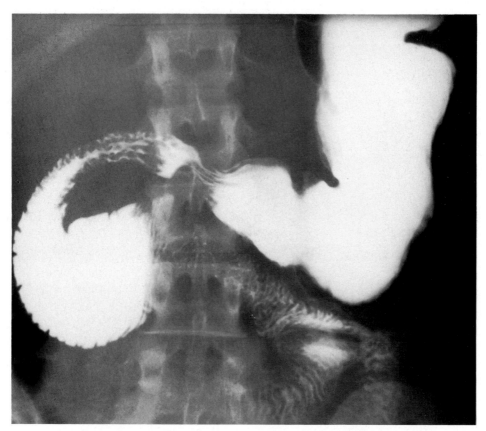

The proximal transverse duodenum is dilated to the level of the spine. The bowel abruptly narrows and appears to be pinched closed by a linear extrinsic mass. The underlying duodenal mucosa is intact. Findings are characteristic of the superior mesenteric artery syndrome.

Narrowing of the third portion of the duodenum can occur as a result of compression by the anteriorly located superior mesenteric artery and posteriorly positioned spine and aorta. This finding often can be observed in asymptomatic individuals, but in certain patients a critical narrowing occurs and results in partial duodenal obstruction. Patients who lose weight rapidly or very asthenic individuals are most often affected. Patients immobilized for long periods (body casts, hyperextension fixation for spinal injuries, extensive burn victims) are also at risk.

Radiologically, the first and second portions of the duodenum are dilated to the level of the extramucosal linear obstruction (superior mesenteric artery). Vigorous peristalsis of the proximal duodenum can often be observed fluoroscopically as these segments attempt to propel duodenal contents beyond the obstruction. Turning the patient into the left decubitus or prone position may reduce the compression on the duodenum, and contrast material can be observed to pass easily into the distal duodenum.

Other conditions causing dilatation of the proximal small bowel include primary or metastatic duodenal tumors (Case 211), pancreatitis (Case 201), pancreatic cancer (Case 220), Crohn's disease (Case 209), abdominal aortic aneurysms, and conditions causing decreased duodenal peristalsis such as scleroderma, dermatomyositis, systemic lupus erythematosus, and idiopathic intestinal pseudo-obstruction.

**Case 237**

## SUPERIOR MESENTERIC ARTERY SYNDROME: CT

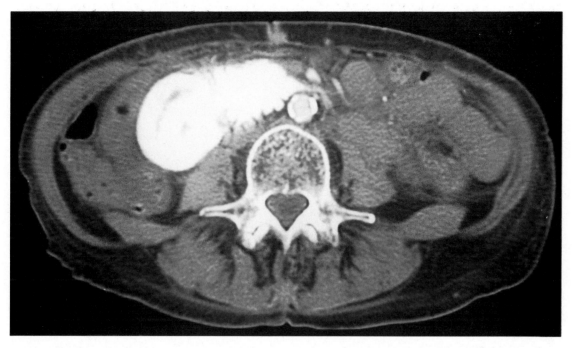

The proximal duodenum is dilated and tapers to a region of high-grade narrowing at the level of the superior mesenteric artery. No mass is present at the level of the duodenal stenosis. Findings are characteristic of the superior mesenteric artery syndrome.

## Case 238

# CYSTIC FIBROSIS

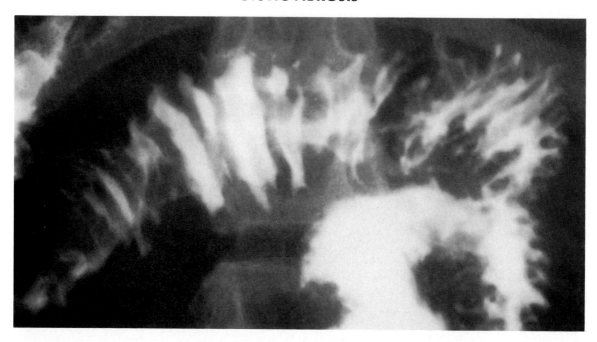

The folds of the transverse duodenum are thickened. This finding alone is nonspecific and could be secondary to any disease causing bowel-wall edema or intramural hemorrhage. This patient had known cystic fibrosis (mucoviscidosis).

Cystic fibrosis manifests in many ways, even within the gastrointestinal tract. Neonates may present with meconium ileus, and a similar syndrome may develop later in life ("meconium ileus equivalent") as a result of the thick colonic contents causing bowel obstruction. Nearly all patients have steatorrhea due to pancreatic exocrine insufficiency. The lack of normal alkaline pancreatic secretions can lead to hyperacidity in the postampullary duodenum, with secondary edematous and thickened folds (as in this case). Thick colonic con-

tents may present as fecal masses that can be mistaken for polyps or cancer and can even cause colonic intussusception. Biliary cirrhosis from long-standing biliary obstruction from mucous debris can also occur. Pancreatic findings include pancreatic calculi and occasional pancreatitis.

Radiologically, the duodenum and colon have findings that are most helpful in suggesting this diagnosis. A featureless, smudged proximal duodenum and thickened folds in the distal duodenum and proximal jejunum are commonly seen. Similar findings can also be seen in Zollinger-Ellison syndrome (Case 184). Hyperplastic-appearing colonic mucosa, best appreciated on post-evacuation films, can suggest the diagnosis and is often seen in older patients with cystic fibrosis.

## Case 239

## AORTOENTERIC FISTULA

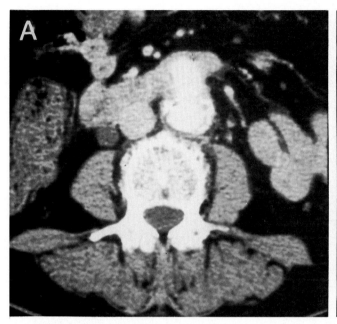
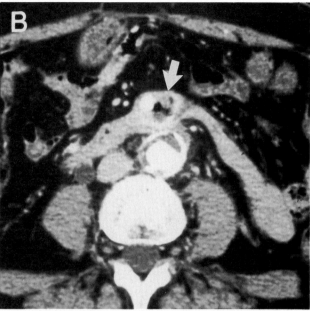

An end-to-side abdominal aortic graft is in place **(A)**, with fluid and gas *(arrow)* within its left limb **(B).** The duodenum is located immediately anterior to the calcified native aorta and graft. The normally visible fat plane between aorta/graft and duodenum is absent. This patient was experiencing gastrointestinal bleeding. Findings are compatible with an aortoenteric fistula. At operation, a 3 × 3-cm defect was present in the fourth portion of the duodenum. The graft was bile-stained and leaking blood into the duodenum.

An aortoenteric fistula is usually a complication of reconstructive aortic surgery after the placement of a prosthetic graft. Perigraft infection is nearly always present and fistulization is a potentially catastrophic complication of the infection. The clinical signs and symptoms of this disorder can be subtle; gastrointestinal bleeding is the most obvious manifestation. The commonest CT findings of aortoenteric fistula include an ectopic gas collection and focal bowel-wall thickening. The fat plane is usually lost between the aorta and the duodenum. The finding of perigraft soft tissue, fluid, or ectopic gas is worrisome for perigraft infection (Low et al., 1990). Although CT can be helpful in excluding this diagnosis, arteriography is often necessary if active gastrointestinal bleeding is occurring. Endoscopy can also be helpful in directly visualizing the duodenal ulcer.

## Case 240

# DUPLICATION (ENTEROGENOUS) CYST

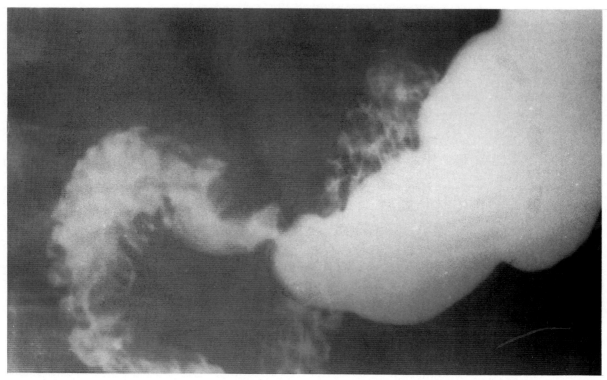

An extramucosal (smooth surfaced) mass indents the superior aspect of the duodenal bulb. Findings are nonspecific. Diagnostic considerations include a duplication cyst, lipoma, ectopic pancreatic rest, hemangioma, and carcinoid tumor. A duplication cyst was removed at operation.

Intestinal duplication occurs as a result of abnormal recanalization of the intestinal tract. Duplications can occur anywhere in the alimentary tract, but they are usually found in the esophagus or ileum. With cysts in the small bowel, patients usually present with symptoms of obstruction during late infancy or early childhood. Peptic ulceration and bleeding can occur when ectopic gastric mucosa is present.

Barium studies usually reveal an extrinsic mass causing narrowing or obstruction of the affected bowel loop. Rarely, communication with the adjacent bowel is seen. Compressibility and pliable shape with palpation and peristalsis are helpful findings that can suggest the diagnosis of either duplication cyst or lipoma. CT or sonography might be helpful in a suspected duplication cyst by identifying a well-defined cylindrical or spherical cystic mass the density of water adjacent to the bowel (Case 357). Treatment is operative resection.

| DIFFERENTIAL DIAGNOSES | CASE NUMBER |
|---|---|
| *FILLING DEFECTS* | |
| Malignant | |
|    Adenocarcinoma | 213 |
|    Leiomyosarcoma | 216 |
|    Lymphoma | 214, 215 |
|    Metastases | 217–219 |
| Benign | |
|    Pseudotumor | 179 |
|    Papilla of Vater | 180, 181 |
|    Prolapsed gastric mucosa | 227, 228 |
|    Polyp | 222, 223 |
|    Brunner's gland hyperplasia | 182, 183 |
|    Villous adenoma | 224 |
|    Leiomyoma | 216 |
|    Lipoma | 225 |
|    Annular pancreas | 235 |
|    Intraluminal duodenal diverticula | 230 |
|    Hematoma | 233 |
|    Edema surrounding a peptic ulcer | 186, 188, 198 |
| *NARROWING* | |
| Malignant | |
|    Adenocarcinoma | 211, 212 |
|    Leiomyosarcoma | 216 |
|    Lymphoma | 215 |
|    Metastases | 218, 220, 221 |
| Benign | |
|    Peptic ulcer disease | 188–190, 198, 199 |
|    Pancreatitis | 202, 203, 206 |
|    Crohn's disease | 208, 209 |
|    Hematoma | 233 |
|    Superior mesenteric artery syndrome | 236, 237 |
|    Annular pancreas | 235 |
| *THICKENED FOLDS* | |
| Peptic ulcer disease/Zollinger-Ellison syndrome | 184, 200 |
| Brunner's gland hyperplasia | 182 |
| Pancreatitis | 201, 202 |
| Giardiasis | 270 |
| Crohn's disease | 209 |
| Cystic fibrosis | 238 |
| Hematoma | 233 |
| Adult celiac disease | 210 |

## SELECTED READINGS

### Normal Anatomy and Variants

Bova JG, Kamath V, Tio FO, Peters JE Jr, Goldstein HM. The normal mucosal surface pattern of the duodenal bulb: radiologic-histologic correlation. *AJR* 1985;145:735–738

Burrell M, Toffler R. Flexural pseudolesions of the duodenum. *Radiology* 1976;120:313–315

*Ferrucci JT Jr, Benedict KT, Page DL, Fleischli DJ, Eaton SB. Radiographic features of the normal hypotonic duodenogram. *Radiology* 1970;96:401–408

*Glick SN, Gohel VK, Laufer I. Mucosal surface patterns of the duodenal bulb. *Radiology* 1984;150:317–322

Johansen AA, Hansen OH. Heterotopic gastric epithelium in the duodenum and its correlation to gastric disease and acid level. *Acta Pathol Microbiol Scand* 1973;81A:676–680

Langkemper R, Hoek AC, Dekker W, Op den Orth JO. Elevated lesions in the duodenal bulb caused by heterotopic gastric mucosa. *Radiology* 1980;137:621–624

Nelson JA, Sheft DJ, Minagi H, Ferrucci JT Jr. Duodenal pseudopolyp—the flexure fallacy. *Am J Roentgenol* 1975;123:262–267

Op den Orth JO. Radiologic visualization of the normal duodenal minor papilla. *Fortschr Geb Röntgenstr Nuklearmed* 1978;128:572–576

*Shousha S, Spiller RC, Parkins RA. The endoscopically abnormal duodenum in patients with dyspepsia: biopsy findings in 60 cases. *Histopathology* 1983;7:23–34

*Smithuis RHM, Vos CG. Heterotopic gastric mucosa in the duodenal bulb: relationship to peptic ulcer. *AJR* 1989;152:59–61

Stevenson GW, Laufer I. Duodenum. In: Laufer I, ed. *Double contrast gastrointestinal radiology with endoscopic correlation.* Philadelphia: WB Saunders, 1979:331–371

Stevenson GW, Somers S, Virjee J. Routine double-contrast barium meal: appearance of normal duodenal papillae. *Diagn Imaging* 1980;49:6–14

### Inflammation: Peptic Disease

Bilbao MK, Frische LH, Rösch J, Benson JA Jr, Dotter CT. Postbulbar duodenal ulcer and ring-stricture. *Radiology* 1971;100:27–35

*Braver JM, Paul RE Jr, Philipps E, Bloom S. Roentgen diagnosis of linear ulcers. *Radiology* 1979;132:29–32

*Bryant LR, Wiot JF, Kloecker RJ. A study of the factors affecting the incidence and duration of postoperative pneumoperitoneum. *Surg Gynecol Obstet* 1963;117:145–150

*Classen M. Endoscopy in benign peptic ulcer. *Clin Gastroenterol* 1973 May;2:315–327

de Roos A, Op den Orth JO. Linear niches in the duodenal bulb. *AJR* 1983;140:941–944

*Edwards RH, Foster JH. Pneumoperitoneum in perforated duodenal ulcer. *Am J Surg* 1962;104:551–554

Eisenberg RL, Margulis AR, Moss AA. Giant duodenal ulcers. *Gastrointest Radiol* 1978;2:347–353

*Ellison EH, Wilson SD. The Zollinger-Ellison syndrome: re-appraisal and evaluation of 260 registered cases. *Ann Surg* 1964;160:512–528

Fraser GM, Pitman RG, Lawrie JH, Smith GMR. The significance of the radiological finding of coarse mucosal folds in the duodenum. *Lancet* 1964;2:979–982

Gelfand DW, Dale WJ, Ott DJ, et al. Duodenitis: endoscopic-radiologic correlation in 272 patients. *Radiology* 1985;157:577–581

*Jones B, Bayless TM, Hamilton SR, Yardley JH. "Bubbly" duodenal bulb in celiac disease: radiologic-pathologic correlation. *AJR* 1984;142:119–122

Lambert R, Mainguet P, Moulinier B. Endoscopy in the management of duodenal ulcer. *Digestion* 1978;18:110–124

Laufer I, Trueman T, deSa D. Multiple superficial gastric erosions due to Crohn's disease of the stomach: radiologic and endoscopic diagnosis. *Br J Radiol* 1976;49:726–728

Legge DA, Carlson HC, Judd ES. Roentgenologic features of regional enteritis of the upper gastrointestinal tract. *Am J Roentgenol* 1970;110:355–360

*Lumsden K, MacLarnon JC, Dawson J. Giant duodenal ulcer. *Gut* 1970;11:592–599

Menuck L, Siemers PT. Pneumoperitoneum: importance of right upper quadrant features. *Am J Roentgenol* 1976;127:753–756

Miller RE. The radiological evaluation of intraperitoneal gas (pneumoperitoneum). *CRC Crit Rev Clin Radiol Nucl Med* 1973;4:61–85

Nelson SW. Some interesting and unusual manifestations of Crohn's disease ("regional enteritis") of the stomach, duodenum and small intestine. *Am J Roentgenol* 1969;107:86–101

Rice RP. Radiologic evaluation of acute abdomen. *CRC Crit Rev Clin Radiol Nucl Med* 1974;4:555–597

*Cited in text.

Rice RP, Thompson WM, Gedgaudas RK. The diagnosis and significance of extraluminal gas in the abdomen. *Radiol Clin North Am* **1982** Dec;20:819–837

Rigler LG. Spontaneous pneumoperitoneum: a roentgenologic sign found in the supine position. *Radiology* **1941**;37:604–607

*Rodriguez HP, Aston JK, Richardson CT. Ulcers in the descending duodenum: postbulbar ulcers. *Am J Roentgenol* **1973**;119:316–322

Schulman A. The cobblestone appearance of the duodenal cap, duodenitis and hyperplasia of Brunner's glands. *Br J Radiol* **1970**;43:787–795

Tallman JM, Clements JL Jr, Gilliam JH III, Weens HS. The multi-channelled pylorus. *Clin Radiol* **1979**;30:337–341

Thompson WM. Duodenal ulcer. In: Taveras JM, Ferrucci JT, eds. *Radiology: diagnosis—imaging—intervention*, vol 4. Philadelphia: JB Lippincott, **1986**:chap 24, 1–8

Thompson WM, Cockrill H Jr, Rice RP. Regional enteritis of the duodenum. *Am J Roentgenol* **1975**;123:252–261

Thompson WM, Kelvin FM, Gedgaudas RK, Rice RP. Radiologic investigation of peptic ulcer disease. *Radiol Clin North Am* **1982** Dec; 20:701–720

Weinberg PE, Levin B. Hyperplasia of Brunner's glands. *Radiology* **1965**;84:259–262

### Neoplasm: Malignant

Balikkian JP, Nassar NT, Shamma'a MH, Shahid MJ. Primary lymphomas of the small intestine including the duodenum: a roentgen analysis of twenty-nine cases. *Am J Roentgenol* **1969**; 107:131–141

Blumgart LH, Kennedy A. Carcinoma of the ampulla of Vater and duodenum. *Br J Surg* **1973**; 60:33–40

Bosse G, Neely JA. Roentgenologic findings in primary malignant tumors of the duodenum: report of 27 cases. *Am J Roentgenol* **1969**;107: 111–118

Dudiak KM, Johnson CD, Stephens DH. Primary tumors of the small intestine: CT evaluation. *AJR* **1989**;152:995–998

Eyler WR, Clark MD, Rian RL. An evaluation of roentgen signs of pancreatic enlargement. *JAMA* **1962**;181:967–971

Freeny PC, Lawson TL. *Radiology of the pancreas.* New York: Springer-Verlag, **1982**:404–407

Frostberg N. A characteristic duodenal deformity in cases of different kinds of peri-vaterial enlarge-

ment of the pancreas. *Acta Radiol* **1938**; 19:164–173

Good CA. Tumors of the small intestine: Caldwell Lecture, 1962. *Am J Roentgenol* **1963**; 89:685–705

Margulis AR. Neoplasms of the pancreas. In: Margulis AR, Burhenne HJ, eds. *Alimentary tract roentgenology*, 2nd ed, vol 2. St. Louis: CV Mosby, **1973**:1154–1181

Olurin EO, Solanke TF. Case of leiomyosarcoma of the duodenum and a review of the literature. *Gut* **1968**;9:672–677

Op den Orth JO. Hypotonic duodenography without the use of a stomach tube. *Radiol Clin Biol* **1973**;42:173–174

Starr GF, Dockerty MB. Leiomyomas and leiomyosarcomas of the small intestine. *Cancer* **1955**;8:101–111

Veen HF, Oscarson JEA, Malt RA. Alien cancers of the duodenum. *Surg Gynecol Obstet* **1976**; 143:39–42

Ziter FMH Jr. Roentgenographic findings in Gardner's syndrome. *JAMA* **1965**;192:1000–1002

### Neoplasm: Benign

Charles RN, Kelley ML Jr, Campeti F. Primary duodenal tumors: a study of 31 cases. *Arch Intern Med* **1963**;111:23–33

Dodds WJ, Lydon SB. Intestinal polyposis syndromes. *CRC Crit Rev Clin Radiol Nucl Med* **1974**;5:295–336

*Feczko PJ. Incidental filling defects (polyps) in the stomach. In: Thompson WM, ed. *Common problems in gastrointestinal radiology.* Chicago: Year Book Medical Publishers, **1989**:183–190

Ring EJ, Ferrucci JT Jr, Eaton SB Jr, Clements JL. Villous adenomas of the duodenum. *Radiology* **1972**;104:45–48

Ushio K, Sasagawa M, Doi H, et al. Lesions associated with familial polyposis coli: studies of lesions of the stomach, duodenum, bones and teeth. *Gastrointest Radiol* **1976**;1:67–80

### Miscellaneous

Anderson JR, Earnshaw PM, Fraser GM. Extrinsic compression of the third part of the duodenum. *Clin Radiol* **1982**;33:75–81

*Balthazar EJ, Einhorn R. Intramural gastrointestinal hemorrhage: clinical and radiographic manifestations. *Gastrointest Radiol* **1976**;1:229–239

Berk RN, Lee FA. The late gastrointestinal manifestations of cystic fibrosis of the pancreas. *Radiology* **1973**;106:377–381

*Blumhagen JD, Maclin L, Krauter D, Rosenbaum

DM, Weinberger E. Sonographic diagnosis of hypertrophic pyloric stenosis. *AJR* **1988**;150: 1367–1370

*Bremner CG. The lesser curve pyloric niche. *Br J Radiol* **1968**;41:291–295

Clifford KMA. Annular pancreas diagnosed by endoscopic retrograde-choledocho-pancreatography (ERCP). *Br J Radiol* **1980**;53:593–595

Cook DE, Walsh JW, Vick CW, Brewer WH. Upper abdominal trauma: pitfalls in CT diagnosis. *Radiology* **1986**;159:65–69

Glazer GM, Buy JN, Moss AA, Goldberg HI, Federle MP. CT detection of duodenal perforation. *AJR* **1981**;137:333–336

Johnson M. Prolapsing gastric mucosa: a review of 117 cases in a private practice. *J Med Assoc Ga* **1952**;41:439–455

*Kiernan PD, ReMine SG, Kiernan PC, ReMine WH. Annular pancreas: Mayo Clinic experience from 1957 to 1976 with review of the literature. *Arch Surg* **1980**;115:46–50

Laudan JCH, Norton GI. Intraluminal duodenal diverticulum. *Am J Roentgenol* **1963**;90:756–760

*Levin EJ, Felson B. Asymptomatic gastric mucosal prolapse. *Radiology* **1951**;57:514–520

*Low RN, Wall SD, Jeffrey RB Jr, Sollitto RA, Reilly LM, Tierney LM Jr. Aortoenteric fistula and perigraft infection: evaluation with CT. *Radiology* **1990**;175:157–162

Mark SM, Moss AA, McCarthy S, McCowin M. CT of aortoenteric fistulas. *Invest Radiol* **1985**;20: 272–275

*Nosher JL, Seaman WB. Association of intraluminal duodenal diverticulum with acute pancreatitis. *Radiology* **1975**;115:21–22

*Roman E, Silva YJ, Lucas C. Management of blunt duodenal injury. *Surg Gynecol Obstet* **1971**; 132:7–14

Taussig LM, Saldino RM, di Sant'Agnese PA. Radiographic abnormalities of the duodenum and small bowel in cystic fibrosis of the pancreas (mucoviscidosis). *Radiology* **1973**;106:369–376

*Toxopeus MD, Lucas CE, Krabbenhoft KL. Roentgenographic diagnosis in blunt retroperitoneal duodenal rupture. *Am J Roentgenol* **1972**; 115: 281–288

Wallace RG, Howard WB. Acute superior mesenteric artery syndrome in the severely burned patient. *Radiology* **1970**;94:307–310

Wiot JF. Intramural small intestinal hemorrhage—a differential diagnosis. *Semin Roentgenol* **1966**; 1:219–233

# Small Bowel

## Case 241

## NORMAL SMALL BOWEL: CONVENTIONAL SMALL BOWEL
## FOLLOW-THROUGH EXAMINATION

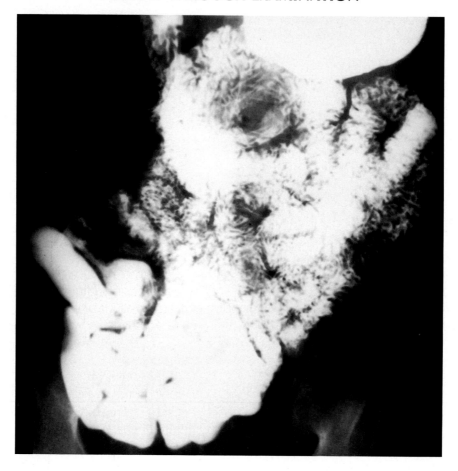

The normal mucosal fold pattern can be seen in the jejunum and ileum. The jejunum has a textured coarse pattern with numerous visible small-bowel folds resembling crinkled tissue paper. The ileum is relatively featureless as a result of fewer valvulae conniventes (folds). The diameter of the small bowel usually measures less than 3 cm, with individual mucosal folds ≤3 mm.

There are several helpful techniques that can be used in examining the small bowel. The method we use most often incorporates examination of the upper gastrointestinal tract and repeat fluoroscopic examination of the small bowel using manual graded compression in multiple oblique projections every 15 to 20 minutes. A posteroanterior overhead film is usually taken after each fluoroscopic examination to document the progress of the barium mixture through the small bowel. After the colon is visualized and the entire small bowel is carefully examined fluoroscopically, two or three overhead films are obtained. A posteroanterior film and both oblique views (right posterior oblique and left posterior oblique) are often useful.

Normal transit time through the small bowel varies widely from 30 minutes to several hours. Unduly slow transit times in otherwise normal individuals can be seen in patients taking narcotics, those with severe pain at the time of the examination, patients with a large amount of retained stool in the colon, and patients recovering from an ileus or bedridden for some time. In the absence of suspected obstruction, orally or intravenously administered metoclopramide (10 mg) can be used to stimulate peristalsis and accelerate transit

through the small bowel. Some radiologists regularly use small amounts of meglumine diatrizoate in the barium mixture to accelerate transit time.

Caution should be exercised in administering barium to patients with a suspected small-bowel obstruction. It is possible for a right-sided colon obstruction to masquerade on an abdominal plain film examination as a mechanical small-bowel obstruction. Barium does not inspissate in the small bowel, but in the colon (particularly proximal to a colonic obstruction) a rock-hard concretion of barium can develop, requiring and complicating surgical removal. In patients with a suspected distal mechanical small-bowel obstruction, many experts recommend excluding a colonic obstruction first by performing a barium enema before the barium meal (small bowel follow through) is given. In many patients contrast material can be refluxed from the colon into the distal small bowel, and a mechanical obstruction can be confirmed. Water-soluble contrast material is hypertonic and rapidly diluted as water is pulled into the small-bowel lumen. Despite difficulties with dilution and mucosal coating, water-soluble agents can be useful in patients who are likely to undergo operation and in whom a proximal small-bowel lesion is suspected. The distal small bowel is usually poorly seen unless a small-bowel decompression tube is positioned in the proximal to mid small bowel. These tubes can be used to instill the contrast material and often a diagnostic study can be done. Hypertonic water-soluble agents should be used with caution in children because of potential problems of hypovolemia and shock.

Case 242

# NORMAL SMALL BOWEL: ENTEROCLYSIS EXAMINATION

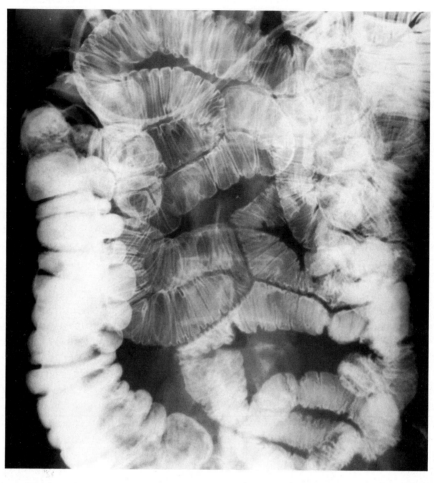

Some experts recommend the routine use of the enteroclysis examination (small-bowel enema) for all patients. We utilize this method of examination in selected patients: those with a suspected partial mechanical obstruction of the small bowel, those with documented gastrointestinal blood loss with negative endoscopic or barium studies of the upper and lower alimentary tract, and those patients in whom clinicians suspect there may be a small-bowel lesion but the conventional small-bowel examination was negative or of suboptimal quality (i.e., multiple overlapping small-bowel loops in the pelvis that were difficult to examine).

The enteroclysis technique is described well in several articles and textbooks (Herlinger, 1978). Generally, a gastrointestinal tube is placed with its tip near the duodenojejunal flexure. Well-suspended barium with excellent coating properties is injected through the tube at a constant rate. After opacification of the small bowel (usually 300 mL of barium is used), a dilute solution of methyl-cellulose is injected to provide a double-contrast effect. Radiographs are taken with the patient in various positions and at an appropriate interval when the bowel is well coated, distended, and ideally translucent.

**Case 243**

## NORMAL SMALL BOWEL

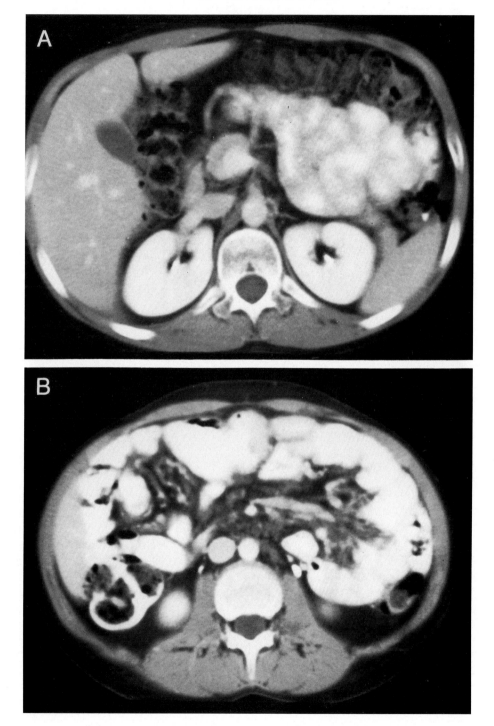

**A.** The normal textured appearance of the jejunum is seen on this CT scan.

**B.** The featureless appearance of the normal ileum is displayed well.

## Case 244

# APPROACH TO DIFFUSE SMALL-BOWEL DISEASE

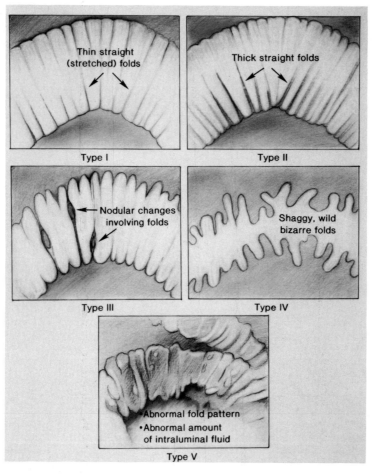

Diffuse disease of the small bowel is often confusing to students. The reasons for this are probably the infrequency with which many of these rare disorders are encountered in everyday clinical practice and a relatively nonspecific radiographic appearance that many of these diffuse diseases exhibit. The following approach and lists of differential diagnoses are borrowed in part from notes obtained at a workshop given by Sidney Nelson, M.D., a distinguished, pioneering gastrointestinal radiologist who, among many other accomplishments, is a marvelous teacher.

If a disease diffusely affects the small bowel, changes will often occur within the wall of the bowel and alter the normal fold pattern. Analysis of the fold pattern can be helpful in understanding that underlying pathologic condition and in developing a reasonable differential diagnosis. Unfortunately, this classification is somewhat arbitrary, because some diseases may have findings that overlap between designated fold types or a disease may present with different fold patterns in different patients. Despite its limitations, this approach may be helpful to the student beginning a study of the small bowel.

**Case 245**

# TYPE I FOLDS (THIN AND STRAIGHT, WITH A DILATED LUMEN)

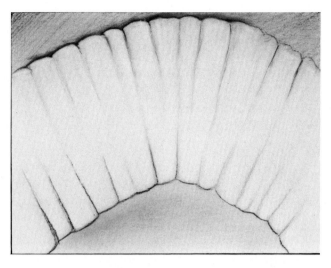

1. Mechanical obstruction (Case 246)
2. Paralytic ileus

3. Scleroderma (Case 250)
4. Sprue (Cases 287–289)

Case 246

# MECHANICAL SMALL-BOWEL OBSTRUCTION

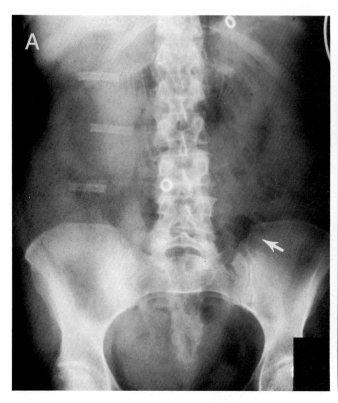
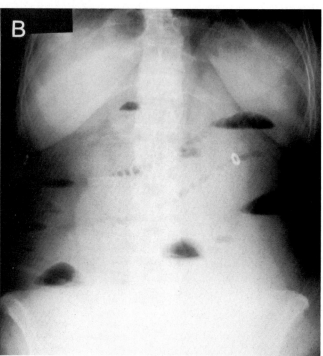

**A.** In this supine abdominal radiograph, multiple, dilated, partially gas-filled small bowel loops are present with no visible gas in the colon. The valvulae conniventes *(arrow)* are thin and straight (type I fold pattern).

**B.** In this upright abdominal radiograph, multiple air-filled levels are seen throughout the small bowel. Many small collections of gas line up within a small-bowel loop and resemble "a string of beads." These are typical findings of a mechanical small-bowel obstruction.

Partial or complete mechanical small-bowel obstruction is a common disease entity that usually manifests clinically with nausea, vomiting, cramping abdominal pain, and distension. The common causes of mechanical obstruction of the small bowel are adhesions (from a prior abdominal surgical procedure or severe intraperitoneal inflammation) (Cases 247 and 248) or hernias (Case 249). Other less frequent causes include an obstructing neoplasm (Cases 327 and 328), intussusception (Cases 290 and 334), stricture (from Crohn's disease [Case 293], prior ischemia, or idiopathic), or volvulus (Cases 348 and 349).

Radiologic evaluation often begins with an abdominal plain film examination. Dilated small-bowel loops are often seen containing air-fluid levels on the film taken in the upright position. It may be difficult to judge the level of obstruction on an abdominal plain film examination; in fact, a proximal colonic obstruction can masquerade as a mechanical small-bowel obstruction radiographically.

**Case 247**

## MECHANICAL SMALL-BOWEL OBSTRUCTION: ADHESIONS

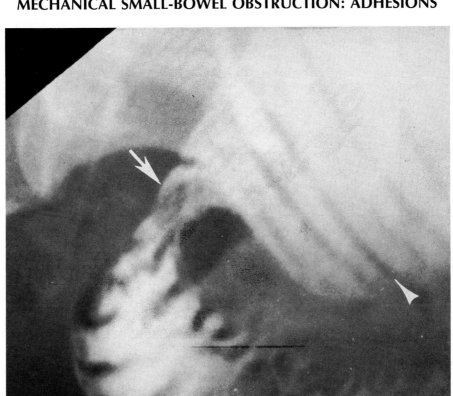

The proximal small bowel is dilated and abruptly narrows from a smooth rounded defect *(arrow)* that eccentrically compresses the lumen and causes partial obstruction. The short and smooth appearance of the defect is characteristic of an adhesion. Notice the straight thin folds in the dilated loop *(arrowhead)*.

Defining the level and cause of obstruction often requires an intraluminal contrast study. A colon examination is often a helpful initial study to exclude a colonic lesion. Usually contrast material can be refluxed into the distal small bowel. The finding of a normal caliber in the distal small bowel and dilated proximal loops confirms the diagnosis of a mechanical small-bowel obstruction. Sometimes the cause of a distal obstruction may be identified (as in this case), but often a conventional small-bowel examination is unsuccessful in elucidating the exact site and cause of obstruction. Some authors think that the enteroclysis examination is more helpful in detecting the site and cause of both partial and complete small-bowel obstructions (Caroline et al., 1984). This technique causes more dilatation of the proximal small bowel than does a conventional small-bowel examination. As a result, a transition point between dilated and normal caliber loops may be more easily detected and indicate the site of the abnormality.

Some adhesive bands will cause more distortion of the small-bowel folds than is seen in this case. The loops may appear angulated and fixed or tethered to either the abdominal wall or another small-bowel loop. Multiple sites of involvement are common but usually produce less severe obstruction and a lower incidence of strangulation than is found with a single adhesive band. Fluoroscopic observation is often helpful because proximal dilatation may be present only transiently and can be missed on overhead radiographs.

**Case 248**

## SMALL-BOWEL OBSTRUCTION: ADHESION

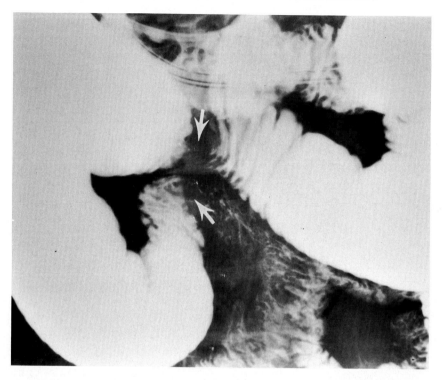

Two short segmental areas of small-bowel narrowing *(arrows)* are present. The focal, smooth, and eccentric appearance of the stricture is consistent with an adhesive band. The proximity of the two affected loops suggests one adhesion that has trapped both bowel loops. The small bowel is dilated to the level of the adhesions, indicating significant obstruction.

**Case 249**

# MECHANICAL SMALL-BOWEL OBSTRUCTION: INGUINAL HERNIA

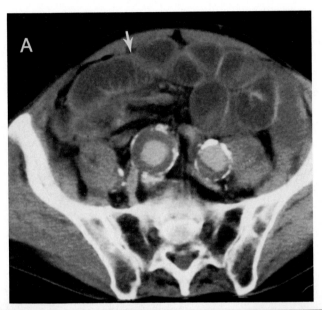

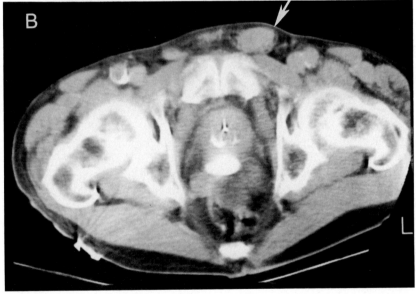

**A.** Multiple, dilated, fluid-filled small-bowel loops are present in the abdomen. Aneurysmal dilatation of both iliac arteries is also seen. Notice the thin, straight small-bowel folds *(arrow)*.

**B.** A loop of small bowel could be traced into the enlarged left inguinal canal *(arrow)* at the site of the obstruction. An incarcerated hernia was repaired surgically.

CT has not been widely used as a primary imaging modality for evaluating patients with a suspected small-bowel obstruction. A recent study confirmed that CT can be used to reliably diagnose intestinal obstruction. In nearly three-quarters of the patients, the cause of the obstruction was identified (Megibow et al., 1991). The diagnosis of mechanical intestinal obstruction should be suspected when a discrepancy in the caliber of the proximal and distal bowel is identified.

## Case 250

## SCLERODERMA

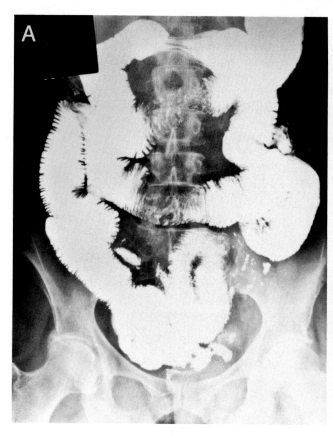
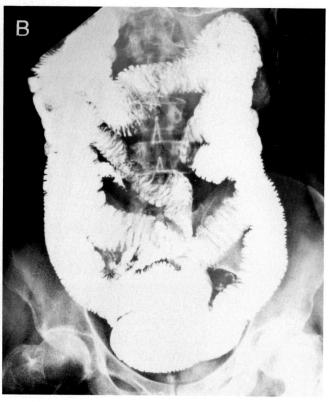

**A** and **B.** Multiple, dilated small-bowel loops are present. The valvulae conniventes are thin and straight (type I folds) and closely stacked together; they have the typical "hidebound" appearance of scleroderma.

Small-bowel changes of scleroderma usually occur relatively late in the course of the disease, usually after the typical skin changes, Raynaud's phenomenon, or arthropathy. Pathologically, atrophy of the mucosa and submucosa is seen, with submucosal fibrosis and round cell infiltration. Mesenteric vascular arteritis may be present.

Radiologically, the small bowel demonstrates delayed transit time, dilatation, and crowding together of the straight and thin mucosal folds. This is referred to as the "hidebound" appearance. Sacculations may be seen on the antimesenteric borders. Pneumatosis cystoides intestinalis can also be seen. It is possible that this latter complication is related to the frequent use of steroid agents among these patients.

Distinguishing scleroderma from sprue is usually easy because there is no hypersecretion in scleroderma and patients with sprue usually have normal small-bowel motility. In mechanical obstruction, the small bowel usually has more peristaltic activity observable at fluoroscopy and may have a considerable amount of retained fluid proximal to the obstruction. Esophageal changes can also be observed in patients with scleroderma (Cases 63 and 64).

## Case 251

# TYPE II FOLDS (THICK, >3 MM, STRAIGHT FOLDS)

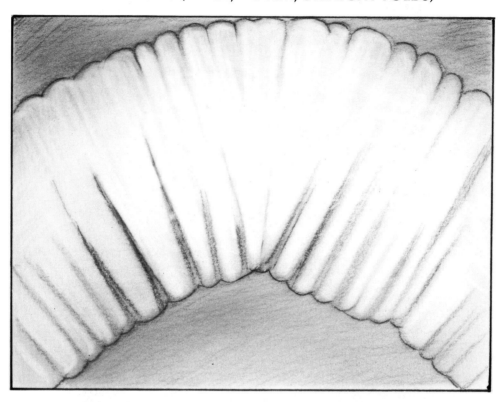

1. Edema
   A. Inflammation
      1) Zollinger-Ellison syndrome (Cases 105 and 200)
      2) Crohn's disease (Case 295)
      3) Radiation enteritis (Cases 252–254)
      4) Giardiasis (Case 270)
   B. Hypoproteinemia (serum albumin level below 2 g/dL) (Cases 283 and 284)
   C. Venous congestion (congestive heart failure)
   D. Proximal to mechanical obstruction (subacute or chronic obstruction) (Cases 246–249)

2. Intramural hemorrhage
   A. Vascular occlusions (both venous and arterial) (Cases 255, 256, 261, and 319)
   B. Hemorrhagic diatheses, including anticoagulant agents (Case 233)
3. Submucosal infiltrates
   A. Whipple's disease (Case 272)
   B. Amyloidosis (Cases 268 and 269)
   C. Eosinophilic gastroenteritis (Case 267)
   D. Lymphoma (Case 271)

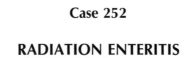

## Case 252

## RADIATION ENTERITIS

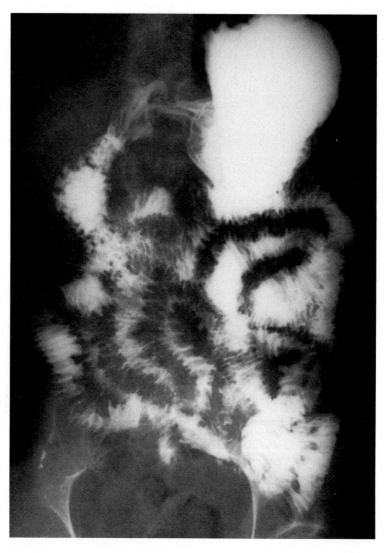

The small bowel has diffusely thickened folds with separation of the loops. This finding is nonspecific (type II fold pattern) but is consistent with acute changes of radiation enteritis.

The small bowel is the portion of the alimentary tract most sensitive to radiation. Usually doses greater than 40 Gy (4,000 rad) are required before radiographic changes occur. Endarteritis obliterans is the underlying pathologic process responsible for the bowel changes. Acute changes can be seen several weeks to a few months after treatment. Fold thickening and serration due to edema are often seen. The affected folds may appear fixed and angulated.

Chronic changes can be seen 6 months after therapy and may develop many years later. These changes are usually due to bowel ischemia from arteriolar damage. Intestinal loops are often narrowed, separated, and straightened and the bowel wall is thickened. Nodularity and thumbprinting may be observed. These changes may become progressively more severe with stenosis, obstruction, perforation, and fistulization. The majority of patients with chronic changes present with obstruction from an adhesion or stenosis rather than from acute ischemia.

## Case 253

# RADIATION ENTERITIS

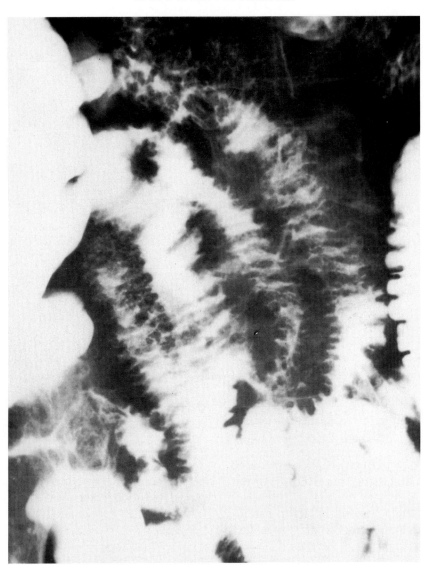

Several distal small-bowel loops are narrowed, with thickened folds and loops that are separated from one another. These findings are consistent with radiation enteritis.

The usual findings in patients with radiation enteritis are fold thickening and bowel-wall thickening (as seen in this case). This is a nonspecific finding and could be seen in ischemia (Case 255), Crohn's disease (Case 295), neoplastic infiltration (lymphoma) (Case 271), intramural hemorrhage (Case 233), or serosal metastases (Case 340).

## Case 254

# RADIATION ENTERITIS

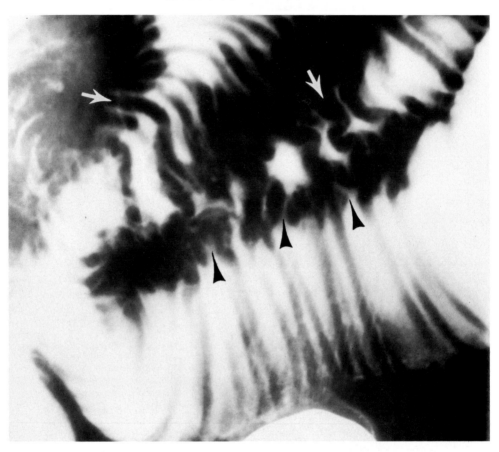

Two angulated loops of small bowel are present with thickening *(arrows)* and "tacking" *(arrowheads)* of the mucosal folds.

Small-bowel obstruction secondary to radiation-induced strictures or adhesions is common and often multiple. The mucosa in the region of a stricture is usually abnormal, with either thickened or absent folds. Angulated loops fixed within the pelvis due to adhesions are often encountered (as in this case).

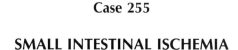

Case 255

# SMALL INTESTINAL ISCHEMIA

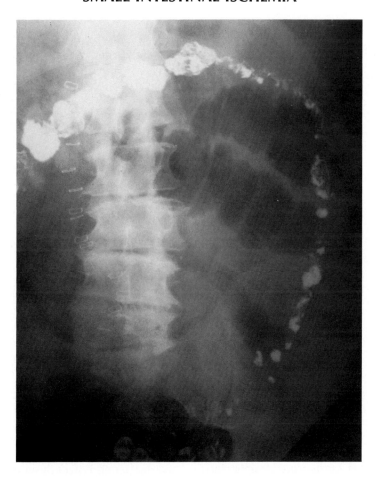

Two small-bowel loops in the left upper abdomen are dilated and contain straight and thickened folds. This finding is nonspecific, but ischemic bowel disease is the most important consideration. At operation, ischemic bowel loops were removed. Residual barium is seen in the colon.

Ischemia of the small bowel and colon remains a difficult diagnosis because of the variable and nonspecific clinical findings. Patients may complain of bloating, gas, nausea, or vomiting. Peritoneal signs usually indicate transmural necrosis and possibly perforation. However, this is generally a late and infrequent finding. Gastrointestinal blood loss may be present.

The pathologic findings depend on the extent and duration of ischemia. Ischemia may be due to arterial embolization, hypoperfusion, or venous thrombosis. Arterial hypoperfusion is believed to be the most frequent cause, often due to either congestive heart failure or prolonged hypotension in association with mesenteric atherosclerotic disease. Histologic findings of bowel ischemia within the first 24 hours include initial submucosal edema and intramural hemorrhage, followed by transmural ischemia, and eventually necrosis. Depending on the severity and depth of bowel-wall injury from the ischemic insult, the three possible results of bowel ischemia are complete healing, stricture formation, and perforation.

Radiologic findings depend on the timing of the examination in relation to the vascular insult. Acutely, most patients will have only an abdominal plain film examination. Many of these studies (up to half) may be normal or have findings of only adynamic ileus (Smerud et al., 1990). Suggestive findings include an isolated, rigid, often dilated and unchanging small-bowel loop with thickened mucosal folds.

**Case 256**

## SMALL-BOWEL ISCHEMIA: PNEUMATOSIS

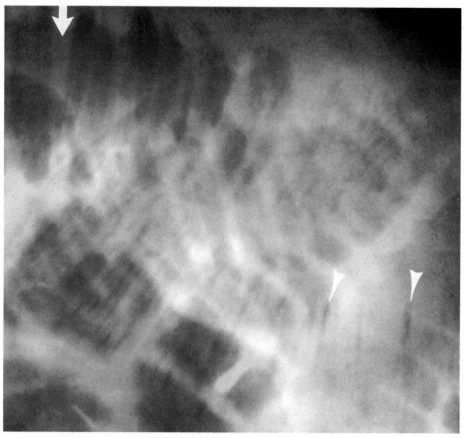

Multiple small-bowel folds *(arrow)* are straight and thickened. In addition, linear intramural pneumatosis *(arrowheads)* is present. At operation, infarcted bowel was resected.

The finding of intramural pneumatosis in a patient with ischemic bowel disease suggests severe ischemia. Urgent operation is usually required to prevent perforation and to decrease the high morbidity and mortality associated with such a complication.

## Case 257

## ISCHEMIA: PNEUMATOSIS INTESTINALIS

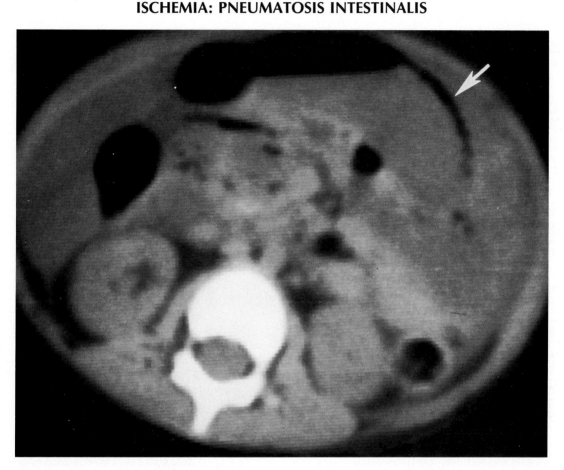

A linear collection of intramural gas *(arrow)* is present within a dilated, fluid-filled small-bowel loop. Infarcted bowel was surgically removed.

The appearance of intramural gas on CT can be either cystic (Case 258) or linear/curvilinear (as seen in this case). CT is more sensitive than abdominal plain films in detecting pneumatosis intestinalis (Kelvin et al.,

*From Smerud MJ, Johnson CD, Stephens DH. AJR*
***1990;**154:99–103. By permission of the American Roentgen Ray Society.*

1984). In addition, other signs of ischemic bowel can be searched for, including portal venous gas (Cases 264 and 265), bowel-wall thickening (Case 262), and patency of the superior mesenteric artery and vein. If a patient with abdominal pain is found to have pneumatosis, it is most important to review the radiologic and clinical findings with the referring physician because of the possibility of bowel ischemia. In some patients, lung window settings are helpful for detecting intramural air at CT.

## Case 258

## ISCHEMIA: PNEUMATOSIS INTESTINALIS

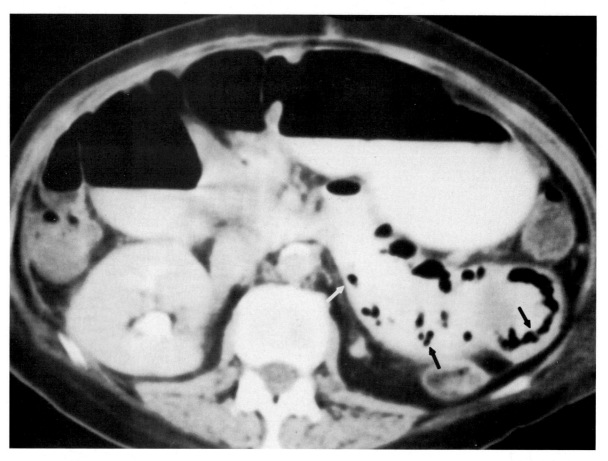

A dilated, contrast-filled small-bowel loop contains multiple, tiny intramural collections of gas *(arrows)*. Notice how intramural gas is most easily identified within the bowel wall by its posterior, dependent location. Ischemic bowel was removed surgically.

Pneumatosis is also usually present within the nondependent wall, but it is sometimes more difficult to distinguish from intraluminal gas.

## Case 259

## JEJUNAL PNEUMATOSIS: INFARCTION

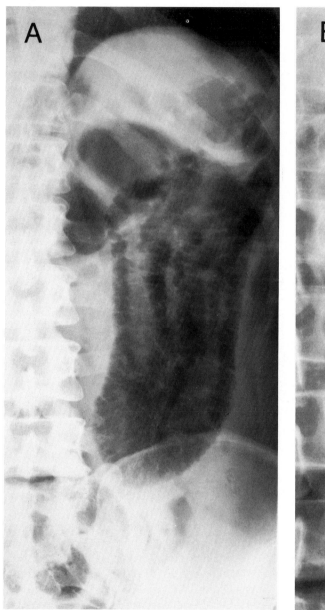

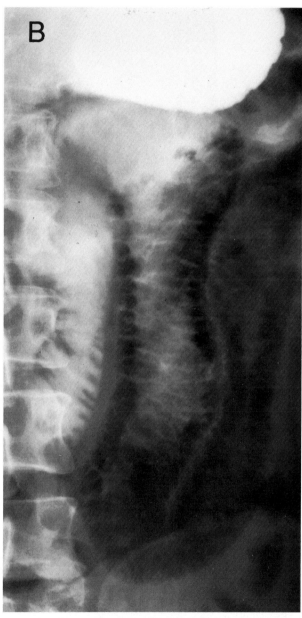

**A.** Extensive cystic pneumatosis is present within the jejunum. These loops were infarcted at the time of operation.

**B.** Intraluminal contrast material is helpful in confirming the intramural location of the gas.

Pneumatosis intestinalis secondary to ischemic or infarcted bowel can have either a cystic or a linear ap-

pearance. Large cystic collections, as seen in this case, are unusual and more commonly associated with nonischemic disease. Clinical correlation is always necessary when pneumatosis intestinalis is encountered so as not to delay treatment or overlook the diagnosis of bowel ischemia.

**Case 260**

## PNEUMATOSIS INTESTINALIS: ISCHEMIA

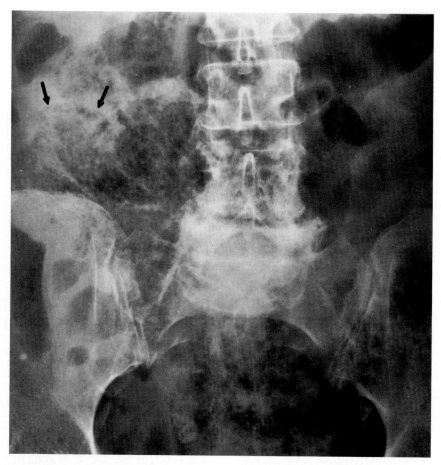

A mottled collection of gas is present in the region of the small bowel. Many of the lucencies resemble tiny cystic gas collections. These lucencies can be identified within the bowel wall *(arrows)*. This patient had abdominal pain and diarrhea. Occlusion of the superior and inferior mesenteric arteries as well as a high-grade stenosis of the celiac trunk was found at arteriography.

Pneumatosis intestinalis can vary in appearance and cause. Intramural gas may appear as small or large cystic lucencies or as linear collections. The cause of intramural gas is usually uncertain on the basis of the radiographic findings, unless large cystic (grape-like) collections are identified. This form of pneumatosis is invariably benign and is usually encountered in the distal colon. Ischemia (as in this case) is the most dreaded cause of pneumatosis. Associated findings of intestinal fold thickening (Cases 255, 256, and 261) or portal venous gas (Cases 264 and 265), or both, are not always present, but when they are discovered this should strongly suggest underlying bowel ischemia.

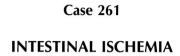

Case 261

# INTESTINAL ISCHEMIA

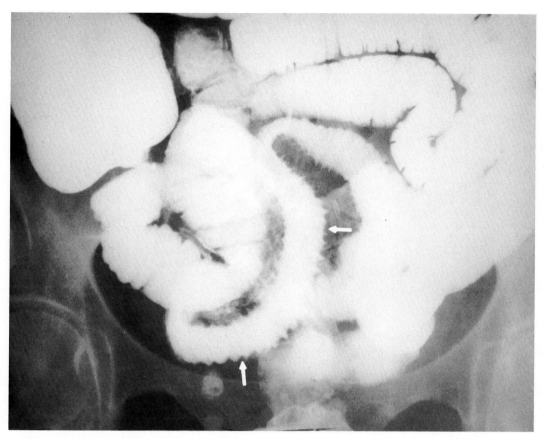

A loop of abnormal distal small bowel is seen in the pelvis. The lumen is slightly narrowed and the folds *(arrows)* and bowel wall are thickened. Diagnostic considerations include: ischemia, Crohn's disease, lymphoma, radiation enteritis, and adjacent inflammatory processes (e.g., appendiceal or pelvic abscess). Infarcted small bowel was surgically removed.

Contrast studies of the small bowel are usually used in evaluating subacute or chronic changes of intestinal ischemia. Subacute changes often involve a segmental region of fold thickening and bowel-wall thickening ("stacked coins" appearance) (as seen in this case and in Case 319). Hemorrhage and intramural edema may cause thumbprinting, luminal narrowing, and blurring of folds. Chronic stricture formation is unusual, but when present it may appear as a focal concentric region of luminal narrowing, often without a recognizable fold pattern. Strictures may vary in length.

## Case 262

## ISCHEMIA: CT

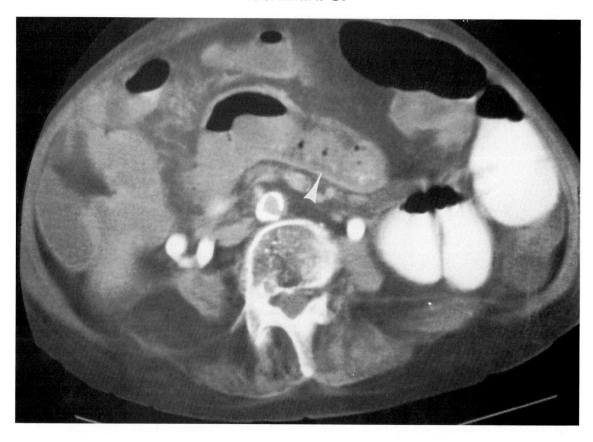

Dilated small-bowel loops are present in the abdomen. The loop in the central portion of the abdomen has thickened walls. A portion of the thickened wall is of low density, near that of water *(arrowhead)*, indicating submucosal edema. An ischemic small-bowel loop was removed at operation.

CT findings in patients with bowel infarction include diffuse or focal bowel-wall thickening, segmental dilatation, mesenteric edema, ascites, intramural gas, and mesenteric or portal venous gas. Only intramural and venous gas are considered specific for ischemia, but even these findings can occasionally be seen in patients without bowel infarction. Edema within the bowel wall is nonspecific and could be secondary to any inflammatory disease within the bowel or adjacent mesentery or to hypoalbuminemia. Despite its nonspecific nature, bowel dilatation with a thickened and edematous wall without apparent cause in a patient with abdominal pain should be regarded as highly suggestive of ischemia.

Case 263

## ISCHEMIC BOWEL: MESENTERIC GAS

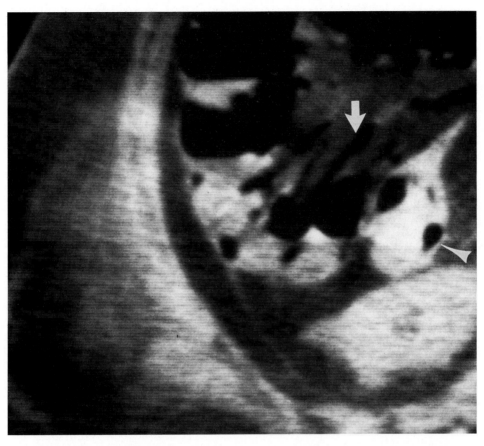

Gas-filled ileocolic veins *(arrow)* are seen within the midabdomen. Pneumatosis intestinalis is also present

*From Smerud MJ, Johnson CD, Stephens DH. AJR* ***1990;***154:99–103. *By permission of the American Roentgen Ray Society.*

*(arrowhead).* Infarcted bowel was removed at operation.

The presence of mesenteric and portal venous gas is usually a sign of advanced ischemia and is often associated with a grave prognosis.

## Case 264

## INFARCTED BOWEL: PORTAL VENOUS GAS

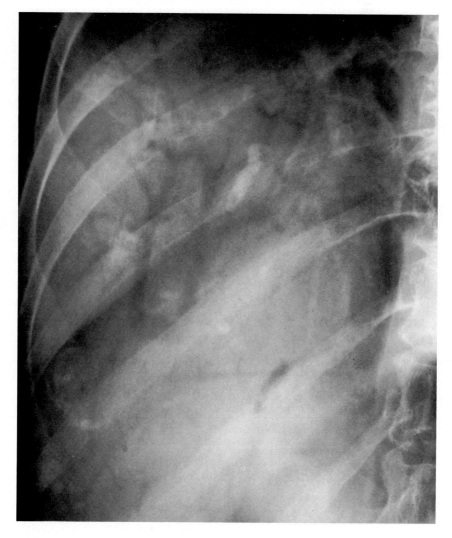

Gas-containing tubular structures are visible within the liver. The peripheral distribution of the gas is typical of portal venous gas.

Portal venous gas is often a late finding in patients with intestinal ischemia. The mucosa is the bowel layer most sensitive to ischemia. As the mucosa breaks down, gas can enter the bowel wall (pneumatosis intestinalis—Cases 256–258) and eventually enter the mesenteric and portal venous system. Although nonischemic causes of portal venous gas have been reported (Gold and Seaman, 1977), portal venous gas is unusual and urgent clinical assessment of the patient is recommended.

## Case 265

## ISCHEMIA: PORTAL VENOUS GAS

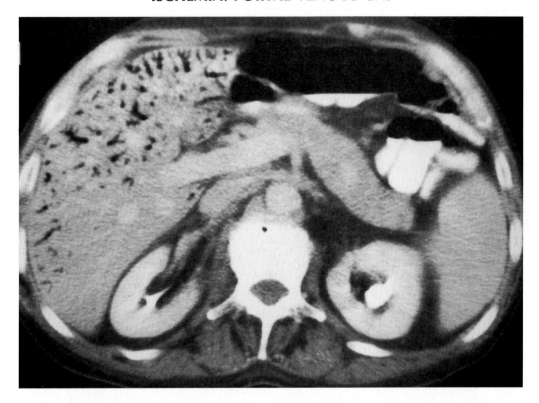

Multiple, gas-filled portal venous branches are visible throughout the periphery of the liver. The nondependent portal veins contain more gas than those in the dependent, posterior right lobe. This is an ominous sign of ischemic bowel disease. At operation, infarcted small bowel was removed.

## Case 266

## ISCHEMIA

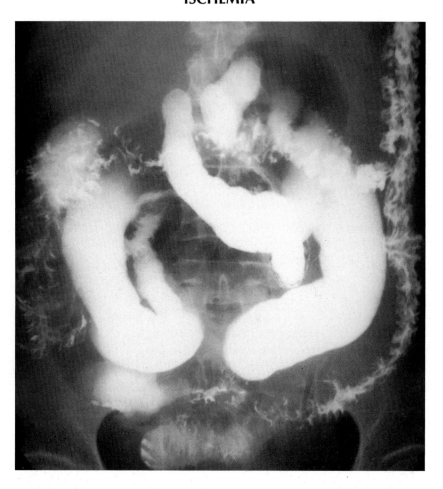

A barium enema examination was performed. The colon was evacuated and the remaining contrast material has refluxed into the ileum, which is dilated and devoid of mucosal markings. Sixty-five centimeters of ischemic ileum was removed at operation. An embolus to the superior mesenteric artery was also removed.

Various morphologic changes can occur in the small bowel from ischemia. This case illustrates bowel dilata-tion, flaccidity, and loss of mucosal markings. Other changes may include narrowing, fold thickening, blurring of the margins of the folds, contour scalloping, and thumbprinting. These findings may all vary in severity and can be seen in combination with one another. The barium examination is unreliable in evaluating the viability of the bowel or the extent of necrosis.

Case 267

## EOSINOPHILIC GASTROENTERITIS

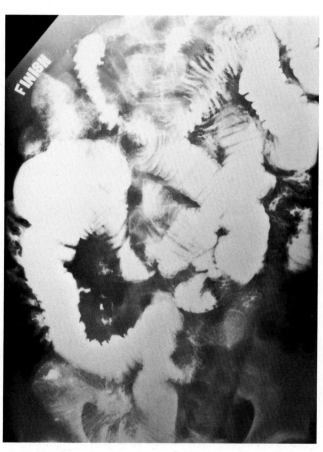

Multiple, dilated small-bowel loops are present, many of which have thickened folds (type II). Although this small-bowel pattern is nonspecific, this patient was found to have eosinophilic gastroenteritis.

Eosinophilic gastroenteritis is a disease of unknown origin, in which the patient presents with abdominal pain, diarrhea, vomiting, and occasionally malabsorption. Usually eosinophilia is present on the peripheral blood smear. Often the clinical course is benign and self-limited, responding to steroid treatments. Some patients will have a history of allergy.

Pathologically, eosinophils and chronic inflammatory cells are present in the bowel wall. Some authorities classify this disease by the depth of eosinophilic involvement in the bowel wall (Marshak et al., 1981). Localized and diffuse bowel involvement occur. Localized eosinophilic granuloma is usually confined to the stomach. Various clinical syndromes have been attributed to the portion of the bowel wall infiltrated by eo-

sinophils. Predominantly mucosal infiltration results in protein loss and malabsorption; intramural disease presents with obstructive symptoms or diarrhea; and serosal eosinophilia results in ascites.

The radiologic findings are similar to those of any other infiltrative small-bowel disease. Thickened (type II), nodular (type III), and bizarre (type IV) fold patterns have been reported. Marked bowel-wall infiltration can result in luminal narrowing and rigidity of the affected segment(s). Any portion of the alimentary tract may be affected, but the stomach and small bowel are the usual sites.

Differential considerations usually include any of the diseases associated with type II through IV fold patterns. Infiltrative diseases such as Crohn's disease, amyloidosis (Case 269), lymphoma (Case 271), and Whipple's disease (Case 272) are important differential considerations.

## Case 268

## AMYLOIDOSIS

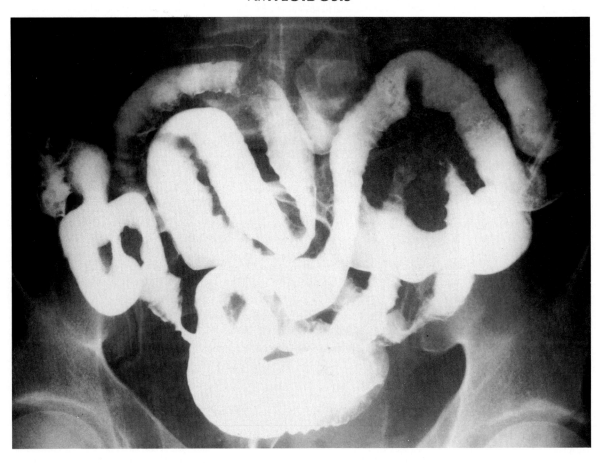

Multiple small-bowel loops have a featureless, atrophic appearance. Thickened (type II) folds are present diffusely. This patient was found to have systemic amyloidosis.

Amyloidosis is caused by deposition of an insoluble fibrillar protein within the extracellular space of various organs. Deposition within arterial walls is often present, resulting in possible ischemia or infarction of the end organ. Several classifications have been devised for this disease. Generally, systemic and localized forms exist. Systemic amyloidosis is most common and can result from a wide variety of causes, including idiopathic, related to a plasma cell dyscrasia (multiple myeloma, light-chain and heavy-chain disease, Waldenström's macroglobulinemia), secondary to chronic infections or inflammatory conditions, and familial types. Amyloid can be deposited throughout the gastrointestinal tract. Patients often complain of weight loss, fatigue, and abdominal pain.

Radiographic findings may be normal, even in patients with debilitating gastrointestinal symptoms (Carlson and Breen, 1986). Diminished motor activity, thickened or atrophic folds, dilatation, and an obstructive pattern may be seen. Changes identical to those of ulcerative colitis can be seen in the colon.

## Case 269

# AMYLOIDOSIS

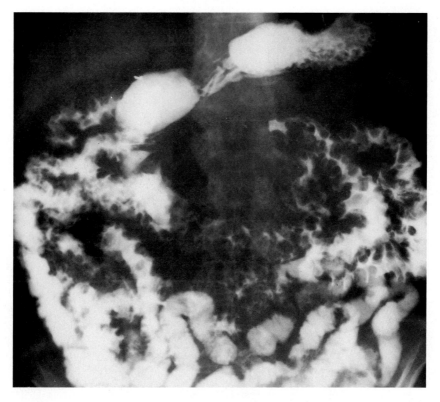

Multiple thickened and nodular (type II and III) folds are present in the proximal small bowel. This patient had known primary (idiopathic) amyloidosis.

The small bowel is that portion of the alimentary tract most often affected with amyloid. Vascular compromise can result in bowel ischemia, infarction, and bleeding. Submucosal amyloid deposition causes polypoid protrusions, fold thickening, and irregular, fine filling defects.

## Case 270

## GIARDIASIS

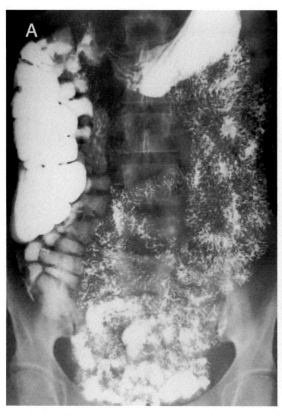

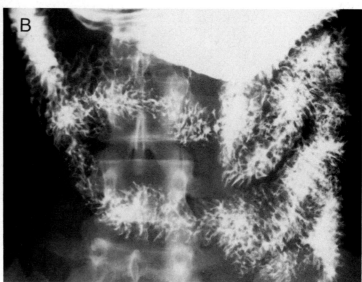

**A** and **B.** The folds of the proximal small bowel are diffusely thickened, with some fold nodularity or contour irregularity. These findings are nonspecific and could be due to any disease causing bowel-wall edema. Localization of the findings within the proximal small bowel suggests giardiasis.

Giardiasis is a disease caused by infection with the protozoan *Giardia lamblia*. Ingested trophozoites attach to the duodenal mucosa and reproduce. Cysts are shed and passed in the stool. The host response to the protozoan varies from an asymptomatic carrier state to severe symptoms of diarrhea and malabsorption. Patients with hypogammaglobulinemia or agammaglobulinemia are believed to be more prone to infection, and often these patients may have changes of nodular lymphoid hyperplasia (Case 278) in the small bowel. The majority of people infected with *G. lamblia* have no clinical or radiographic manifestations of their infection.

Radiographically, the proximal small bowel usually shows inflammatory changes, including fold thickening, increased secretions, irritability, and spasm or rapid transit. Tiny nodular lesions are frequently seen due to hypertrophied lymphoid follicles. A sprue-like pattern may be seen in the distal jejunum and ileum, with reversal of the normal fold pattern. These changes revert to normal after treatment with quinacrine or metronidazole.

Differential considerations include other inflammatory diseases of the proximal small bowel, including Whipple's disease (Case 272), eosinophilic gastroenteritis (Case 267), and pancreatitis (Case 201). Amyloidosis (Case 269), lymphangiectasia (Case 279), and ischemia (Case 261) could also present with similar radiographic findings.

**Case 271**

# LYMPHOMA: INFILTRATIVE FORM

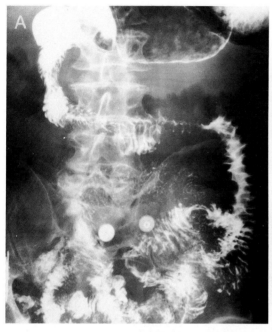

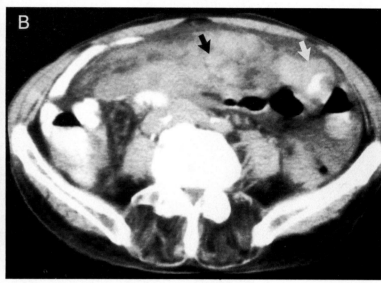

**A.** Diffuse fold thickening (type II and III) is present throughout the small bowel. This appearance is nonspecific.

**B.** Adenopathy *(black arrow)* is present within the small-bowel mesentery. A small-bowel loop with thickened wall is visible *(white arrow)*. This patient was found to have diffuse small-bowel lymphoma.

CT is often included in the evaluation of patients with nonspecific complaints. In patients with lymphoma affecting the small bowel, CT can be helpful in suggesting the diagnosis. Bowel abnormalities vary from thickened folds (as in this patient) to circumferential, long segments of bowel-wall thickening (Case 322). Mesenteric adenopathy is displayed well at CT, and although nonspecific it is a supportive finding of lymphoma.

## Case 272

## WHIPPLE'S DISEASE

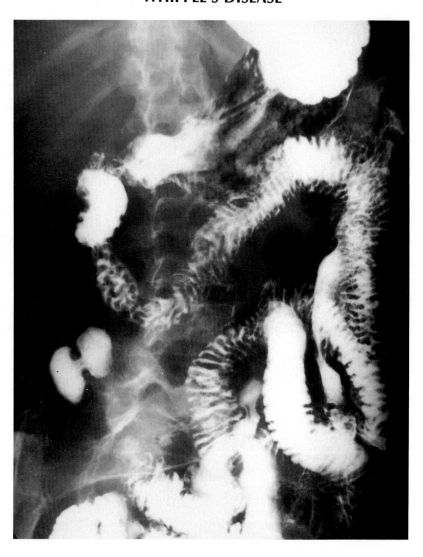

Thickened folds (type II) are present throughout the proximal small bowel. Although this finding is nonspecific, the patient was found to have Whipple's disease.

The cause of Whipple's disease is uncertain. It is characterized clinically by malabsorption, arthritis or arthralgias, lymphadenopathy, abdominal tenderness, and increased skin pigmentation. Histologically, a periodic acid-Schiff-positive glycoprotein is deposited within macrophages in the lamina propria and lymph nodes of the small bowel. Gram-positive rods and granules have also been identified during the active phase of the disease, but no organism has yet been cul-

tured. Treatment usually consists of a long-term course of antibiotics.

Radiologically, fold thickening and nodularity are commonly seen in the proximal small bowel. Sometimes the pattern may appear wild and bizarre. Hypersecretion, dilatation, and diffuse small-bowel involvement are usually absent, which helps to differentiate this disease from sprue. In the immunocompromised patient, infection with *Mycobacterium avium-intracellulare*, *Giardia*, or *Cryptosporidium* can produce identical radiographic findings and should be considered (Berk et al., 1884; Vincent and Robbins, 1985).

## Case 273

## WHIPPLE'S DISEASE

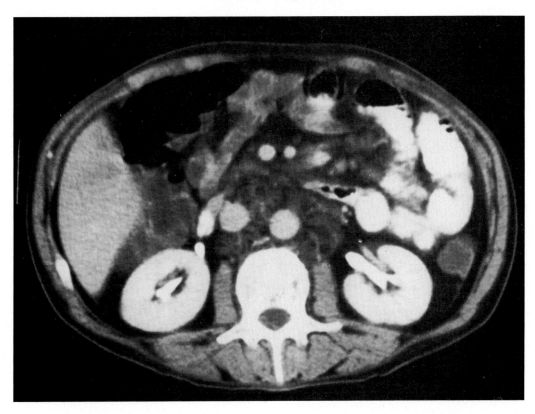

Multiple, low-density lymph nodes are present within the retroperitoneum and small-bowel mesentery. This patient was known to have Whipple's disease.

Whipple's disease is often associated with abdominal lymphadenopathy, but this finding is rarely appreciated on small-bowel examinations. The lymph nodes usually have a low density on CT because of the deposition of fat and fatty acids within the nodes. Occasionally, only mesenteric lymphadenopathy is present.

Other diseases can be associated with low-density lymphadenopathy, including tuberculosis, testicular neoplasms, epidermoid carcinoma of the genitourinary tract, and rarely lymphoma. Sacroiliitis, a component of this systemic illness, may also be detectable on CT scans of the abdomen. The sacroiliac joints may be affected either unilaterally or bilaterally and the articular symptoms may precede the gastrointestinal symptoms (usually diarrhea) by 5 years or more.

## Case 274

# TYPE III FOLDS (NODULAR CHANGES INVOLVING FOLDS)

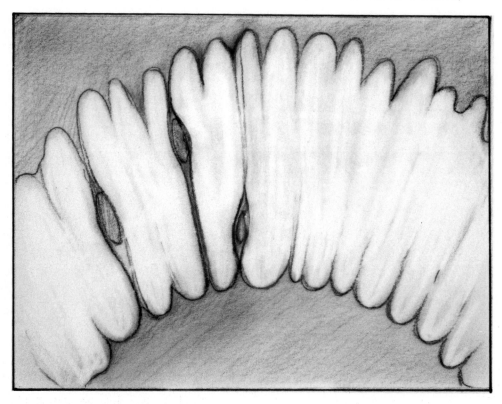

1. Crohn's disease (Cases 275, 276, and 292)
2. Lymphoma (Cases 277 and 324)
3. Polyposis syndromes (Cases 373–377)
4. Nodular lymphoid hyperplasia (Case 278)

5. Whipple's disease (Case 272)
6. Lymphangiectasia (Cases 279 and 280)
7. Metastases (Cases 281 and 333–338)

Case 275

## CROHN'S DISEASE: EARLY NONSTENOTIC PHASE

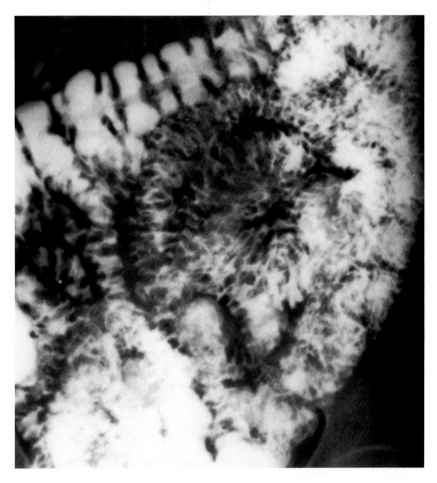

Thickened, somewhat nodular (type II and III) folds are present throughout the small bowel. These findings are nonspecific but consistent with early nonstenotic Crohn's disease.

Crohn's disease is a chronic disorder of unknown origin. The disease involves the small bowel in at least 80% of patients (Marshak, 1975). The clinical activity of the disease (abdominal pain, diarrhea, fever, weight loss, anemia) correlates poorly with radiologic changes. It is interesting that in the absence of an operation, the longitudinal extent of disease does not progress to involve previously normal bowel. The location of the involved small-bowel segment does affect a patient's prognosis. Crohn's disease confined to the distal small bowel has the best long-term prognosis, whereas ileocolic involvement has the highest incidence of complications (abscess, fistula) (Glick, 1987). The terminal ileum is usually involved (spared in only 5% of all patients) (Mekhjian et al., 1979). Recurrent disease after resection of a diseased small-bowel segment invariably occurs about the anastomosis. Recurrences are usually detectable radiographically within 2 years after operation (Glick, 1987).

Superficial mucosal changes include ulceration (aphthoid, linear, transverse) (Cases 276 and 292), thickened folds, and enlarged lymphoid follicles. Some authors report the frequent finding of mucosal granularity (Glick and Teplick, 1985), but this has not been widely seen in our practice.

## Case 276

# CROHN'S DISEASE: APHTHOUS ULCERS

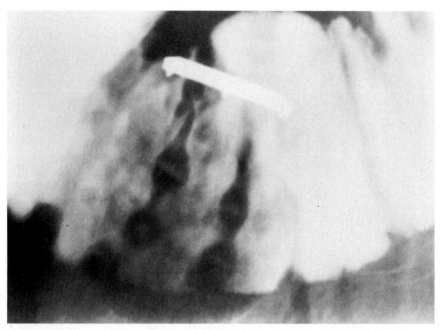

Multiple discrete ulcerations are present in the distal small bowel. The central barium collections (ulcer crater) and mounds of edema are characteristic of aphthous ulcers. A compression device with metallic marker is seen.

These tiny mucosal ulcers are believed to be the first mucosal lesions of Crohn's disease (Lichtenstein, 1987). These lesions may coalesce and form longitudinal and transverse ulcerations that are typical of more advanced disease (Case 292). Discrete ulcers are not specific for Crohn's disease and can be seen in various infectious disorders that affect the terminal ileum (*Yersinia,* amebiasis, tuberculosis).

## Case 277

# LYMPHOMA: MULTIPLE NODULES

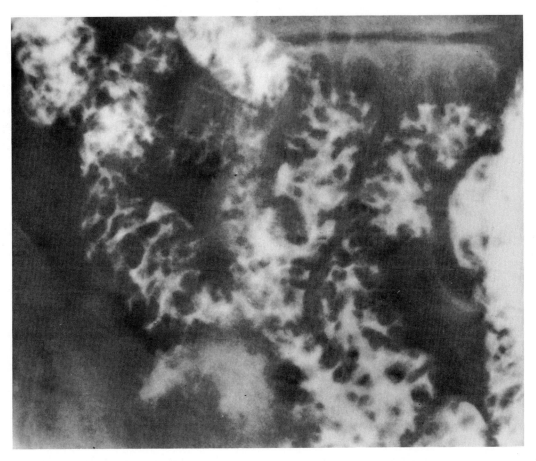

Multiple nodules of various sizes are present throughout these small-bowel loops. The smooth surface of these nodules suggests their submucosal location. Non-Hodgkin's lymphoma was found.

Multiple nodules and fold thickening are manifestations of lymphoma diffusely involving the small bowel. In addition to the diffuse form, 10% to 20% of patients with gastrointestinal lymphoma will have multiple focal lesions (Koehler, 1989). These lesions may appear to be of submucosal origin and their surface may be ulcerated. The polyposis syndromes (Cases 373–377) would be a differential consideration, but usually these

patients have their disease diagnosed before a small-bowel examination is performed. A prior history of malignancy (e.g., melanoma) is often known in patients with metastatic tumors of the small bowel (Case 281). Metastases are usually not as numerous as the diffuse nodularity seen in this patient. Nodular lymphoid hyperplasia has small (<4 mm) nodules of uniform size (Case 278). Lymphangiectasia (Case 279) is usually diagnosed by early adulthood, whereas non-Hodgkin's lymphoma generally occurs during the 5th and 6th decades of life.

## Case 278

## NODULAR LYMPHOID HYPERPLASIA

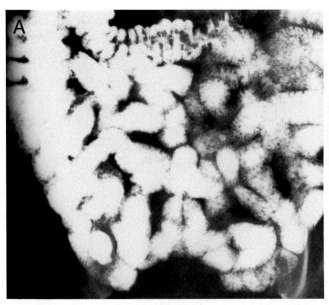 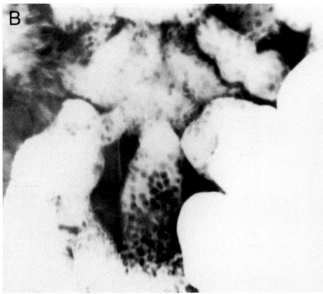

**A** and **B.** Multiple, tiny, nodular filling defects are present throughout the small bowel. All the nodules are uniform size and shape.

Nodular lymphoid hyperplasia is usually associated with an immunologic disorder, primarily a deficiency of IgA and IgM. Occasionally, this disease may be present without an immunologic disorder. Malabsorption and an intestinal infection *(Giardia lamblia, Strongyloides,* or *Monilia)* are often associated conditions. There is an increased incidence of gastric and colonic cancers (in all patients with enteropathic immunoglobulin deficiencies), especially in children (Hermans et al., 1966).

Radiographically, innumerable tiny nodules are seen in the involved portions of the small bowel. The nodules are usually less than 4 mm in diameter and uniform size. They may be centrally umbilicated and resemble an aphthous ulcer (Cases 276 and 363). The main differential consideration is lymphoma; however, usually these nodules are larger, vary in size, and may ulcerate (Case 277). Normal lymphoid nodules can regularly be seen in patients of any age but are usually encountered in children and young adults (Case 362). These nodules are uniform size, nearly always less than 4 mm in diameter, and primarily involve the distal small bowel and proximal colon.

## Case 279

## INTESTINAL LYMPHANGIECTASIA

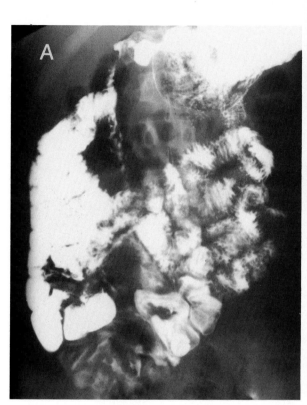

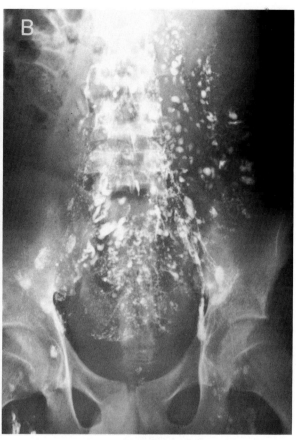

**A.** Thickened folds and tiny nodules are present within the proximal small bowel. Dilution of barium due to excess intraluminal fluid is seen in the distal small bowel.

**B.** A lymphangiogram demonstrates multiple, dilated, and bulbous lymphatic channels within the small-bowel mesentery. Findings are characteristic of lymphangiectasia.

Intestinal lymphangiectasia is a disorder of abnormal lymph flow, with loss of lymphatic fluid (most importantly protein) into the alimentary tract. Patients often present with hypoalbuminemia, hypoproteinemia, and occasionally malabsorptive symptoms. Diarrhea, vomiting, and abdominal pain are often present. Lymphangiectasia is often a congenital condition or it may be acquired later in life from inflammatory or neoplastic lymphatic obstruction.

Pathologically, lymph channels are dilated in the lamina propria and submucosa of the bowel wall, with associated enlarged and distorted villi. Submucosal edema is often present due to hypoalbuminemia. It is believed that these lymph channels rupture into the gut lumen and are responsible for the protein loss. Treatment may be difficult, but some patients respond to a low-fat diet using medium-chain triglycerides which do not require lymphatic transport for absorption. Lymphatic abnormalities elsewhere in the body are often found.

Radiologically, thickened and sometimes nodular small-bowel folds are present diffusely throughout the small bowel. Increased secretions are usually present. Differentiation of this disorder from other diseases that diffusely affect the small bowel may be impossible. Whipple's disease (Case 272) usually affects the proximal small bowel most severely, and in amyloidosis (Cases 268 and 269), lymphoma (Case 271), and mastocytosis, increased secretions are absent. A reversal of the fold pattern is often present in celiac disease (Case 289), and nodularity is atypical. Eosinophilic gastroenteritis (Case 267) and constrictive pericarditis may present with identical radiographic findings.

**Case 280**

## INTESTINAL LYMPHANGIECTASIA

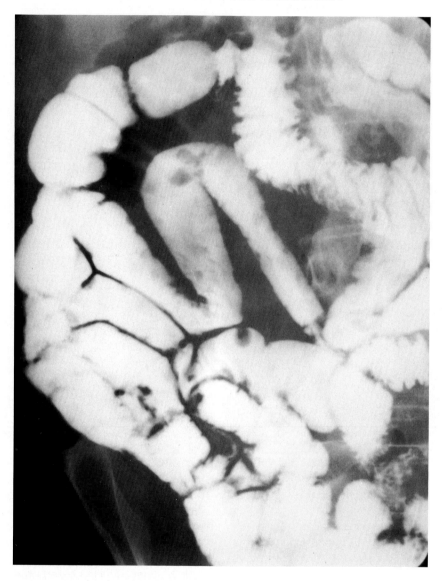

Multiple, polypoid filling defects are present in the distal small bowel. These were found to represent dilated lymphatic bullae within the small-bowel lumen.

The nodular filling defects that may be seen in lym-phangiectasia can vary considerably in size. Large filling defects (as seen in this case) can be several millimeters in diameter, whereas tiny defects may appear as sandlike lucencies.

### Case 281

### METASTASES

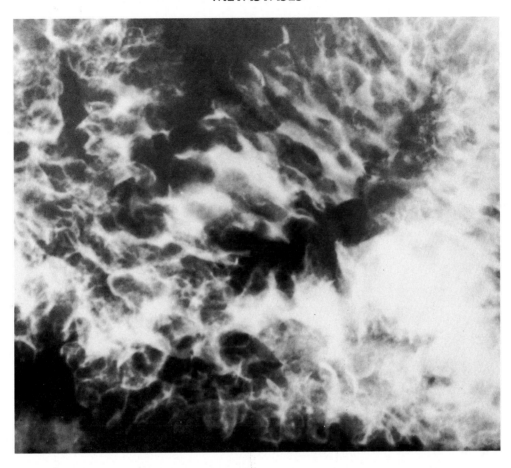

The small bowel is involved with diffusely nodular folds (type III fold pattern). This patient was found to have metastases from melanoma.

Diffuse hematogenous seeding of the gastrointestinal tract with metastatic tumor can result in nodular changes within the bowel wall. A history of melanoma would make this radiographic appearance nearly diagnostic of metastases. Other considerations include diffuse lymphoma (Case 277), Crohn's disease (Cases 275 and 276), Whipple's disease (Case 272), lymphangiectasia Cases 279 and 280), and amyloidosis (Case 269). Nodular lymphoid hyperplasia (Case 278) has smaller nodules (usually <4 mm diameter) of uniform size. Whipple's disease affects the proximal small bowel most severely. Patients with Crohn's disease usually have segmental areas of intervening normal small bowel, often with luminal stenoses and fistulae.

## Case 282

# TYPE IV FOLDS (SHAGGY, WILD, BIZARRE MUCOSAL FOLDS)

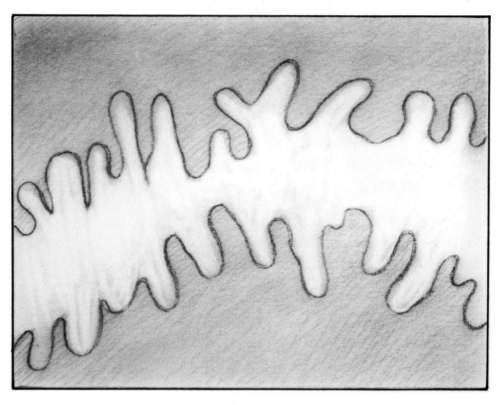

1. Edema (e.g., hypoproteinemia, cirrhosis)
   (Cases 283 and 284)
2. Gastroenteritis

3. Whipple's disease

## Case 283

## HYPOPROTEINEMIA

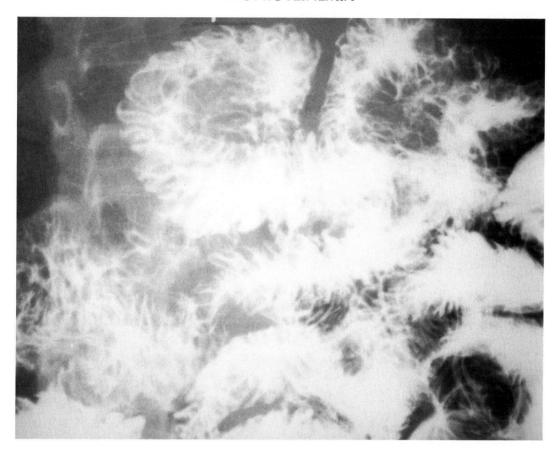

The folds of the small bowel are diffusely thickened. Classification of the fold type is difficult, but it could be classified as wild and bizarre (type IV). This patient had chronic active hepatitis and secondary hypoalbuminemia.

Intestinal edema due to hypoproteinemia (usually the serum albumin level is ≤2 g/dL) can be idiopathic or secondary to various diseases, including cirrhosis, Crohn's disease, ulcerative colitis, Ménétrier's disease, Whipple's disease, lymphangiectasia, lymphoma, carcinoma, constrictive pericarditis, congestive heart failure, and exudative skin lesions. Cirrhosis of the liver is the most often encountered underlying disease.

Various radiographic changes can be seen, including diffusely thickened folds (type II), or even a wild and bizarre pattern (fold pattern type IV). Haustral thickening of the right colon may also be seen. Ascites may be present.

## Case 284

# HYPOPROTEINEMIA

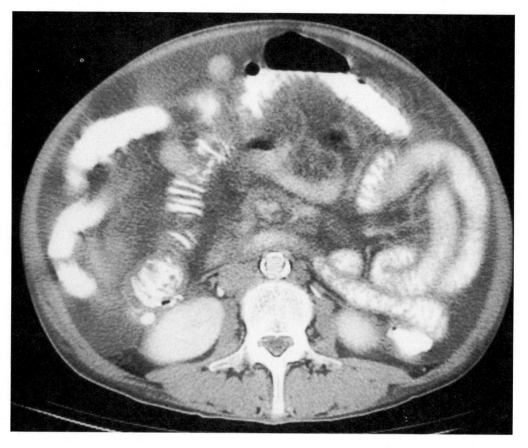

Diffuse ascites is present in the abdominal cavity. Small-bowel fold thickening and increased mesenteric markings are present. These findings are nonspecific but consistent with hypoproteinemia.

CT findings in patients with hypoalbuminemia include not only edematous changes within the bowel and mesentery but also edema within other body tissues. These edematous changes include soft tissue stranding and a generalized increased density within the subcutaneous and mesenteric fat.

**Case 285**

## TYPE V FOLDS: ANY ABNORMAL FOLD PATTERN PLUS AN ABNORMAL AMOUNT OF INTRALUMINAL FLUID

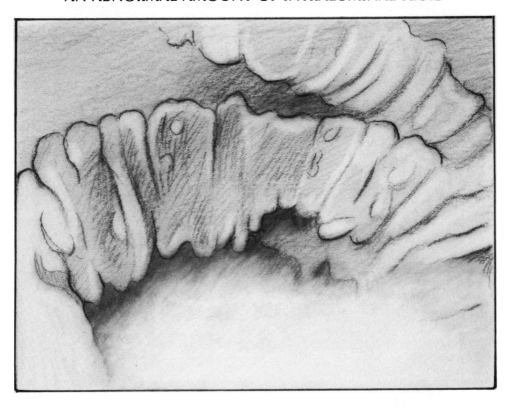

1. Proximal to mechanical obstruction (Cases 246 and 249)
2. Sprue (Cases 286–288)
3. Zollinger-Ellison syndrome (Cases 105 and 200)
4. Acute caustic ingestion

**Case 286**

# CELIAC DISEASE (SPRUE)

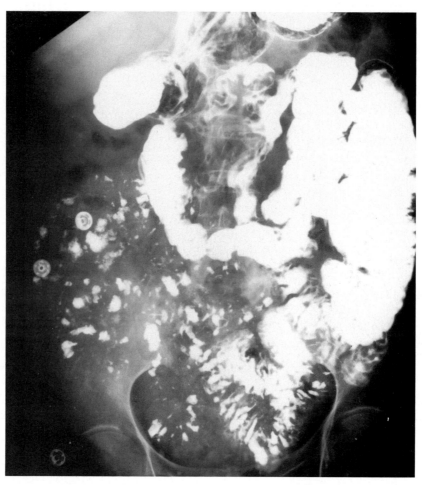

Flocculation and segmentation of barium indicate the presence of excessive fluid in the distal small bowel. The normal jejunal fold pattern is also absent. These loops appear featureless. A few small-bowel loops in the pelvis have thickened folds (type II). Celiac disease was diagnosed from the results of a small-bowel biopsy.

The term "sprue" is given to three diseases with common radiographic and pathologic manifestations. Childhood and adult (nontropical) sprue are probably the same disease, secondary to a gluten (a water-insoluble protein found in various cereals and grains, including wheat, rye, oats, and barley) sensitivity. The cause of tropical sprue is unknown, but patients do not respond to dietary gluten restriction. These patients often respond to folate therapy, antibiotic (usually tetracycline) therapy, or both.

Pathologically, villous atrophy is usually seen with elongation of the crypts of Lieberkühn and infiltration of the lamina propria with inflammatory cells. Changes are often more marked in the proximal small bowel.

This case demonstrates many of the radiologic features of excess intraluminal fluid ("hypersecretion") that are commonly encountered in patients with sprue. Barium may become radiolucent and separated into clumps (segmentation) or tiny pieces (flocculation) as a result of dilution. This is most commonly seen in the distal small bowel. Small-bowel folds in patients with sprue may remain normally thin or they may become thickened. Thickened folds are usually secondary to intramural edema from hypoalbuminemia. The gastrointestinal loss of albumin is the result of the malabsorption which is typically present in these patients.

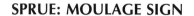

**Case 287**

# SPRUE: MOULAGE SIGN

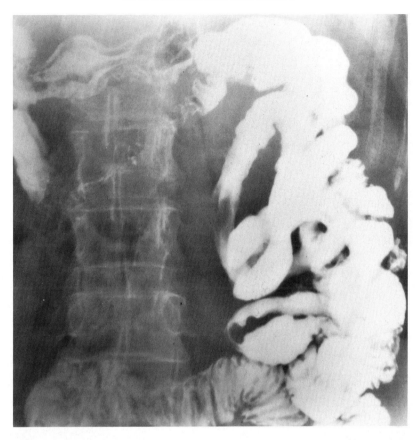

The jejunum is devoid of most of its normal mucosal markings. The tubular featureless appearance of these loops has been referred to as the moulage sign. This patient was known to have celiac disease.

Excessive intraluminal fluid obscures and prevents adequate mucosal coating of the proximal small bowel and results in the "moulage sign." Moulage refers to a molded or casted structure. The jejunum in this patient resembles a tubular cast of small bowel because of its paucity of mucosal folds.

## Case 288

## CELIAC DISEASE

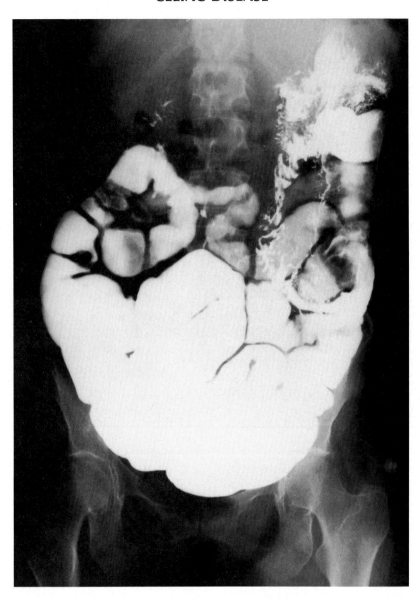

The normal, jejunal fold pattern has been lost. The gray granular appearance of several small-bowel loops indicates excess intraluminal fluid. Mild dilatation of several loops is also present. These findings are typical of celiac disease.

Modern barium remains in suspension longer than previous preparations. As a result, segmentation and flocculation of barium are less frequently encountered today. Reversal of the small-bowel fold patterns ("ilealization of the jejunum" and "jejunization of the ileum") (Case 289), mild dilatation, and dilution of barium (as seen in this case) are radiographic findings usually encountered. The transit time of contrast material through the small bowel is usually normal.

## Case 289

## CELIAC DISEASE

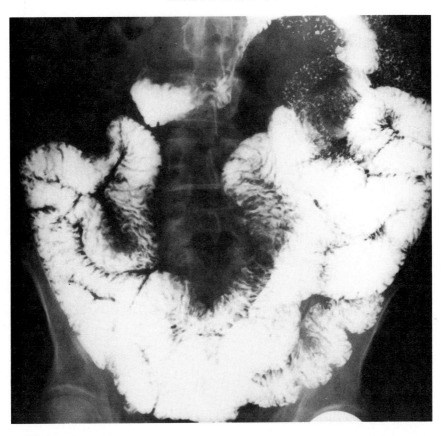

The ileum has a fold pattern that mimics the jejunum. The jejunum has fewer folds than normally expected. There is no excess fluid or bowel dilatation.

This typical example of the reversed fold pattern is generally encountered in patients with celiac disease. This "jejunization of the ileum" is believed to be an adaptive response to the loss of absorptive surface area in the proximal small bowel (Bova et al., 1985). The jejunal folds have been shown to decrease in number, a feature particularly evident on enteroclysis examinations. Three folds or less per inch in the jejunum on an enteroclysis examination is strong evidence for this disease (Herlinger and Maglinte, 1986).

## Case 290

## SPRUE: INTUSSUSCEPTION

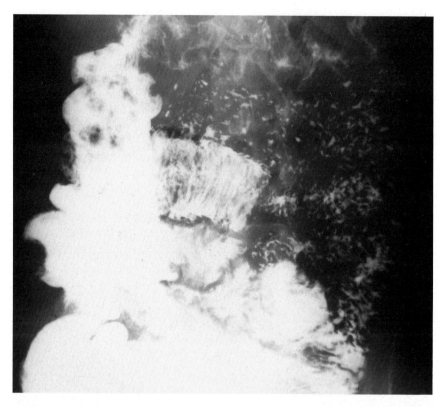

The typical coiled-spring appearance of a jejunal intussusception is present in the upper abdomen. This patient had known celiac disease.

Intussusceptions occur often in patients with celiac disease. One report (Cohen and Lintott, 1978) noted this disorder in 20% of patients. Intussusceptions are usually asymptomatic, transient, and self-reducing. As with any intussusception, careful fluoroscopy should be performed to exclude a small-bowel mass as a lead point for the intussusception.

**Case 291**

## CELIAC DISEASE: SEGMENTAL ULCERATION

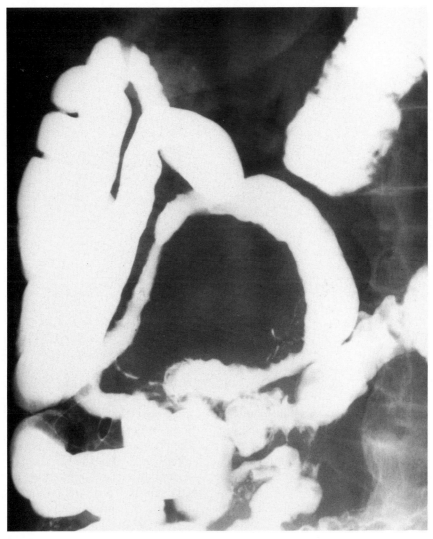

Several small-bowel loops appear featureless, and other loops are narrowed with nodular and thickened folds. The narrowed segments may be ulcerated. These findings are due to segmental ulceration in this patient with known sprue.

Segmental ulceration in patients with sprue is an unusual complication of the disease. Patients often present with worsening of their malabsorptive symptoms and abdominal pain. Bleeding and perforation can occur as a result of the nonspecific ulcers. The ulcers are morphologically nonspecific, often multiple, and usually involve the jejunum. They can be difficult to detect radiologically. Spasm, irritability, and persistent areas of narrowing can make it difficult to differentiate these changes from lymphoma. As a result, the involved loops are usually resected. In some patients, the nonspecific ulcers may precede the development or recognition of intestinal lymphoma (Baer et al., 1980).

## Case 292

# CROHN'S DISEASE: NONSTENOTIC COBBLESTONING

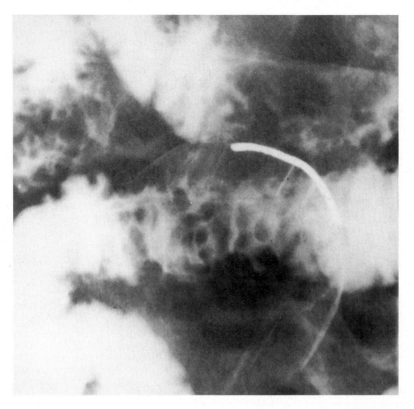

A cobblestone mucosal pattern affects a nonstenotic segment of small bowel. This pattern is typical of Crohn's disease. Longitudinal and transverse ulcerations, in conjunction with bowel-wall edema, produce a cobblestone mucosal pattern. A metallic marker on a compression device is present.

Patients with Crohn's disease often have the insidious onset of abdominal cramping, diarrhea, weight loss, low-grade fever, anorexia, and anemia. Patients are usually treated conservatively with rest, dietary changes, and antidiarrheal and anti-inflammatory agents. Approximately one-third to one-half of patients can be successfully managed without operation (Glick, 1987). Surgical treatment is usually reserved for the complications of the disease—fistulae, obstruction, and abscess.

Extraintestinal manifestations of Crohn's disease include arthritis (and ankylosing spondylitis), erythema nodosum, pyoderma gangrenosum, and rarely primary sclerosing cholangitis. An increased incidence of cholesterol gallstones and oxalate renal stones can occur in patients with ileal disease as a result of abnormalities in the enterohepatic bile acid circulation.

**Case 293**

## CROHN'S DISEASE: STRING SIGN

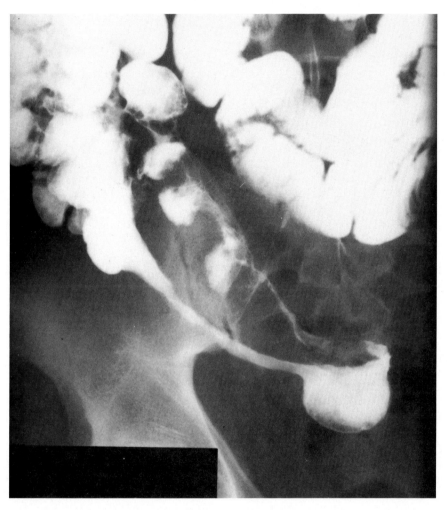

A long segment of narrowed ileum (string sign) is present with areas of bowel-wall asymmetry. This appearance is pathognomonic of Crohn's disease.

The string sign of Crohn's disease may or may not represent a fixed stricture. This region of narrowing may be inconstant due to marked spasm, and proximal small-bowel dilatation may be lacking. Fixed narrowing from transmural fibrosis is usually associated with a short segmental stricture and dilatation of proximal loops (Glick, 1987). The terminal ileum is often affected.

Small-bowel ischemia can cause featureless stric-tures; however, multiple skip areas are usually absent. A patient's age and history can also be helpful. Patients with ischemia are often older and have an acute onset of abdominal pain and adynamic ileus. Patients with Crohn's disease are usually young adults with a chronic history of abdominal pain and diarrhea. Other inflammatory disorders such as tuberculosis (Case 306), actinomycosis, histoplasmosis, and blastomycosis can present with findings that are indistinguishable from Crohn's disease. *Yersinia* and *Salmonella* can produce superficial erosions and fold thickening, but strictures are uncommon.

**Case 294**

## CROHN'S DISEASE: ASYMMETRIC BOWEL-WALL INVOLVEMENT

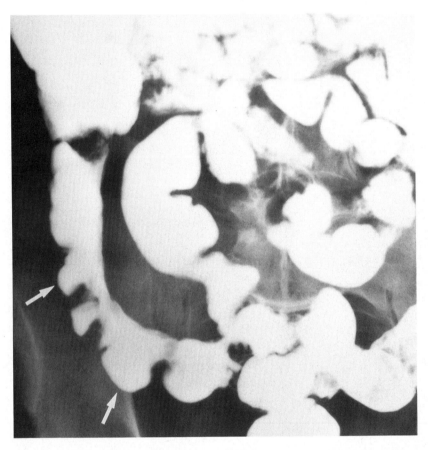

An abnormal loop of distal small bowel is present in the right lower quadrant *(arrows)*. The loop is separate from others, and the medial wall is flattened and featureless. Pseudodiverticula are present along the lateral wall. These findings are due to circumferential asymmetric bowel-wall involvement—a characteristic finding of Crohn's disease.

Circumferential asymmetry of the bowel lumen can be a helpful radiographic finding in Crohn's disease.

This finding may be due to skip areas of fibrosis or ulceration with folding and sometimes dilatation of the opposite wall. Other causes of eccentric small-bowel changes include serosal metastases (mass effect and tethered folds are usually seen) (Case 340), scleroderma (usually diffusely affects the small bowel with sacculations on the antimesenteric border) (Case 457), and chronic ischemic changes (in older patients with known vascular or heart disease).

**Case 295**

## CROHN'S DISEASE: BOWEL-WALL THICKENING

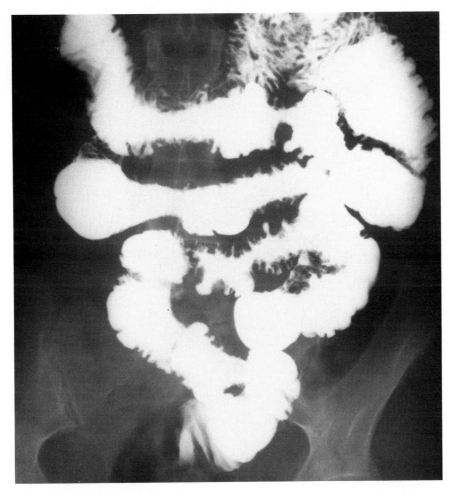

Typical changes of Crohn's disease are present with mucosal-fold thickening, ulceration, nodularity, asymmetric bowel-wall involvement, regions of narrowing, and separation of small-bowel loops.

Advanced changes of Crohn's disease are often secondary to transmural inflammation and fibrosis. Transmural inflammation leads to bowel-wall thickening and bowel-loop separation (as seen in this case). Fistulae and abscesses also result from transmural disease. Fibrosis nearly always accompanies the healing phase of the disease. Patchy discontinuous regions of fibrosis result in circumferential asymmetry of the bowel wall.

**Case 296**

## CROHN'S DISEASE: SHORT STENOSES

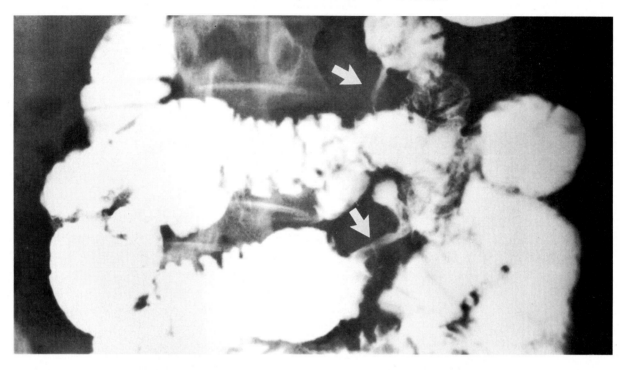

Two regions of high-grade stenosis *(arrows)* are present in the proximal small bowel. The abrupt edges and ulcerated mucosa of the lesions resemble neoplasm (metastases, carcinoma, lymphoma), but Crohn's disease can also have this appearance.

Stenotic Crohn's disease can affect both long and short segments of the bowel. Proximal dilatation of the small bowel usually indicates significant obstruction by the lesion. Complete obstruction from Crohn's is rarely encountered. In some patients, particularly those with a solitary short stenosis, it may be impossible to exclude neoplasm radiologically. These patients usually require resection of the diseased bowel.

**Case 297**

## CROHN'S DISEASE: FISTULA FORMATION

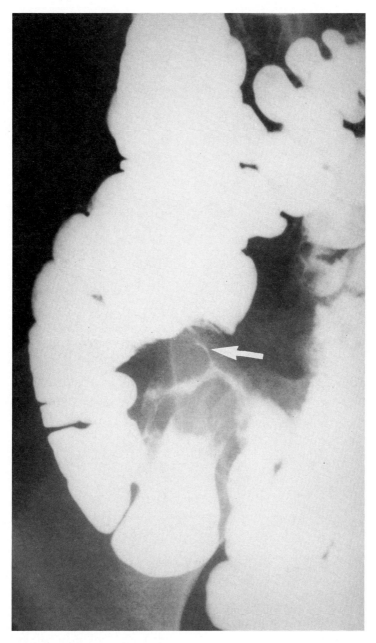

The terminal ileum is narrowed and a fistulous communication *(arrow)* exists between the distal ileum and colon. Inflammatory changes with tethered folds are present along the medial aspect of the cecum.

Fistula formation is a common finding in patients with transmural disease. Fistulae can communicate with other small-bowel loops, colon, genitourinary tract, retroperitoneum, mesentery, and skin. Fistulae can occasionally be multiple and are often incorporated within an inflammatory mass of bowel and mesentery. Abscess formation often accompanies fistulization and sinus tracts.

Case 298

## CROHN'S DISEASE: FISTULA FORMATION

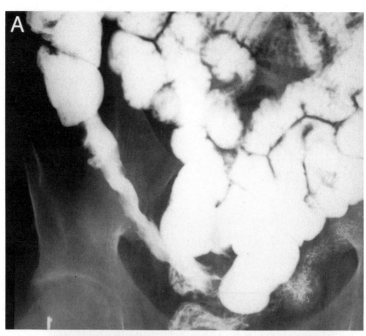

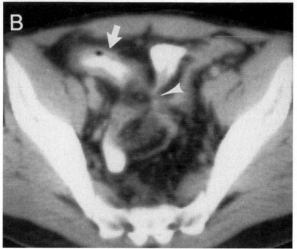

**A.** The terminal ileum has irregular contours. Considerable mass effect displaces adjacent small-bowel loops toward the midline. A fistula is not seen. Findings are typical of Crohn's disease.

**B.** The wall of the terminal ileum *(arrow)* is thickened. Considerable soft-tissue stranding and thickening *(arrowhead)* are present between the ileum and sigmoid colon. A fistulous communication can be suspected between these two organs. At operation, a fistulous tract was excised.

Fistulous tracts may not always fill during an intraluminal examination with contrast material. CT can provide unique information regarding extraluminal disease extent. A fistula can be suspected when a soft-tissue tract is identified containing air or contrast material. The full extent and exact location of the fistula may be revealed best at CT. Bowel-wall thickening, mesenteric inflammation, and abscess can be directly imaged at CT.

**Case 299**

## CROHN'S DISEASE: PSOAS ABSCESS

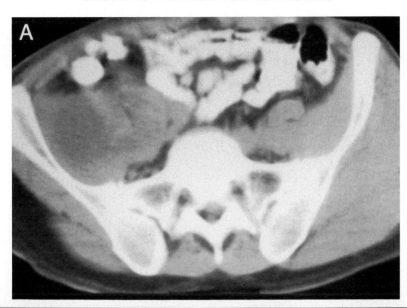

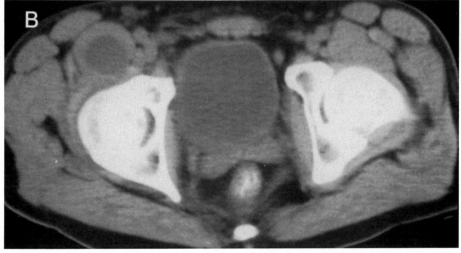

**A** and **B.** The right iliacus muscle and psoas muscle are enlarged and contain a central low-density region. These findings are consistent with an abscess, which was surgically drained.

The development of an abscess in a patient with Crohn's disease is common, occurring in up to one-quarter of all patients (Keighley et al., 1982). The diagnosis is important because percutaneous or surgical drainage is usually required for cure. Transmural inflammation and fistulae can lead to an abscess within any abdominal compartment or organ. CT is generally recognized as the best modality in detecting these ab-

scesses and in planning possible percutaneous drainage. The efficacy of percutaneous abscess drainage is often dependent on the presence of an enteric communication. If an intestinal communication is present, either long-term drainage or operation is often required. Percutaneous drainage is often curative if an enteric fistula is absent. If safe access to the abscess is possible, there is little risk to the patient, and in some patients a single-stage rather than a two-stage operation can be performed by percutaneously draining the abscess preoperatively (Safrit et al., 1987).

**Case 300**

# CROHN'S DISEASE: MESENTERIC FIBROFATTY CHANGES

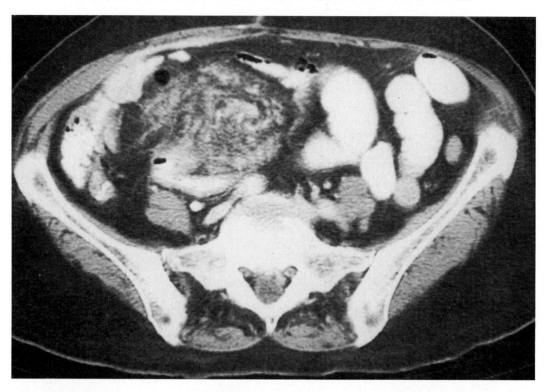

A mass composed of fat and soft tissue stranding is present in the right lower quadrant. A loop of distal small bowel has mildly thickened walls just posterior to the mass. This is the typical appearance of fibrofatty mesenteric changes associated with Crohn's disease.

The fibrofatty changes seen in the mesentery in patients with Crohn's disease are referred to by surgeons and pathologists as "creeping fat." Enlarged and normal-sized lymph nodes are often visible. The mass may be of homogeneous fat density or may contain streaks and poorly defined soft tissue changes within it. Soft tissue changes (as in this case) within the mass are often associated with acute inflammation. This fibrofatty proliferation has been reported to cause ureteral compression and obstruction when the retroperitoneum is affected (Megibow et al., 1981).

## Case 301

## CROHN'S DISEASE: CT

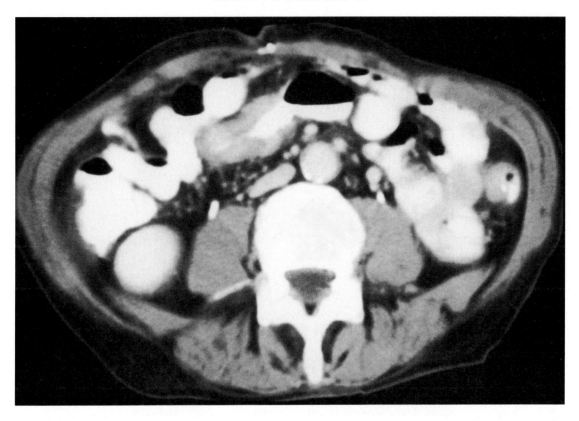

Marked homogeneous segmental bowel-wall thickening is present in the distal small bowel in this patient with Crohn's disease. This finding is not specific for Crohn's disease and could be due to neoplasm (lymphoma, metastasis, carcinoma).

Case 302

# CROHN'S DISEASE: CT

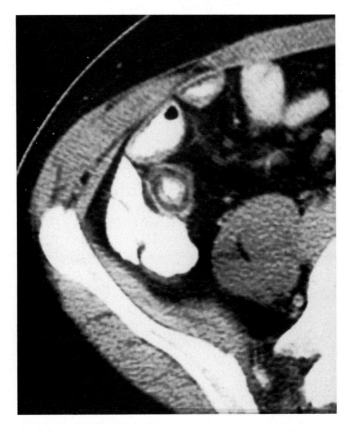

The terminal ileum has a markedly thickened wall that contains a central ring the density of fat. This CT "target sign" is nonspecific and could be due to any inflammatory disorder affecting the ileum. This patient had known Crohn's disease.

CT findings of active Crohn's disease include bowel-wall thickening, mesenteric fibrofatty proliferation, abscess, mesenteric inflammation, and lymphadenopathy. In Crohn's disease, bowel-wall thickening is usually greater than 1 cm and is the commonest CT finding. The wall thickening in active disease may be the density of soft tissue or contain a central low-density ring. Fat within the bowel wall has been shown to accumulate in the submucosa of patients with either ulcerative colitis or Crohn's disease. Active inflammation is not present when this finding is identified. The cause of the fat deposition is unknown, although long-term corticosteroid treatment may be responsible (Jones et al., 1986).

## Case 303

# GRAFT-VERSUS-HOST DISEASE

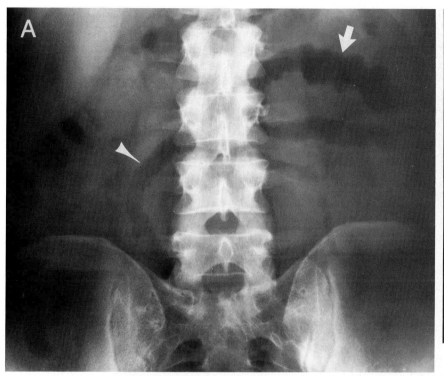
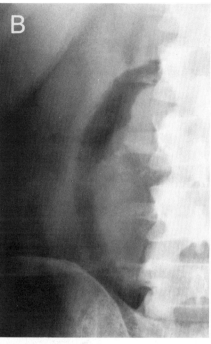

**A.** Several abnormal small-bowel loops are present on this plain film radiograph. The mucosal folds are markedly thickened *(arrow)* or nearly absent *(arrowhead)*. Separation of small-bowel loops suggests bowel-wall thickening.

**B.** Close-up view of a single small loop shows an atrophic, mildly narrowed loop with luminal irregularity. This patient had undergone bone marrow transplantation. The radiographic findings were attributed to graft-versus-host disease.

Graft-versus-host disease occurs in more than half of all patients receiving a bone marrow transplant (Fisk et al., 1981). The skin, liver, and gastrointestinal tract are most often affected. Severe mucosal inflammation, destruction, and atrophy occur, resulting in a profuse secretory diarrhea. Graft-versus-host disease can affect stomach, small bowel, and colon—small bowel usually is affected most severely.

Radiographic changes include fold thickening, effacement, and featureless (atrophic) loops that have been referred to as "ribbon bowel" (Case 304). The changes are not specific to graft-versus-host disease; identical findings may be seen in patients with enterovirus infection.

## Case 304

## GRAFT-VERSUS-HOST DISEASE

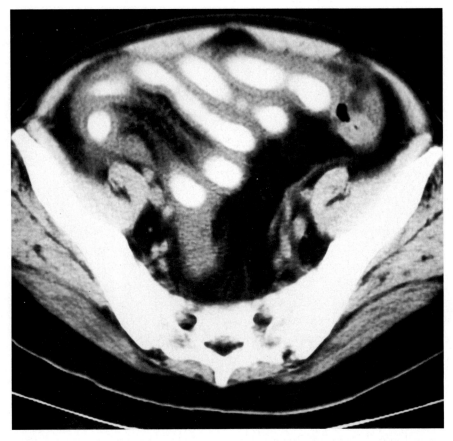

Diffuse wall thickening is seen throughout the small bowel. Normal mucosal folds were not visible. The small bowel has a "ribbon bowel" appearance. This patient had received a bone marrow transplant. Acute graft-versus-host disease was confirmed at endoscopic biopsy.

The featureless appearance of these small-bowel loops is characteristic of graft-versus-host disease but nonspecific. Other conditions—including ischemia, enterovirus infection, celiac disease, or radiation enteritis—could cause similar radiographic features. A feature unique to bone marrow transplant patients is prolonged coating of the affected bowel segments with barium for several days after the examination (Jones et al., 1988). The cause of this finding is unknown.

## Case 305

## TUBERCULOSIS ADENOPATHY

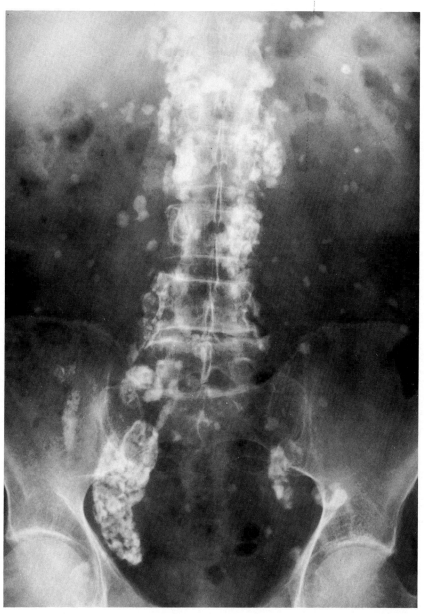

Multiple, calcified, retroperitoneal and mesenteric lymph nodes are present in the abdomen. Affected lymph nodes are more numerous in the upper abdomen. This patient was known to have had tuberculosis in the past.

Tuberculosis is frequently associated with lymphadenopathy and peritonitis. Lymphadenopathy is commonly seen at CT in these patients, particularly in the upper abdomen (mesenteric and peripancreatic nodes). Nodal calcification is unusual in patients with active disease and is probably found most often in patients with chronic or healed infection. Ascites may be present in some patients with tuberculous peritonitis.

## Case 306

## ILEOCECAL TUBERCULOSIS

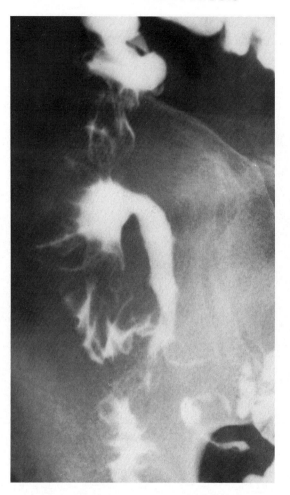

The terminal ileum is narrowed with fine contour irregularities. The cecum is contracted. The ileocecal valve is widely patent. Tuberculosis was found at laparotomy.

Tuberculosis involving the gastrointestinal tract is now a rare disease in this country, but it continues to be common in other parts of the world. Many patients with gastrointestinal tuberculosis will have a normal chest radiograph. Tuberculosis can affect any part of the gastrointestinal tract, but the distal small bowel and cecal region are most often affected. Pathologically, granulomas form in the bowel wall. These granulomas can ulcerate or form a localized mass. Nodal and peritoneal involvement are common. Chronic infection leads to fibrosis and luminal narrowing. Clinical symptoms are vague—weight loss and malaise—often suggesting the possibility of an underlying malignancy.

Radiologically, findings on barium examinations of the small bowel can mimic Crohn's disease. Ulcerations, luminal narrowing, multiple segmental regions of involvement, bowel-wall thickening, fistulae, and a localized mass are typical. The cecum may be shrunken and deformed (acutely as a result of spasm and chronically from fibrosis). The ileocecal valve may be patulous and incompetent.

Differential considerations usually include Crohn's disease and amebiasis. Amebic changes (Case 458) rarely occur above the terminal ileum. It is probably impossible to distinguish Crohn's disease (Cases 292–298) from tuberculosis on the basis of the radiologic findings. Lesions elsewhere in the alimentary tract can mimic and can be indistinguishable from carcinoma.

Case 307

# ABDOMINAL TUBERCULOSIS

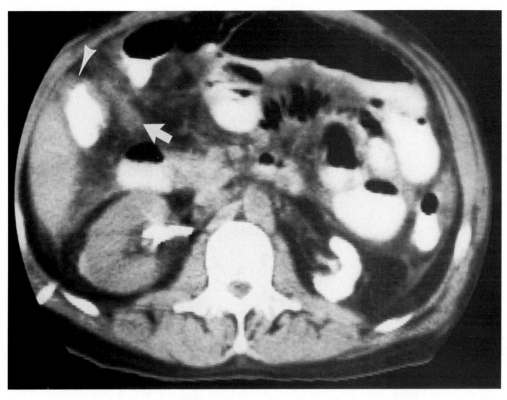

The mesenteric fat is of increased density due to soft-tissue stranding and variable-sized masses *(arrow)*. The anterior pararenal fascia is thickened. The wall of the right colon is thickened *(arrowhead)*. The left kidney is shrunken and homogeneously hyperdense (no intravenous contrast material was administered), consistent with tuberculous nephropathy (putty kidney). A nephrostomy tube is present within the right kidney and collecting system. Findings in the peritoneal cavity were shown to be due to tuberculous peritonitis.

Tuberculosis in the United States today is usually found among immunosuppressed individuals, alcoholics, drug abusers, diabetics, cancer patients, and those on steroid therapy. Tuberculous peritonitis is a relatively rare manifestation of this disease, occurring in less than 4% of all patients with tuberculosis (Carrera et al., 1976). Ascites, mesenteric soft-tissue stranding, and mesenteric adenopathy are usual radiographic findings. Adenopathy in patients with tuberculosis involves predominantly the upper abdomen within the mesentery and the peripancreatic nodal groups. Low-density centers within the nodes can occasionally be identified. Infection with either *Mycobacterium tuberculosis* or *M. avian* can yield similar radiographic findings. Infection with *M. avian* is more common among patients with AIDS. The diagnosis of tuberculosis requires a high level of awareness in the correct clinical setting. CT-directed biopsy and culture of enlarged lymph nodes can be helpful in establishing the correct diagnosis.

## Case 308

## ASCARIASIS

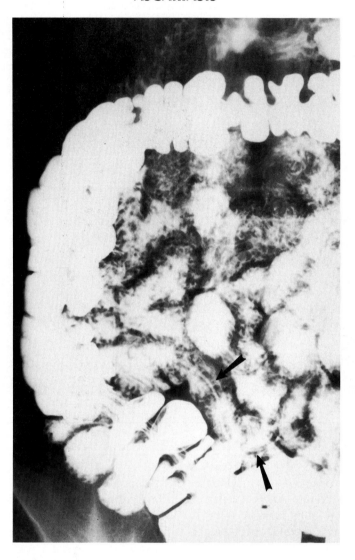

An elongated filling defect *(arrows)* is present in the distal small bowel. These changes are typical of ascariasis. A thin white line traverses the length of the worm, representing ingested barium.

Ascariasis is a common roundworm infection encountered most frequently in tropical climates. Infection is acquired by ingesting contaminated water, food, or soil. Ingested eggs hatch in the small bowel, penetrate the intestinal mucosa, and are carried to the lungs by the portal system or intestinal lymphatics. The worms perforate the alveoli, travel up the bronchi, and are swallowed. Worms grow, reproduce, and shed infectious eggs, usually within the distal small bowel. In-

volved organ systems include: respiratory (pneumonia, bronchitis, hemoptysis, and asthma), gastrointestinal (nausea, vomiting, distension, and tenderness), and biliary (jaundice, cholecystitis, cholangitis, pancreatitis, and hepatic abscess).

Radiographically, identification of the typical, elongated filling defect is characteristic. Mucosal folds may be thickened. Occasionally, the mass of worms can be large enough to cause partial or complete intestinal obstruction. A worm may be identified at sonography or endoscopic retrograde cholangiopancreatography in the biliary tree or pancreatic duct.

Case 309

## PEUTZ-JEGHERS SYNDROME

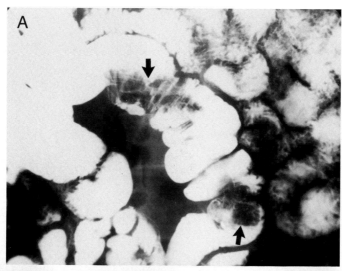

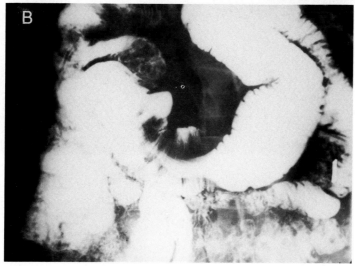

**A.** Two large lobulated polyps *(arrows)* are present in the mid small bowel. These hamartomas were surgically removed in this patient with Peutz-Jeghers syndrome.

**B.** Transient intussusception with the typical coiled-spring appearance was observed. A polyp was the lead point.

Hamartomatous polyps are most often found in the small bowel in patients younger than age 30 years—the majority of these patients have Peutz-Jeghers syndrome. The small-bowel polyps are often cauliflower-like, found in groups, and located within the jejunum. Patients may present with bleeding, pain, or obstruc-

tion from intussusception. Usually these lesions are benign, but adenocarcinomas have been reported in the gastrointestinal tract (usually stomach, duodenum, or colon) (Dodds, 1976). Ovarian cysts and tumors are found in a minority (5%) of female patients with Peutz-Jeghers syndrome (Dozois et al., 1970).

Peutz-Jeghers syndrome is inherited as an autosomal dominant disease. Hamartomas most often affect the small bowel, but approximately one-quarter of patients will have similar polyps in the stomach. Colonic polyps in these patients are adenomatous (Dodds, 1976). Brown pigmented spots on the perioral mucous surfaces are typical.

## Case 310

## ⸺ LEIOMYOMA

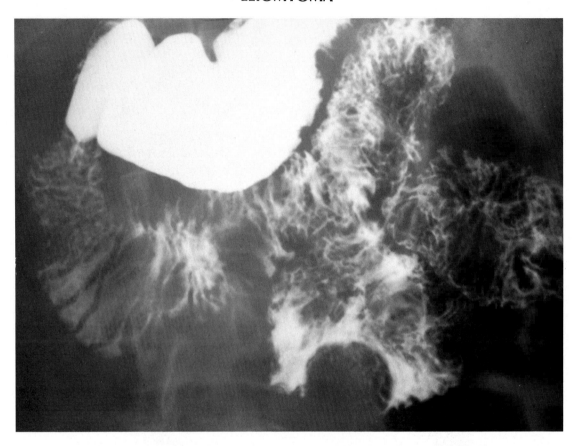

A well-marginated, smooth-surfaced filling defect is present in the jejunum. At operation, a leiomyoma was removed.

Smooth muscle tumors of the small bowel are most frequent within the jejunum. They are encountered less often than smooth muscle neoplasms of the esophagus or stomach. The radiographic appearance of these tumors depends on their location within the bowel wall. Subserosal leiomyomas may be undetected unless adja-

cent small-bowel loops are displaced by the mass. Submucosal tumors will appear as typical intramural lesions elsewhere in the gastrointestinal tract. Some may grow intraluminally and appear as a polypoid mass. Gastrointestinal bleeding is the usual symptom. The bleeding usually occurs as short repeated episodes of melena or dark red stool. Even in the absence of active bleeding, these tumors may be detectable at angiography because of their hypervascularity.

## Case 311

## LIPOMA

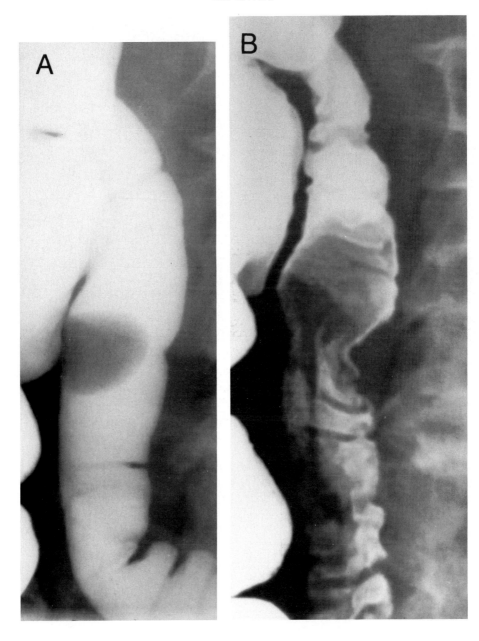

**A.** A smooth-surfaced, well-defined filling defect is present in the ileum.

**B.** The mass has changed in shape with peristalsis and compression. A lipoma was removed surgically.

Lipomas are the third most frequently occurring benign small-bowel tumor. They can be encountered anywhere in the alimentary tract. In the small bowel they are usually seen distally. Most are asymptomatic.

Symptoms, when present, are often due to an intussusception. Occasionally, obstruction or bleeding can develop. These tumors have no malignant potential.

Radiographically, the smooth surface and compressible nature of these masses suggest the diagnosis. The fatty density of these tumors is diagnostic at CT (Case 312 B).

## Case 312

## MULTIPLE INTESTINAL LIPOMAS

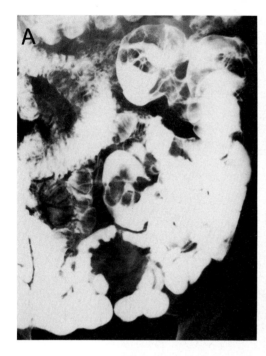
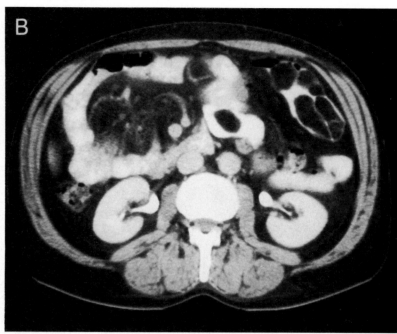

**A.** Multiple, well-defined, smooth-surfaced filling defects are present within several small-bowel loops.

**B.** Multiple masses the density of fat are present within several loops of small intestine. The density of these masses is diagnostic of lipomas.

CT is usually not a primary screening tool for small-bowel tumors, but it can be helpful in confirming a diagnosis if a lesion that resembles a lipoma is found on conventional barium studies. If the typical fat density of

*B, From Ormson MJ, Stephens DH, Carlson HC. AJR 1985;144:313–314. By permission of the American Roentgen Ray Society.*

these tumors is identified at CT, the diagnosis of a lipoma can be made unequivocally. Rarely, multiple lipomas will be present (as in this case). No surgical therapy is necessary if patients are asymptomatic. Intestinal lipomatosis can be distinguished from a liposarcoma by the homogeneous fat density and absence of intratumoral soft tissue density in lipomas. Multiple small-bowel lesions can be found in patients with lymphoma, a polyposis syndrome, hemangiomas, neurofibromas, and metastases. At CT, the tumors in all these other conditions are the density of soft tissue.

**Case 313**

## HEMANGIOMA

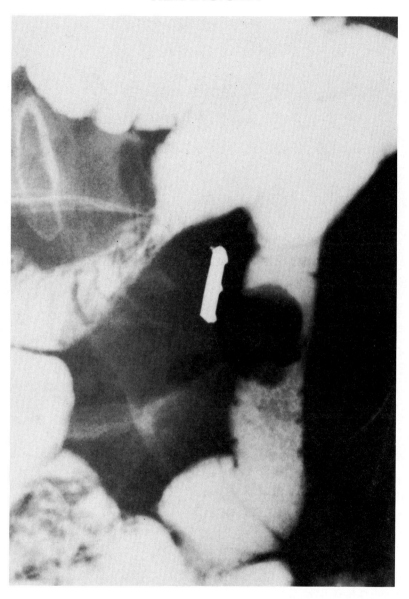

A smooth-surfaced filling defect is present in the small bowel. This extramucosal mass could be due to any intramural tumor. A hemangioma was removed surgically. A compression device containing a metallic marker is present.

Hemangiomas are rare tumors of the small bowel that usually affect the jejunum. Bleeding, intussusception, and rarely obstruction are the most frequently associated symptoms. Pathologically, multiple thin-walled vessels are seen either intraluminally or within the wall of the small bowel. Patients with Turner's syndrome, tuberous sclerosis, Blue-Rubber-Bleb syndrome, and Rendu-Osler-Weber syndrome have an increased incidence of this disorder.

Radiologically, hemangiomas usually present as focal masses but occasionally can be diffuse malformations. Many are multiple, small compressible lesions and can be easily overlooked during a small-bowel examination. Larger malformations may contain multiple phleboliths that are detectable on a plain film radiograph.

## Case 314

## DIFFUSE HEMANGIOMATOSIS

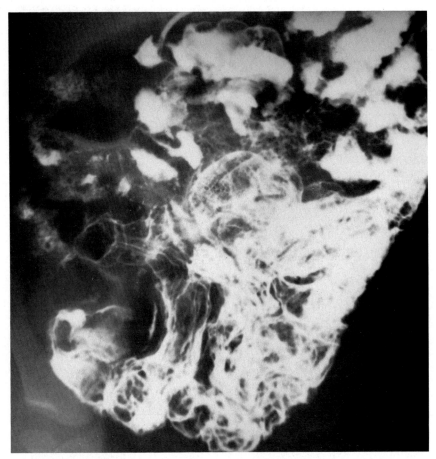

Multiple submucosal and intraluminal filling defects are present within the distal small bowel. Diffuse hemangiomatosis was surgically confirmed.

Diffuse hemangiomatosis is a rare cause of gastrointestinal bleeding; it usually occurs in infants. Intussusception, obstruction, and malabsorption can also cause symptoms. This condition may be associated with other syndromes, including Klippel-Trenaunay-Weber syndrome (varicose veins, cutaneous hemangiomas, soft tissue and bone hypertrophy), Maffucci's syndrome (enchondromas, subcutaneous cavernous hemangiomas),

and diffuse hemangiomatosis. There is a spectrum of disease ranging from small submucosal nodules to diffuse intestinal-wall involvement with associated extension into the mesentery, retroperitoneum, and other adjacent tissues. Bowel-wall phleboliths may suggest a diagnosis but are an unusual radiographic finding. Angiography can be helpful in detecting and classifying vascular abnormalities of the alimentary tract. Dynamic CT has also been reported to be diagnostic in this condition (Bank et al., 1987).

## Case 315

# INFLAMMATORY FIBROID POLYP

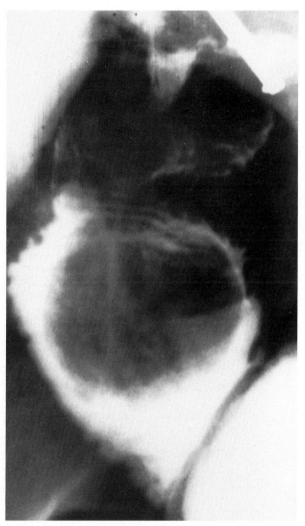

A round filling defect is present in the ileum. An inflammatory fibroid polyp was surgically removed.

These polyps are rarely encountered and are not true neoplasms histologically. They have been called by various names: infective granuloma, fibroma, hemangiopericytoma, neurinoma, plasma cell granuloma, and Vanek tumor. Histologically, many cell types are found, including fibroblasts, endothelial cells, histiocytes, leukocytes, and small blood vessels. This mixture of cells resembles reparative tissue. The cause of these tumors is unknown, but they can lead to intussusception and obstruction. Radiologically, they are indistinguishable from other polypoid small-bowel tumors.

Case 316

# CARCINOID TUMOR

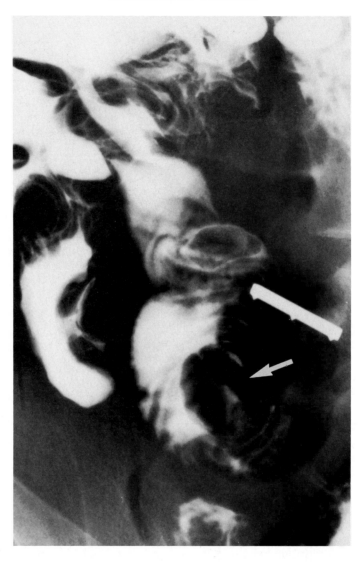

An ulcerated submucosal mass *(arrow)* is present in the distal ileum. At operation a primary ileal carcinoid tumor was removed. A compression device containing a metallic marker is present.

Carcinoid tumors are neuroendocrine neoplasms derived from Kulchitsky cells that can be found throughout the intestinal tract. Their neural-crest origin and biochemical behavior have led to their classification as an APUD (amine precursor uptake and decarboxylation) tumor. These tumors usually produce 5-hydroxytryptamine (serotonin). 5-Hydroxyindoleacetic acid is a useful biologic marker produced by the degradation of serotonin; it can be measured in the serum or urine

of these patients. Malignant transformation usually occurs in tumors ≥1 cm in diameter (Moertel et al., 1961). Carcinoids are usually found in the distal small bowel; nearly 40% are within 2 feet of the ileocecal valve. About 30% of patients have more than 1 tumor. Nearly one-third of patients will also have a second primary malignancy (Moertel et al., 1961).

Radiographic features of the primary tumor are usually those of an intramural neoplasm, usually 2 to 3 cm in diameter. Ulceration may be present. Often the primary neoplasm is not detected radiographically, and evidence of mesenteric metastases is generally found (Case 317).

**Case 317**

## CARCINOID TUMOR

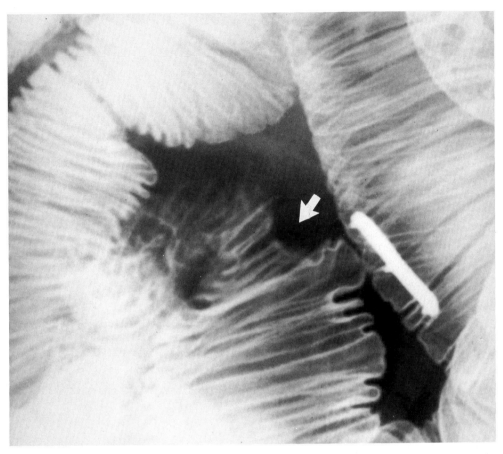

Kinking of a small-bowel loop as well as a submucosal mass *(arrow)* is present on this enteroclysis small-bowel examination. This patient had a known carcinoid tumor. A compression device with metallic marker is present.

Carcinoid tumors initially spread by direct invasion through the bowel wall into the mesentery. A fibrotic reaction ensues within the mesentery, with kinking and obstruction of the bowel. Usually obstruction is only partial, and patients may complain of symptoms attrib-

utable to partial mechanical obstruction for many years. Advanced disease with mesenteric metastases may result in separation of small-bowel loops, tethering of small-bowel folds, encasement, and luminal narrowing. The radiographic findings of mesenteric metastases are not specific for carcinoid tumors. Similar findings can also be seen with other malignancies. Kinking and tethered folds can also be caused by adhesions and a localized inflammatory process.

Case 318

# CARCINOID TUMOR

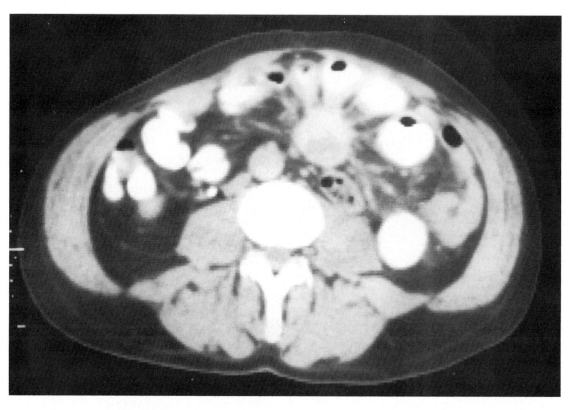

A partially necrotic mesenteric mass is associated with marked thickening and stranding of mesenteric tissues. This combination of a mesenteric mass and desmoplastic stranding is typical of a carcinoid tumor.

CT evaluation of patients with known or suspected carcinoid tumors can be helpful. The primary tumor is often not detected, but the extent of mesenteric dis-

ease, retroperitoneal adenopathy, and hepatic metastases can be assessed. The metastases in the small-bowel mesentery often have a typical "starburst" appearance, with linear stranding radiating from a central mesenteric mass (as seen in this case). Liver metastases are hypervascular, often containing regions of central necrosis. Retroperitoneal adenopathy is frequently encountered but rarely found without hepatic or mesenteric metastasis.

*From Dudiak KM, Johnson CD, Stephens DH.* AJR *1989;152:995–998. By permission of the American Roentgen Ray Society.*

## Case 319

## CARCINOID: INTESTINAL ISCHEMIA

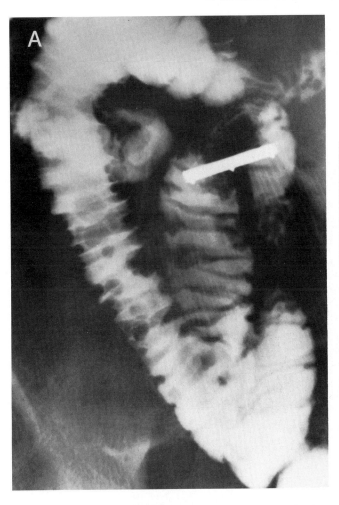

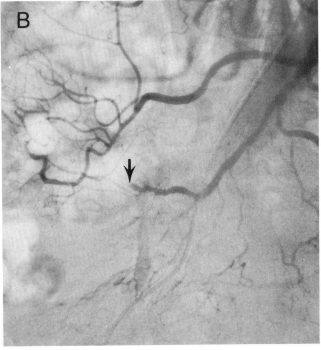

**A.** A loop of ileum has numerous straight and thickened folds. Intramural edema and hemorrhage from ischemia could cause these changes, although this appearance is nonspecific. A compression device with a metallic marker is present.

**B.** Occlusion and irregularity of the distal branches of the ileocolic artery *(arrow)* are shown. At operation metastatic carcinoid tumor had encased and occluded these affected vessels.

Carcinoid tumor often metastasizes to regional and distant lymph nodes. Tumor extension can cause arterial encasement and occlusion, with associated bowel ischemia and infarction. This is a common cause of death in patients with small-bowel carcinoids. Angiography is usually required to establish the diagnosis of bowel ischemia. Common angiographic findings include arterial irregularity, kinking, encasement, and occlusion.

## Case 320

## NON-HODGKIN'S LYMPHOMA

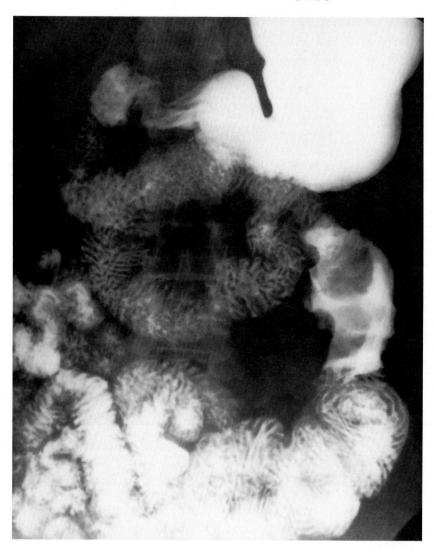

A circumferential ulcerated mass involves a relatively long segment of proximal small bowel. The lumen is larger than the adjacent normal small-bowel lumen, exemplifying "aneurysmal dilatation."

Small-bowel lymphoma constitutes 20% of all malignant small-bowel tumors (Dragosics et al., 1985). The vast majority of tumors are of the non-Hodgkin variety. Usual symptoms include nausea, vomiting, weight loss, and abdominal pain. Although there are no known predisposing factors, patients with conditions such as AIDS, celiac sprue, Crohn's disease, and systemic lupus erythematosus have a higher risk of the disease developing.

There are several radiologic classifications for lymphoma. The traditional classification includes: multiple nodules (Case 277), infiltrating form (Case 324), polypoid (Case 323), and endo-exoenteric (Cases 321 and 322) with excavation and fistula formation. An abbreviated classification recently proposed (Rubesin et al., 1990) includes primary form, lymphoma complicating sprue, and mesenteric nodal form. The traditional classification describes only primary small-bowel lymphoma, whereas the latter classification emphasizes secondary forms of the disease. This case is an example of the primary endo-exoenteric lymphoma with excavation.

## Case 321

# CAVITATED LYMPHOMA

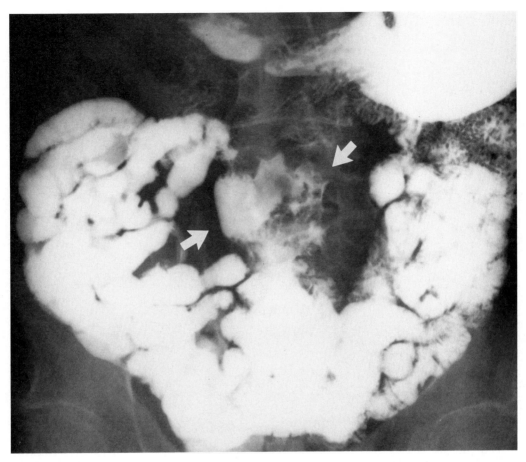

A large mass *(arrows)* is present within the small bowel mesentery. A large ulcerated region occupies the central portion of this mass. This could be considered an "aneurysmal" or a cavitary lesion, typical of primary lymphoma.

Non-Hodgkin's lymphoma is generally a large and bulky tumor. These tumors do not incite the usual desmoplastic reaction found with other neoplasms. Little resistance occurs as the tumor infiltrates the muscularis propria. The tumor can easily grow and expand within the bowel wall and mesentery. Ulceration, necrosis, and excavation lead to the opacified cavity seen in this case. The lack of desmoplastic containment of the tumor explains why some of these tumors perforate or develop fistulae. Obstruction is a rare occurrence.

## Case 322

## EXCAVATED LYMPHOMA

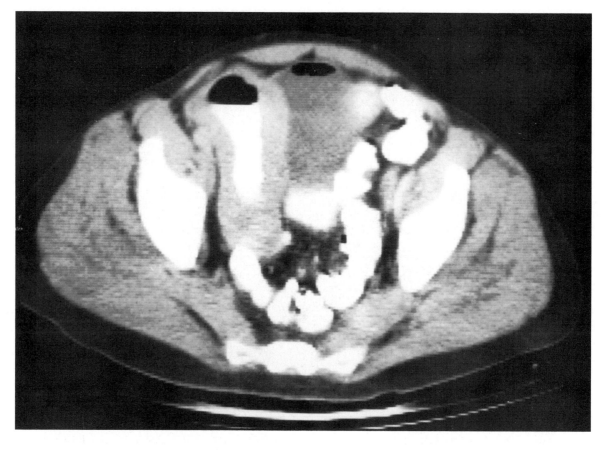

A large lesion encases a distal small-bowel loop. Marked bowel-wall thickening is present. The lumen is dilated. This appearance at CT is typical of lymphoma in the small intestine.

*From Dudiak KM, Johnson CD, Stephens DH. AJR* **1989;**152:995–998. By permission of the American Roentgen Ray Society.

**Case 323**

## LYMPHOMA: POLYPOID MASS

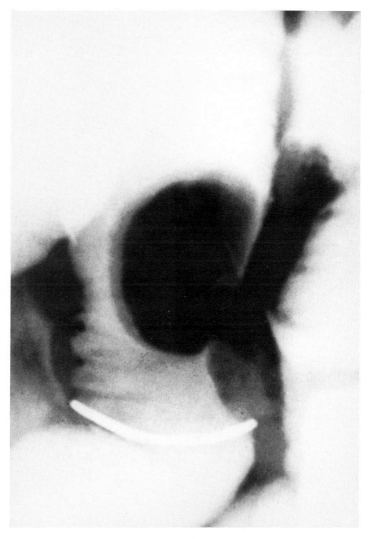

An intraluminal polypoid mass is present within the small bowel. A polypoid lymphomatous mass was surgically excised.

Solitary intraluminal masses are unusual manifestations of lymphoma. It is believed that the mass arises within the submucosa of the bowel wall and as a result of peristalsis, it forms a predominantly intraluminal mass, sometimes attached to the bowel wall by a pseudopedicle. The mass could become the lead point for an intussusception.

## Case 324

# POLYPOID LYMPHOMA

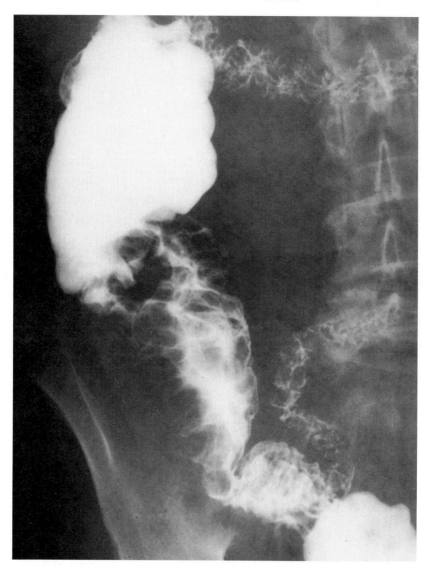

A long segment of terminal ileum is involved with multiple, submucosal, polypoid filling defects. The lumen is increased in diameter. The submucosal location and long length of the lesion are typical of lymphoma.

This form of lymphoma often involves the distal ileum and can cross the ileocecal valve and affect the cecum.

## Case 325

## LYMPHOMA

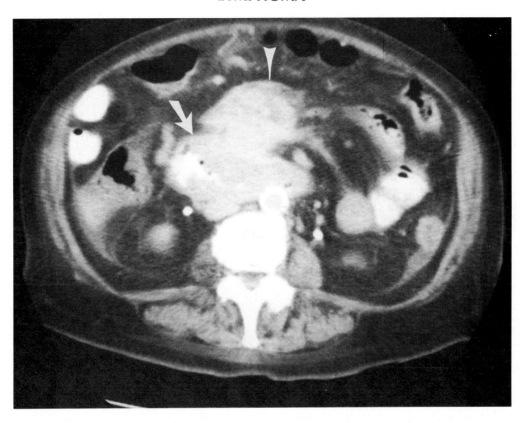

Marked wall thickening *(arrow)* affects a distal small-bowel loop. In addition, adjacent adenopathy *(arrowhead)* encases mesenteric vessels. Mesenteric or, less

often, retroperitoneal adenopathy, or both, may be present in any form of primary small-bowel lymphoma. In this case, lymphoma within the bowel wall appears to be the site of origin of the tumor, with secondary spread to mesenteric lymph nodes.

*From Dudiak KM, Johnson CD, Stephens DH. AJR 1989;152:995–998. By permission of the American Roentgen Ray Society.*

Case 326

# LYMPHOMA: INVASIVE MESENTERIC FORM

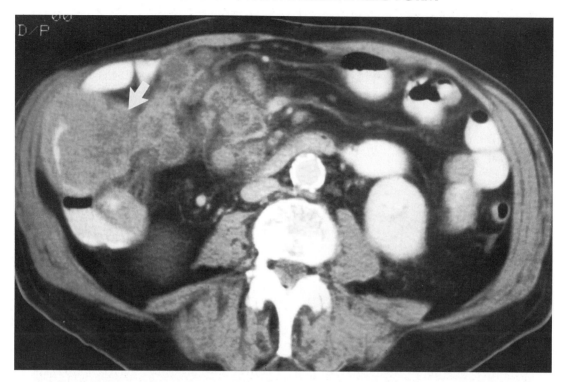

Centrally necrotic mesenteric lymphadenopathy is seen in the right side of the abdomen. These lymph nodes coalesce and form a mass *(arrow)* that displaces and narrows the terminal ileum.

In some patients the bulk of the tumor is extraluminal, within mesenteric lymph nodes. This mass can become quite large and cause narrowing, displacement, angulation, and local bowel invasion. This is an example of the mesenteric-nodal form of non-Hodgkin's lymphoma.

**Case 327**

# HODGKIN'S LYMPHOMA

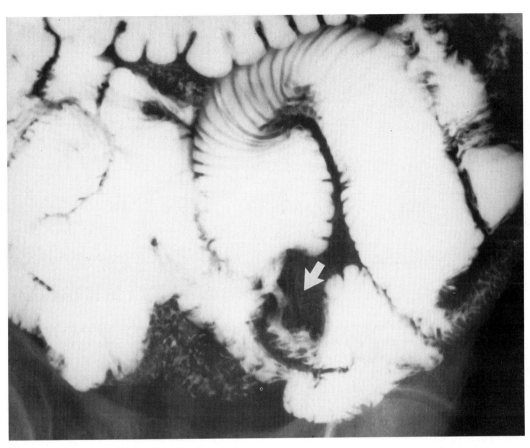

A focal region of ulcerative constriction *(arrow)* is present in the mid small bowel. The loop proximal to the stenosis is dilated, indicating partial mechanical obstruction.

Hodgkin's lymphoma of the small bowel is less common than non-Hodgkin's lymphoma. Unlike non-Hodgkin's lymphoma, these tumors can incite a desmoplastic reaction, producing luminal narrowing and at times obstruction. Other patterns of lymphoma can also be seen: diffuse fold thickening and irregularity, long segmental regions of involvement, and ulceration. "Aneurysmal ulceration," perforation, and fistulization are distinctly uncommon. In this patient, a primary carcinoma (Case 328) could have an identical appearance.

Case 328

# ADENOCARCINOMA

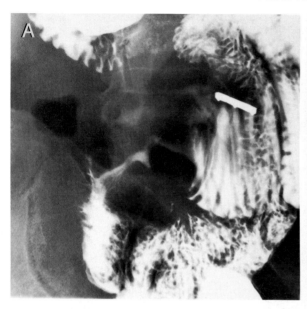

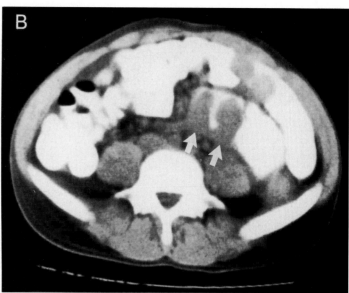

**A.** An ulcerative annular constrictive lesion is present in the mid small bowel. The abrupt margins and narrowed lumen are typical of a primary adenocarcinoma. The tumor is partially obstructive with mild proximal-bowel dilatation. A compression device with a metallic marker is present.

**B.** A lobulated soft tissue mass *(arrows)* narrows the small-bowel lumen and thickens its wall. The focal, short segment of bowel-wall thickening is typical of adenocarcinoma at CT.

*From Dudiak KM, Johnson CD, Stephens DH.* AJR *1989;152:995–998. By permission of the American Roentgen Ray Society.*

Primary small-bowel adenocarcinoma is most commonly found in the proximal small bowel, usually the duodenum. Patients are often symptomatic: abdominal pain, obstruction, bleeding, or anemia.

There is an increased incidence of this tumor in patients with adult celiac disease and a small increased risk with regional enteritis. Radiographically, a focal region of narrowing with mucosal ulceration is usually seen on barium studies. Detection of these lesions can be difficult at CT if the tumor is less than 2 cm in diameter. Focal circumferential bowel-wall thickening in the proximal small bowel is characteristic of an adenocarcinoma at CT.

**Case 329**

## ADENOCARCINOMA

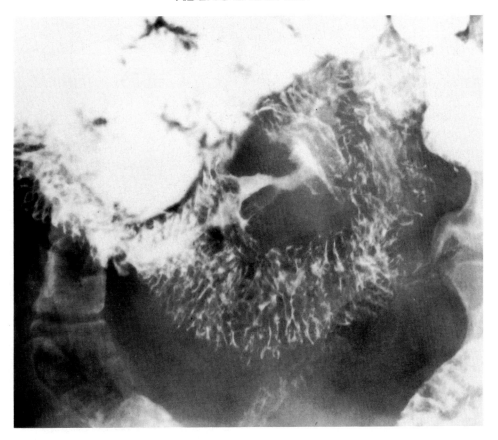

A typical "apple core" lesion is present in the jejunum. Notice the absence of normal mucosal markings through this lesion. The contour of the lesion is irregular and the mucosal surface has a smudged appearance due to ulceration. The short annular nature of the lesion is characteristic of an adenocarcinoma.

## Case 330

# LEIOMYOSARCOMA

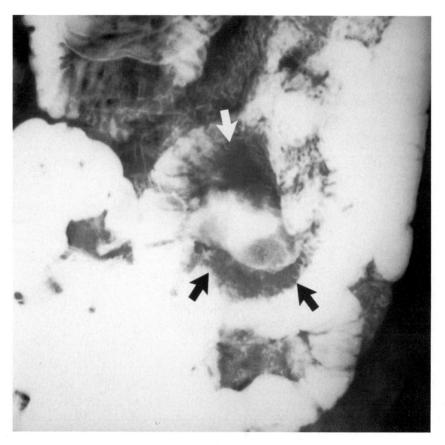

An ulcerated mass *(arrows)* is present in the proximal small bowel. Ulcerated lumen is expanded compared to adjacent small-bowel loops. Differential considerations included lymphoma, leiomyosarcoma, or metastasis. At operation, a leiomyosarcoma was removed.

Smooth muscle tumors can be divided by their gross pathologic features into intramural, exoenteric, endoenteric, and dumbbell growths. The exoenteric growths are most commonly encountered and can incorporate bowel lumen (as seen in this case). Ulcer-

ation, necrosis, degeneration, hemorrhage, fistula, and infection can often be found in these tumors. These tumors metastasize by hematogenous and peritoneal seeding. Nodal metastases are distinctly uncommon. In the absence of metastases, the size of the primary tumor is the most important predictor of malignancy. Debulking of even grossly incurable tumors is often performed because patients may have prolonged periods of remission after such a procedure.

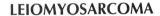

## Case 331

## LEIOMYOSARCOMA

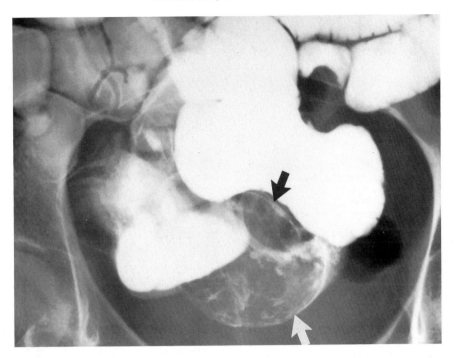

A large intraluminal filling defect *(arrows)* is present within the small bowel. A leiomyosarcoma was surgically removed.

Smooth muscle tumors may grow predominantly intraluminally. Other masses that could present as an intraluminal filling defect include adenomas, lipomas (Cases 311 and 312), hemangiomas (Case 313), hamartomas (Case 309), and foreign bodies. Lipomas may be suspected because of their soft and changeable shape. Hamartomas could be suspected in patients with Peutz-Jeghers syndrome. Pathologic distinction between benign and malignant smooth muscle tumors can be difficult. Large tumors (>5 cm) are more frequently sarcomatous.

**Case 332**

# LEIOMYOSARCOMA

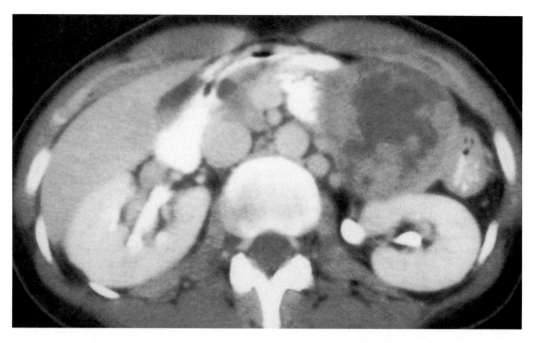

A large mixed-density mass is present in the upper abdomen. The low attenuation central zone is due to necrosis—a common finding for leiomyosarcomas at CT (Dudiak et al., 1989). This surgically proven leiomyosarcoma was an exophytic mass arising from the small bowel.

CT is particularly helpful in this case because the nature of the mass can be suggested, and hepatic metastases can be identified if present. Surgical removal of smooth muscle tumors is a preferred treatment option because these tumors are radioresistant and unresponsive to current chemotherapeutic agents.

### Case 333

## METASTASES: SUBMUCOSAL NODULES

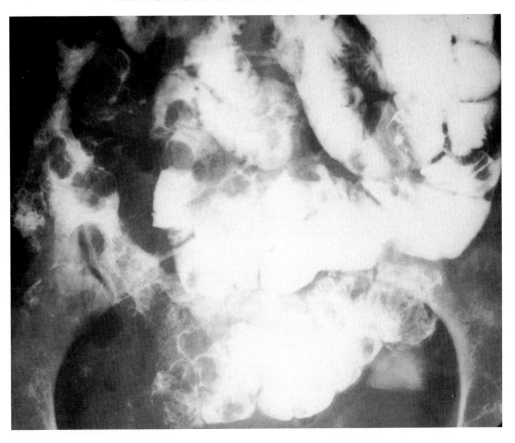

Multiple filling defects are present throughout the small bowel. They are smooth surfaced (indicating their intramural location) and uniform size. The sheer number and size of the lesions suggest metastases—in this patient, secondary to melanoma.

Metastatic melanoma metastasizes widely and usually spreads hematogenously to the gastrointestinal tract. The small bowel is involved in 50% of cases at autopsy, followed by the colon and stomach (Reintgen et al., 1984). The metastatic lesions may appear as nodules (as in this case and Case 334), plaques, or polypoid masses (Case 336). Central necrosis is common and may result in a bull's-eye lesion (target appearance) (Case 335) or large ulceration within a mass (Case 339).

Differential considerations include metastases from other sources, including Kaposi's sarcoma, lymphoma, other hematogenously seeded metastases, and polyposis syndromes. Fortunately, the diagnosis of melanoma is usually known by the time intestinal metastases develop.

## Case 334

## SMALL BOWEL METASTASES: MELANOMA

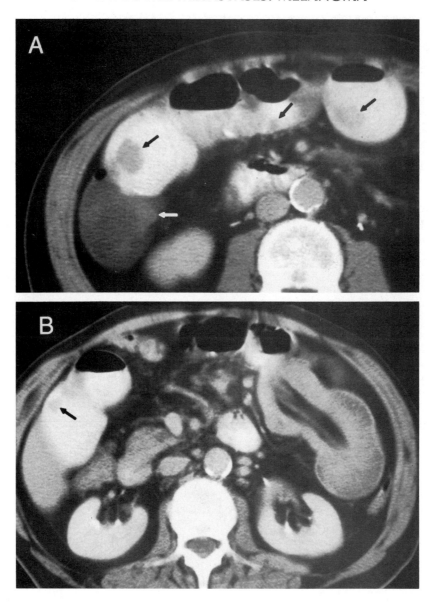

**A.** Multiple intraluminal filling defects *(arrows)* are seen in several bowel loops. Findings are typical of multiple, diffuse small-bowel metastases. This patient had a history of melanoma.

**B.** An intussusception is present in a small-bowel loop on the left side of the abdomen. The typical appearance of intraluminal mesenteric fat and vessels is diagnostic of this condition. There is also a small soft-tissue nodule *(arrow)* in another bowel loop.

Hematogenous seeding of the small bowel is most often seen in patients with melanoma, breast or lung cancer, and Kaposi's sarcoma. If a hematogenous metastasis grows to circumferentially engulf the bowel, it can resemble a primary adenocarcinoma (Cases 328 and 329). Melanoma metastases can present as multiple masses (as in this case), a solitary large mass (Case 336), or a bulky ulcerated lesion(s) (Case 337). Intraluminal masses can act as a lead point for an intussusception (as in this case), causing obstruction, bleeding, ischemia, perforation, and pain.

**Case 335**

## METASTASES: TARGET LESION

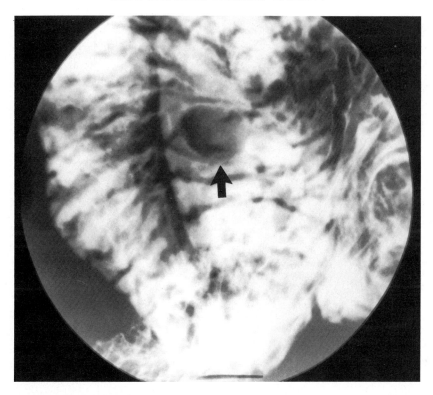

An intraluminal mass *(arrow)* is present within the small bowel. The mass contains a central ulceration (target lesion). Other lesions of similar appearance were also present in this patient with metastatic melanoma.

Ulcerated metastases are common in patients with melanoma, but nearly any metastases or primary tumor could present in this fashion. Primary small-bowel tumors such as leiomyosarcomas and lymphomas can have this appearance, but usually the mass and ulceration are larger. Kaposi's sarcoma, eosinophilic granuloma, and ectopic pancreatic tissue can also present as a target lesion.

**Case 336**

## METASTASES: SOLITARY POLYPOID LESION

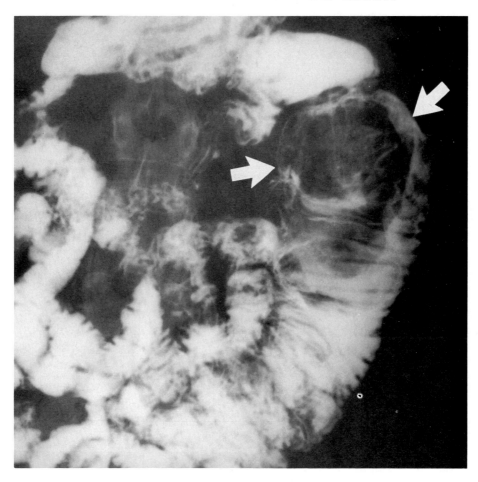

A large, intraluminal polypoid mass *(arrows)* is present within the proximal small bowel. Metastatic melanoma was confirmed at operation.

Intraluminal (as in this case) or ulcerated (Case 337) submucosal metastases can bleed, obstruct, or intussuscept (Case 334). Renal adenocarcinomas have a propensity to directly invade adjacent organs and present as bulky, intraluminal masses (Case 219). Often the retroperitoneal duodenum is involved. Any submucosal tumor can extrude into the lumen as a polypoid mass. Lipomas (Case 311), leiomyomas (Case 310), and leiomyosarcomas (Case 331) are the commonest primary small bowel tumors to protrude intraluminally as polypoid masses. The history of melanoma in this patient is helpful in making the correct diagnosis.

## Case 337

## METASTASES

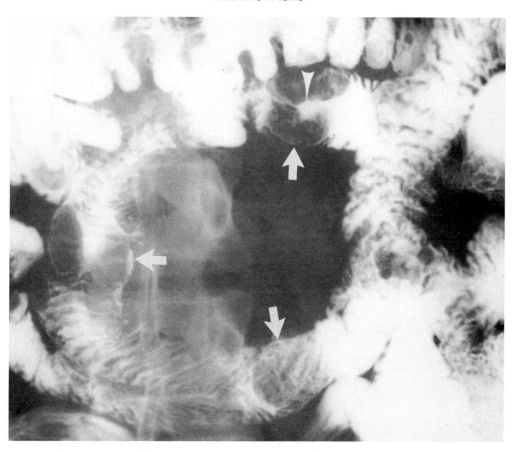

Multiple masses *(arrows)* are present within a small-bowel loop. The central portion *(arrowhead)* of some of these masses appears ulcerated. There is also a large mesenteric mass that displaces the small-bowel loop around it. Tethered folds adjacent to the mesenteric mass are also present. At operation, multiple metastases from a primary tumor of unknown origin were found.

Mesenteric metastases usually displace and indent adjacent small-bowel loops. An associated desmoplastic reaction is often present and causes luminal narrowing, kinking, fixation, and shortening. Ascites is also often present.

## Case 338

## METASTASES: INTUSSUSCEPTING MASS

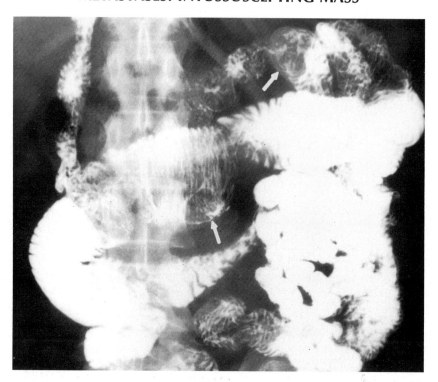

An intussusception involves a proximal small-bowel loop. In addition, several nodular masses *(arrows)* are also present. At operation, multiple metastases (adenocarcinoma) were found within the small bowel, including a metastasis acting as the lead point for the intussusception.

In adults, intussusceptions are usually secondary to a polypoid intraluminal mass (primary or secondary neoplasm). Spontaneous intussusceptions without a leading mass are frequently encountered in adults with celiac disease (Case 290). Obstruction and bowel ischemia are important complications of an intussusception. Patients often complain of nausea, vomiting, and colicky abdominal pain.

**Case 339**

## METASTASIS: EXCAVATED MASS

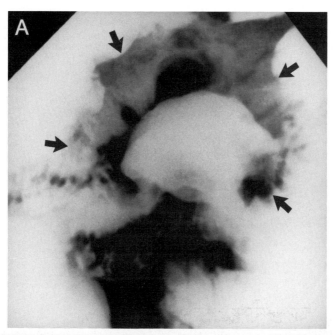

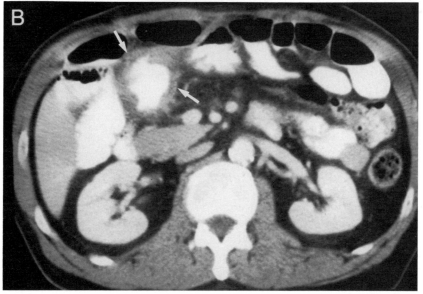

**A.** A large ulcerated mass *(arrows)* is present within the small bowel. The ulceration resembles the "aneurysmal" ulcer often seen in patients with lymphoma.

**B.** The mass *(arrows)* described above is seen at CT. A rind of soft tissue surrounds the ulcer. At operation, metastatic colon cancer was removed.

Some metastases will arise in the bowel wall and grow into the mesentery. Some authors refer to this as exoenteric growth, in which the tumor grows and destroys the bowel wall, forming a large cavitated mass devoid of mucosal markings. Tumors most likely to present in this manner include lymphoma (Cases 320–322), leiomyosarcoma (Case 332), and occasionally colon cancer.

## Case 340

## SEROSAL METASTASES

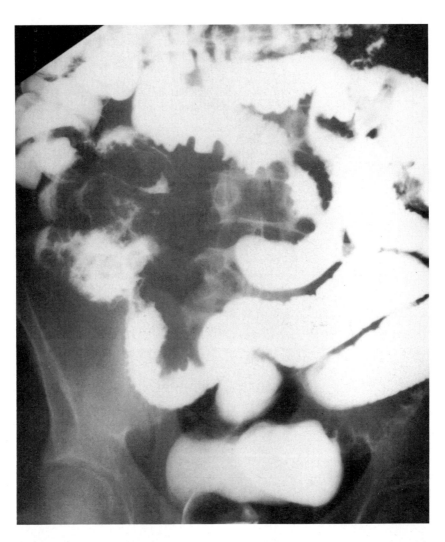

The small-bowel loops in the ileocecal region are displaced by a mesenteric mass. Many of the small-bowel folds appear tethered and thickened in response to the mesenteric abnormality. An inflammatory or infectious process or neoplasm could cause these changes. At operation, an appendiceal adenocarcinoma with serosal and mesenteric metastases was found.

Tumors that spread by intraperitoneal seeding will often implant and grow in three regions: the pouch of Douglas (the most dependent position in the pelvis), the ileocecal region, and the superior aspect of the sigmoid colon. Meyers (1981) described the anatomic regions and usual locations of metastatic implants. Serosal implants will displace adjacent bowel loops, narrow bowel lumen(s), cause angulation and kinking of loops, thicken small-bowel folds, and result in fold tacking and tethering (from direct invasion and mesenteric retraction). Primary tumors arising from the gastrointestinal tract or ovaries often spread by intraperitoneal seeding.

Case 341

## CALCIFIED METASTASES

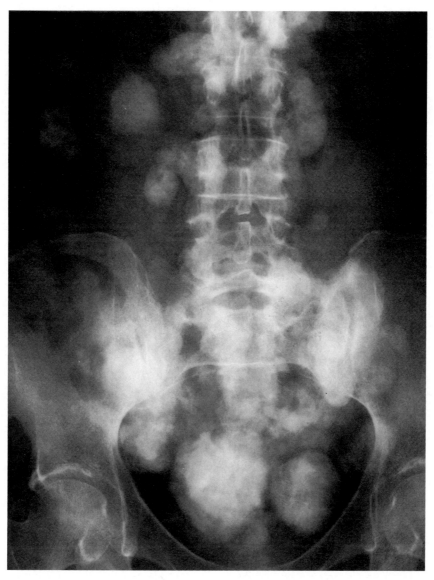

Multiple calcified masses are present throughout the abdomen. These masses represent calcified peritoneal metastases in this patient with a known cystadenocarcinoma of the ovary.

Metastatic mucinous tumors of the abdomen are the tumors that are most likely to calcify. These include cystadenocarcinomas of the ovary or appendix and well-differentiated adenocarcinomas of gastrointestinal origin. Subtle sandlike or curvilinear calcifications throughout the peritoneal cavity are seen most often. Occasionally, these tumors will form a jellylike (mucous) peritoneal rind (pseudomyxoma peritonei) that can also calcify (Case 398).

## Case 342

## PNEUMATOSIS INTESTINALIS

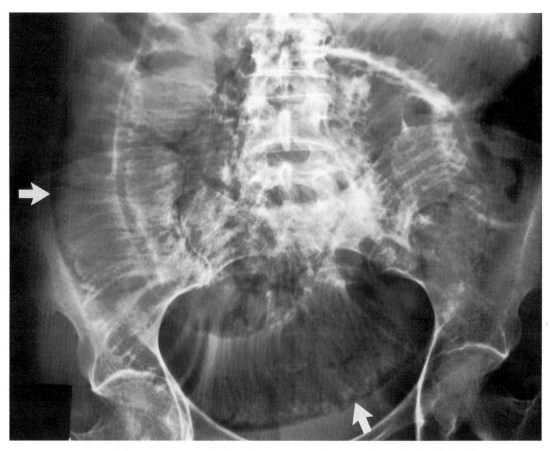

Extensive intramural gas *(arrows)* is present within the small bowel. This patient with scleroderma had been hospitalized several times for intestinal pseudo-obstruction. She recovered uneventfully. The pneumatosis was considered benign, secondary to her scleroderma and steroid medication.

Pneumatosis intestinalis, or air within the wall of the small bowel, can result from several causes. Commonly associated conditions include: steroid medications, scleroderma, chronic obstructive lung disease, and ischemic bowel. The exact cause is often not known, but many theories suggest that a slow-healing mucosal ulceration develops, followed by dissection of gas into the bowel wall. Alternatively, some authors have suggested that in patients with obstructive lung disease, air can dissect from the alveoli into the medi-

astinum, to retroperitoneum, and eventually to small-bowel mesentery and bowel wall. Patients are usually asymptomatic and do not require treatment for this condition unless they have ischemic bowel disease. Patients with ischemic bowel may have associated portal venous gas and bowel-wall thickening, and usually they require urgent surgical exploration.

Radiologically, a lucent rim that follows the contours of the bowel wall (as in this case) is pathognomonic. The air collections may appear cystlike or linear. Cystic pneumatosis (Case 466) is usually secondary to nonischemic disease states, whereas linear pneumatosis can be seen with any of the diseases listed above, including ischemic bowel (Cases 256 and 257). Occasionally, the intramural air collections escape into the peritoneal cavity and cause asymptomatic pneumoperitoneum.

Case 343

# SMALL BOWEL DIVERTICULOSIS

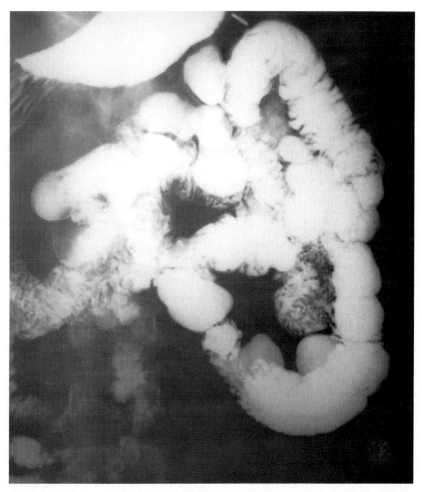

Diverticula are present throughout the small bowel and are most numerous in the jejunum.

Small-bowel diverticula are often encountered incidentally during the course of a small-bowel examination. The majority are singular or few in number, and most affect the proximal small bowel, especially the duodenum. Tiny diverticula can also be seen frequently arising from the terminal ileum. In our experience, most diverticula are incidental findings and rarely cause clinical symptoms. Occasionally, significant stasis occurs in one or more diverticula, resulting in bacterial overgrowth, macrocytic anemia, and vitamin B$_{12}$ deficiency. Malabsorption can be problematic as a result of bile acid deconjugation by the abundant bacteria and subsequent fat malabsorption. Bacterial exotoxins can also damage the intestinal lining and impair absorption. Bleeding (Taylor, 1969), perforation (Eckhauser et al., 1979), diverticulitis (Giustra et al., 1977), enterolith formation, and pneumoperitoneum (Dunn and Nelson, 1979) are other rarely reported complications.

## Case 344

## MECKEL'S DIVERTICULUM

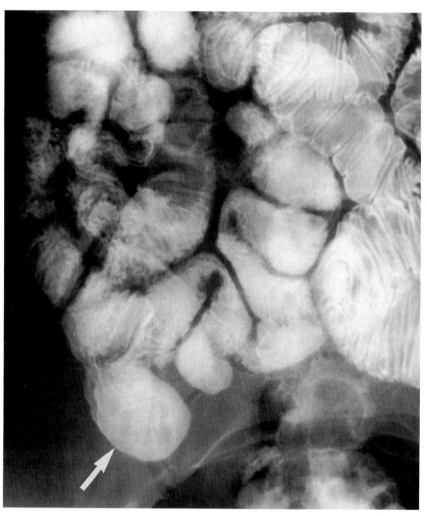

A diverticulum *(arrow)* arising from the distal small bowel is present in the right lower portion of the abdomen. This location is typical of Meckel's diverticulum.

Meckel's diverticulum is an outpouching of the small bowel representing the remnant of the omphalomesenteric duct (a connection between the yolk sac and the midgut). These diverticula are usually located within the distal 3 feet of the small bowel and approximately two-thirds contain heterotopic gastric mucosa. Symptoms can develop at any age, but most patients seek medical attention before age 3 years. Signs and symptoms usually include melena and abdominal pain. Ul-

ceration, perforation, intussusception, or enterolith formation have all been reported to occur in Meckel's diverticulum (Dalinka and Wunder, 1973).

Radiographic evaluation may include an abdominal plain film. Calcified enteroliths as well as free air or findings of a mechanical small-bowel obstruction may be seen. Barium examination of the small bowel may reveal the diverticulum; however, this entity is identified less frequently than the expected incidence (3%) for the general population. Some investigators believe an enteroclysis small-bowel examination is more sensitive in detecting this entity (Maglinte et al., 1980).

**Case 345**

## MECKEL'S DIVERTICULUM

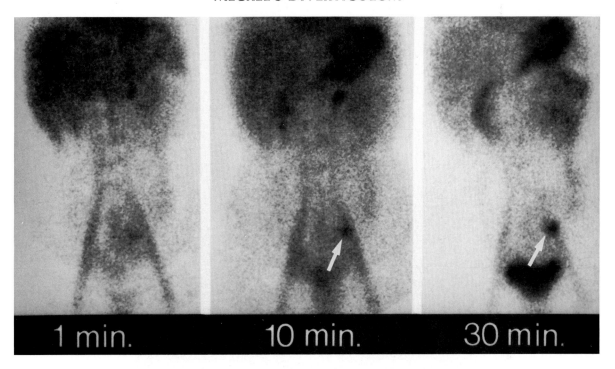

1 min.  10 min.  30 min.

A region of abnormally increased tracer *(arrows)* is visible in the left lower portion of the abdomen on this technetium pertechnetate study. This finding is consistent with a Meckel diverticulum containing ectopic gastric mucosa; however, usually tracer is identified in the right lower quadrant in this condition.

Technetium pertechnetate scans are useful in identifying patients with a Meckel diverticulum because it is taken up and secreted by gastric mucosa. Some controversy exists as to which cell type specifically accumulates the tracer. Because many Meckel's diverticula contain ectopic gastric mucosa, they can be identified with this examination. Organs that normally take up pertechnetate include stomach, salivary glands, early image blood pool, and urinary tract (because a small amount of tracer is cleared by the kidneys). Uptake can also occur in other organs with gastric mucosa, including Barrett's esophagus, duplication cysts, and ectopic islands of gastric mucosa in the small bowel.

## Case 346

## INVERTED MECKEL'S DIVERTICULUM

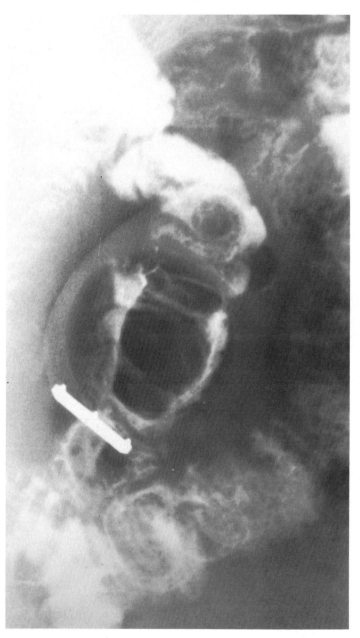

An oblong, sausage-shaped filling defect is present within the lumen of the distal small bowel. A compression device with a metallic marker is present. Differential considerations include polypoid tumors (lipoma, leiomyoma, leiomyosarcoma, hamartoma, adenoma, lymphoma), foreign bodies, and an inverted Meckel diverticulum. An inverted Meckel diverticulum was excised.

Other complications that can occur from Meckel's diverticulum include ulceration, bleeding, perforation, obstruction, intussusception, and enterolith formation (Dalinka and Wunder, 1973).

**Case 347**

## MALROTATION (NONROTATION)

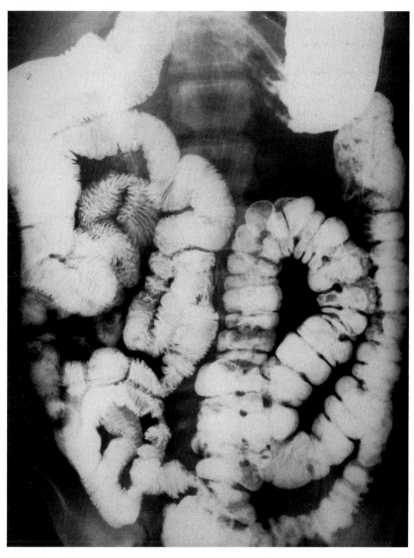

All of the small bowel occupies the right side of the abdomen. The colon resides on the left side of the abdomen. Findings are those of nonrotation of the alimentary tract.

Normally, the intestines undergo a rotation of 270° during fetal life. Rotation involves two major segments of intestine: the duodenal-jejunal region which migrates to its normal position early in fetal life and the cecocolic segments which enter the abdominal cavity and rotate into their normal positions later. Abnormalities of rotation can interrupt this sequence of events at

any stage of development, resulting in nonrotation (small bowel resides in the right portion of the abdomen, colon on the left); incomplete rotation (normal small-bowel rotation but the cecum is located in the left portion of the abdomen, epigastrium, or high on the right side); and incomplete mesenteric fixation (mobile cecum). Midgut volvulus or small-bowel obstruction from mesenteric bands is an important complication of malrotation (Case 348). Congenital diaphragmatic hernias and omphaloceles are also sequelae of nonrotation.

Case 348

## MALROTATION: LADD'S BANDS

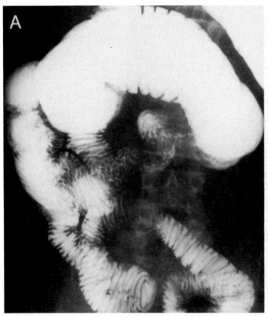

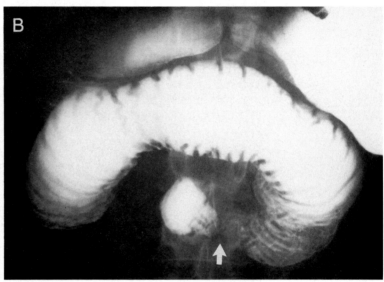

**A.** The small bowel occupies the right side of the abdomen, typical of nonrotation. The duodenum is dilated.

**B.** The stomach and duodenum are dilated and there is a low-lying duodenal-jejunal flexure. A region of high-grade narrowing *(arrow)* is present in the proximal jejunum.

The combination of nonrotation and a proximal small-bowel obstruction suggests Ladd's bands, midgut volvulus, or both.

Patients with malrotation have incomplete fixation of the small bowel or colon, or both, to the posterior peritoneum. This patient was found to have peritoneal bands (Ladd's bands), which attempt to fix the gut to the abdominal wall. These bands can compress and obstruct the small bowel (as in this case). The duodenum or proximal jejunum are the usual sites of obstruction by these bands.

## Case 349

# MALROTATION MIDGUT VOLVULUS

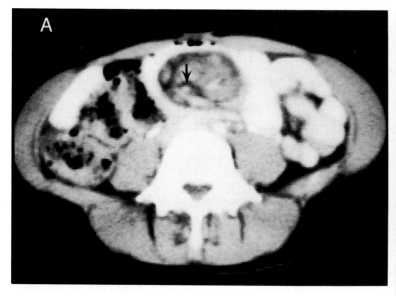

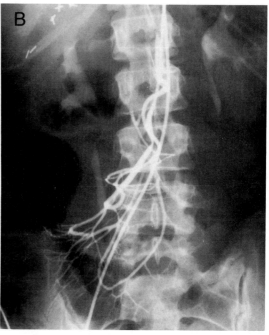

**A.** CT scan shows small bowel encircling the superior mesenteric artery *(arrow)* in a whorl-like pattern. Mesenteric fat parallels the bowel lumen as it encircles the superior mesenteric artery.

**B.** Selective superior mesenteric arteriogram demonstrates twisting and deformity of the superior mesenteric artery. These findings are diagnostic of midgut volvulus.

Patients with rotational anomalies of the gut lack normal posterior peritoneal attachments. Normal peritoneal attachments prevent the small bowel and colon from moving or twisting into an abnormal location or position. In the absence of sufficient fixation, the small bowel can twist about the superior mesenteric artery, leading to bowel obstruction and ischemia. Symptoms of obstruction usually develop. Urgent surgical repair is often required in order to prevent ischemia or to resect infarcted bowel loops. Intermittent or partial obstruction can lead to bowel congestion, edema, and symptoms of malabsorption.

Case 350

# GALLSTONE ILEUS

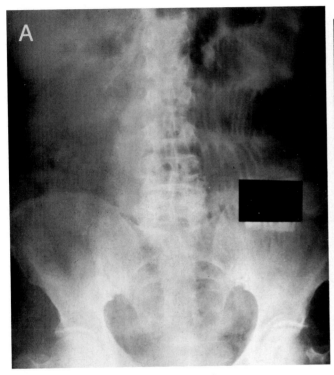

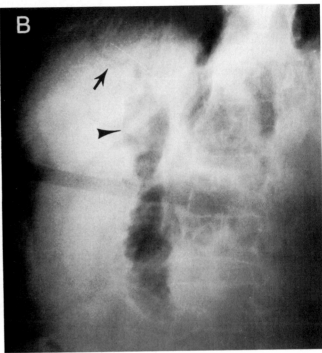

**A.** Multiple, dilated small-bowel loops are present with little visible colonic gas. Findings are consistent with a mechanical small-bowel obstruction.

**B.** A few linear gas lucencies representing the biliary tree *(arrow)* and gallbladder *(arrowhead)* are visible in the right upper quadrant. The combination of biliary gas and mechanical small-bowel obstruction is highly suggestive of gallstone ileus if no prior biliary operation has been performed. An obstructing radiolucent gallstone causing ileal obstruction was removed at laparotomy.

Gallstone ileus is a syndrome of mechanical small-bowel obstruction by gallstone(s). Classically, elderly women without prior biliary or abdominal disease present with acute intestinal obstruction. Symptoms of acute cholecystitis are unusual, but many patients will have a history of gallstones and recurrent cholecystitis (Hudspeth and McGuirt, 1970). Gallstones can erode into the stomach, small bowel, or colon. Stones in the small bowel most often cause obstruction at the ileocecal valve (the narrowest point). Obstructing stones usually are not spontaneously passed and require surgical lithotomy. Cholecystectomy and fistula repair are usually performed, but not acutely.

Radiographically, the triad of air within the biliary tree, ectopic calcified gallstone, and mechanical small-bowel obstruction is considered characteristic of this entity. Even the findings of biliary air and small-bowel obstruction should be regarded as consistent with gallstone ileus.

**Case 351**

## GALLSTONE ILEUS

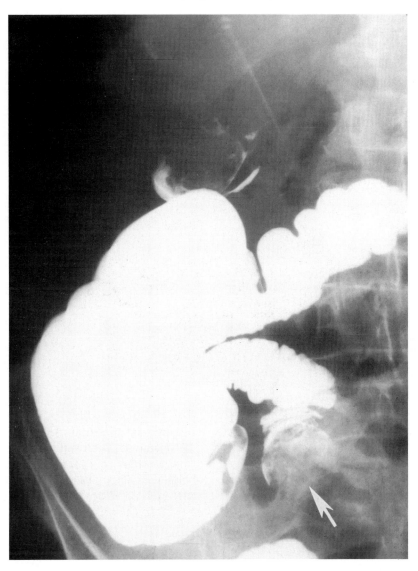

A cholecystocolonic fistula demonstrated during a barium enema examination is present as well as a smooth filling defect in the terminal ileum. Findings are those of gallstone ileus. The filling defect *(arrow)* in the ileum represents the ectopic obstructing gallstone.

Ectopic gallstones in patients with gallstone ileus may not be visible without using intraluminal contrast material during the radiographic examination. Patients with a suspected mechanical small-bowel obstruction should first have an enema with contrast material. This study will exclude a proximal colonic obstruction, and often contrast material can be refluxed into the distal ileum. A radiolucent gallstone can often be identified because stones usually obstruct near the ileocecal valve. Once an obstructing stone is found, operation is indicated because these gallstones rarely pass spontaneously. Many gallstones will pass through the ileocecal valve without causing symptoms. Cholecystocolonic fistulae often cause diarrhea and steatorrhea because of the diversion of bile from the small bowel and of bacterial overgrowth in the proximal small bowel from colonic bacteria infecting the biliary tract.

Case 352

# PARASTOMAL HERNIA

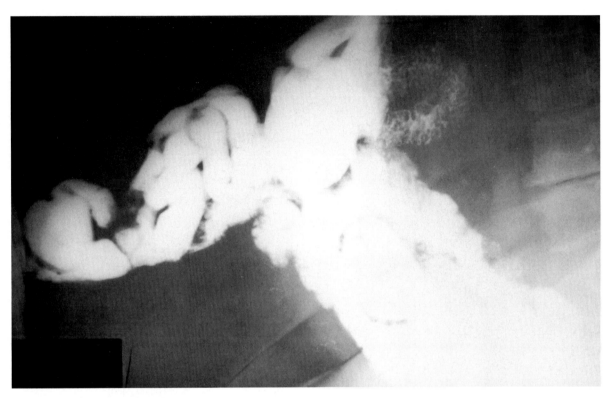

An ileostomy is present on this lateral abdominal radiograph. Several small-bowel loops have herniated through the abdominal-wall defect into a "parastomal" location.

Parastomal hernias are often found after an operation involving ileostomy or colostomy. The diagnosis may not be obvious when the patient is examined in the su-

pine or prone position. A lateral radiograph with the ostomy tract in profile is usually helpful in displaying the anatomy. Often the diagnosis of a hernia is clinically apparent, but a radiographic examination can be helpful in determining the size of the hernia and its contents and to evaluate for obstruction.

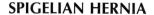

Case 353

# SPIGELIAN HERNIA

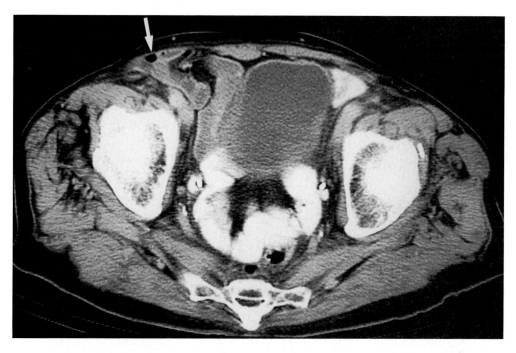

A herniated loop of bowel *(arrow)* is seen entering the subcutaneous space lateral to the rectus abdominus muscles. This location is typical of a spigelian hernia.

A spigelian hernia is a type of ventral hernia in which the abdominal wall defect arises along the linea semilunaris, a connective tissue structure that runs from the costal cartilages to the symphysis pubis, just lateral to the rectus abdominus muscles. These hernias most often occur as a result of increased intra-abdominal pressure (e.g., in heavy laborers, patients with chronic obstructive lung disease, those with urinary or gastric retention, and in multiparous women).

## Case 354

## PARADUODENAL HERNIA

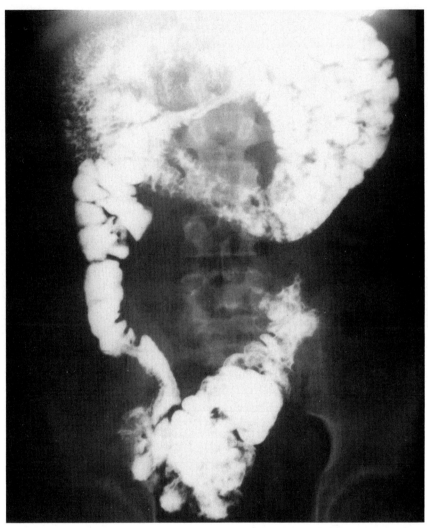

The majority of the small bowel is located in the upper abdomen and appears to be confined within a sac-like structure. Findings are typical of a paraduodenal hernia.

Paraduodenal hernias are the most frequent type of internal hernias. Other types include herniation through the foramen of Winslow, pericecal, intersigmoid, and transmesenteric or mesocolic. Most occur as a congenital anomaly of intestinal rotation and peritoneal attachment. Paraduodenal hernias usually (75%) occur on the left as a result of bowel herniating through a peritoneal reflection created by the inferior mesenteric artery. Bowel resides lateral to the ascending limb (4th portion) of the duodenum. Less commonly (25%), paraduodenal hernias occur on the right through the fossa beneath the superior mesenteric artery. Radiographically, a mass of small-bowel loops is usually located in the left upper quadrant, appearing to be encapsulated within a sac. Stasis of intraluminal barium and bowel dilatation may be present.

## Case 355

## PARADUODENAL HERNIA

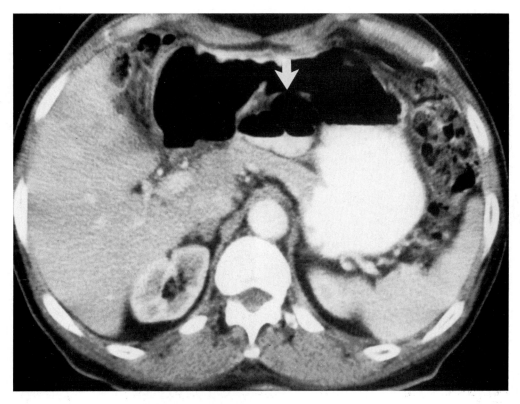

A loop of bowel *(arrow)* is located between the stomach and the body of the pancreas. This is a typical location for an internal hernia. This patient was found to have a left paraduodenal hernia. Conceivably, a foramen of Winslow hernia could have a similar appearance but would be much less common.

Case 356

## BOCHDALEK HERNIA

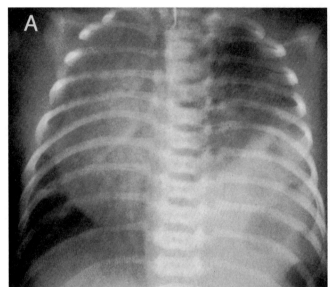

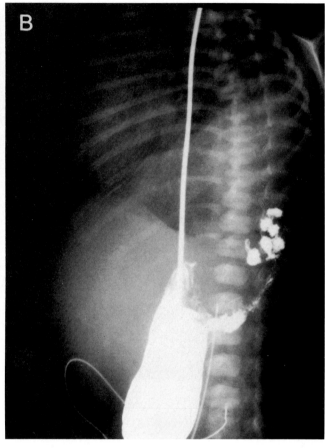

**A.** Chest radiograph shows opacification of the left lower lung, which contains several gas collections within it. These gas bubbles could be due to bowel loops that have herniated into the thorax. The cardiothymic silhouette is displaced to the right.

**B.** Contrast material has been instilled into the stomach via a nasogastric tube. Small bowel loops are seen to enter the thorax, traversing a posteriorly located diaphragmatic defect. The location of this diaphragmatic defect is typical of a Bochdalek hernia.

Bochdalek hernias are most commonly seen in infants. They occur as a result of incomplete closure of the pleuroperitoneal canal. The defect is always posterior and usually on the left. If the defect is large, nearly all of the abdominal contents can reside in the thorax. This can result in pulmonary developmental abnormalities and an associated high infant mortality.

## Case 357

## DUPLICATION CYST

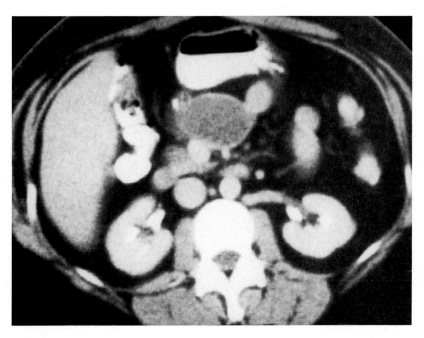

A well-circumscribed mass the density of water is located within the mesentery. Diagnostic considerations include duplication cyst, mesenteric cyst, obstructed blind loop, or diverticulum. At operation, an enterogenous cyst was removed.

## Case 358

# IDIOPATHIC INTESTINAL PSEUDO-OBSTRUCTION

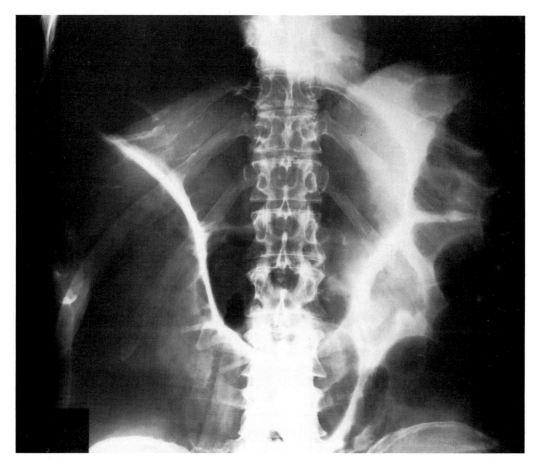

Massive gaseous distension of the colon is present. The pelvis is not visible but a low mechanical obstruction, pseudo-obstruction, or colonic ileus could have this radiographic appearance. No obstruction was present at barium enema.

Chronic idiopathic intestinal pseudo-obstruction is a rare disorder with radiographic findings of a mechanical obstruction, without an obstructing lesion or known cause of paralytic ileus. Gastrointestinal abnormalities may involve either the neural or the smooth muscular elements of the hollow viscera. Often the entire alimentary tract is affected. Esophageal complaints are uncommon but may include dysphagia. Peristaltic abnormalities may range from feeble contractions to findings that mimic achalasia. The duodenum is often dilated (megaduodenum), with associated delayed gastric emptying. Dilatation and delayed transit are present in the small bowel. Radiographic findings of mechanical obstruction may be present. The colon is often dilated and redundant and may contain diverticula. The diagnosis of chronic idiopathic intestinal pseudo-obstruction is usually one of exclusion; this requires eliminating a mechanical obstruction and the various causes of adynamic ileus.

| DIFFERENTIAL DIAGNOSES | CASE NUMBER |
|---|---|
| *THICKENED SMALL-BOWEL FOLDS (TYPE II FOLDS)* | |
| Hypoproteinemia | 283, 284 |
| Proximal to a mechanical obstruction | 350 |
| Ischemia | 255, 256, 261, 319 |
| Intramural hemorrhage | 233 |
| Whipple's disease | 272 |
| Amyloidosis | 268, 269 |
| Radiation enteritis | 252–254 |
| Giardiasis | 270 |
| Eosinophilic gastroenteritis | 267 |
| Lymphoma | 271 |
| Crohn's disease | 275, 295 |
| Zollinger-Ellison syndrome | 184 |
| *MULTIPLE FILLING DEFECTS (TYPE III FOLDS)* | |
| Nodular lymphoid hyperplasia | 278 |
| Lymphoma | 277 |
| Lymphangiectasis | 279, 280 |
| Crohn's disease | 275, 276, 292 |
| Metastases | 281, 333, 334 |
| Polyposis syndrome | 309 |
| Giardiasis | 270 |
| *EXCESSIVE FLUID IN THE LUMEN* | |
| Proximal to a mechanical obstruction | 246 |
| Celiac disease (sprue) | 286, 288 |
| Zollinger-Ellison syndrome | 105, 200 |
| *SOLITARY FILLING DEFECT* | |
| Benign tumors | |
|    Lipoma | 311 |
|    Hemangioma | 313, 314 |
|    Adenoma | 224 |
|    Leiomyoma | 310 |
|    Hamartoma | 309 |
| Malignant tumors | |
|    Carcinoid | 316, 317 |
|    Lymphoma | 323, 324 |
|    Adenocarcinoma | 328 |
|    Leiomyosarcoma | 331 |
|    Metastasis | 335, 336 |
| Gallstone | 351 |
| Duplication cyst | 240, 357 |
| *LUMINAL NARROWING* | |
| Adhesions/bands | 247, 248, 348 |
| Crohn's disease | 293–298, 301 |
| Adenocarcinoma | 329 |
| Lymphoma | 325–327 |
| Metastases | 337, 338 |

| DIFFERENTIAL DIAGNOSES | CASE NUMBER |
|---|---|
| Intramural hemorrhage | 233 |
| Tuberculosis | 306 |
| Ischemia | 261 |
| Radiation enteritis | 254 |

## SELECTED READINGS

### Normal Anatomy

Thoeni RF. Radiologic examination. In: Margulis AR, Burhenne HJ, eds. *Alimentary tract radiology*, 4th ed, vol 1. St. Louis: CV Mosby Company, **1989**:729–757

### Type I Folds

Bluestone R, MacMahon M, Dawson JM. Systemic sclerosis and small bowel involvement. *Gut* **1969**;10:185–193

*Caroline DF, Herlinger H, Laufer I, Kressel HY, Levine MS. Small-bowel enema in the diagnosis of adhesive obstructions. *AJR* **1984**;142:1133–1139

*Herlinger H. A modified technique for the double-contrast small bowel enema. *Gastrointest Radiol* **1978**;3:201–207

Horowitz AL, Meyers MA. The "hide-bound" small bowel of scleroderma: characteristic mucosal fold pattern. *Am J Roentgenol* **1973**;119:332–334

*Megibow AJ, Balthazar EJ, Cho KC, Medwid SW, Birnbaum BA, Noz ME. Bowel obstruction: evaluation with CT. *Radiology* **1991**;180:313–318.

Poirier TJ, Rankin GB. Gastrointestinal manifestations of progressive systemic scleroderma based on a review of 364 cases. *Am J Gastroenterol* **1972**;58:30–44

Rice RP. The plain film of the abdomen. In: Taveras JM, Ferrucci JT, eds. *Radiology: diagnosis—imaging—intervention*, vol 4. Philadelphia: JB Lippincott, **1986**:chap 2, 1–21

### Type II Folds

#### Radiation Enteritis

Mendelson RM, Nolan DJ. The radiological features of chronic radiation enteritis. *Clin Radiol* **1985**; 36:141–148

Rogers LF, Goldstein HM. Roentgen manifestations of radiation injury to the gastrointestinal tract. *Gastrointest Radiol* **1977**;2:281–291

Roswit B. Complications of radiation therapy: the alimentary tract. *Semin Roentgenol* **1974**;9:51–63

#### Ischemia

Alpern MB, Glazer GM, Francis IR. Ischemic or infarcted bowel: CT findings. *Radiology* **1988**; 166:149–152

Federle MP, Chun G, Jeffrey RB, Rayor R. Computed tomographic findings in bowel infarction. *AJR* **1984**;142:91–95

*Gold RP, Seaman WB. Splenic flexure carcinoma as

a source of hepatic portal venous gas. *Radiology* **1977**;122:329–330

Joffe N, Goldman H, Antonioli DA. Barium studies in small-bowel infarction: radiological-pathological correlation. *Radiology* **1977**;123:303–309

*Kelvin FM, Korobkin M, Rauch RF, Rice RP, Silverman PM. Computed tomography of pneumatosis intestinalis. *J Comput Assist Tomogr* **1984**; 8:276–280

Marshak RH, Lindner AE, Maklansky D. Ischemia of the small intestine. *Am J Gastroenterol* **1976**; 66:390–400

Scott JR, Miller WT, Urso M, Stadalnik RC. Acute mesenteric infarction. *Am J Roentgenol* **1971**; 113:269–279

*Smerud MJ, Johnson CD, Stephens DH. Diagnosis of bowel infarction: a comparison of plain films and CT scans in 23 cases. *AJR* **1990**;154:99–103

### Eosinophilic Gastroenteritis

Burhenne HJ. Eosinophilic (allergic) gastroenteritis. *Am J Roentgenol* **1966**;96:332–338

Dodds WJ, Geenen JE, Stewart ET. Eosinophilic enteritis. *Am J Gastroenterol* **1974**;61:308–312

Goldberg HI, O'Kieffe D, Jenis EH, Boyce HW. Diffuse eosinophilic gastroenteritis. *Am J Roentgenol* **1973**;119:342–351

MacCarty RL, Talley NJ. Barium studies in diffuse eosinophilic gastroenteritis. *Gastrointest Radiol* **1990**;15:183–187

*Marshak RH, Lindner AE, Maklansky D, Gelb A. Eosinophilic gastroenteritis. *JAMA* **1981**;245: 1677–1680

### Amyloidosis

*Carlson HC, Breen JF. Amyloidosis and plasma cell dyscrasias: gastrointestinal involvement. *Semin Roentgenol* **1986**;21:128–138

Gilat T, Revach M, Sohar E. Deposition of amyloid in the gastrointestinal tract. *Gut* **1969**;10:98–104

Kyle RA, Greipp PR. Amyloidosis (AL): clinical and laboratory features in 229 cases. *Mayo Clin Proc* **1983**;58:665–683

Seliger G, Krassner RL, Beranbaum ER, Miller F. The spectrum of roentgen appearance in amyloidosis of the small and large bowel: radiologic-pathologic correlation. *Radiology* **1971**;100: 63–70

Tada S, Iida M, Matsui T, et al. Amyloidosis of the small intestine: findings on double-contrast radiographs. *AJR* **1991**;156:741–744

*Cited in text.

### Whipple's Disease

*Berk RN, Wall SD, McArdle CB, et al. Cryptosporidiosis of the stomach and small intestine in patients with AIDS. *AJR* 1984;143:549–554

Clemett AR, Marshak RH. Whipple's disease: roentgen features and differential diagnosis. *Radiol Clin North Am* 1969 April;7:105–111

Li DKB, Rennie CS. Abdominal computed tomography in Whipple's disease. *J Comput Assist Tomogr* 1981;5:249–252

Philips RL, Carlson HC. The roentgenographic and clinical findings in Whipple's disease: a review of 8 patients. *Am J Roentgenol* 1975;123:268–273

Rice RP, Roufail WM, Reeves RJ. The roentgen diagnosis of Whipple's disease (intestinal lipodystrophy): with emphasis on improvement following antibiotic therapy. *Radiology* 1967;88:295–301

Rijke AM, Falke TH, de Vries RR. Computed tomography in Whipple disease. *J Comput Assist Tomogr* 1983;7:1101–1102

*Vincent ME, Robbins AH. *Mycobacterium avium-intracellulare* complex enteritis: pseudo-Whipple disease in AIDS. *AJR* 1985;144:921–922

### Giardiasis

Hodgson JR, Hoffman HN II, Huizenga KA. Roentgenologic features of lymphoid hyperplasia of the small intestine associated with dysgammaglobulinemia. *Radiology* 1967;88:883–888

Marshak RH, Ruoff M, Lindner AE. Roentgen manifestations of giardiasis. *Am J Roentgenol* 1968;104:557–560

### Type III Folds

Clemett AR, Fishbone G, Levine RJ, James AE, Janower M. Gastrointestinal lesions in mastocytosis. *Am J Roentgenol* 1968;103:405–412

*Glick SN. Crohn's disease of the small intestine. *Radiol Clin North Am* 1987 Jan;25:25–45

*Glick SN, Teplick SK. Crohn disease of the small intestine: diffuse mucosal granularity. *Radiology* 1985;154:313–317

*Hermans PE, Huizenga KA, Hoffman HN II, Brown AL Jr, Markowitz H. Dysgammaglobulinemia associated with nodular lymphoid hyperplasia of the small intestine. *Am J Med* 1966;40:78–89

*Koehler RE. Neoplasms. In: Margulis AR, Burhenne HJ, eds. *Alimentary tract radiology*, 4th ed, vol 1. St. Louis: CV Mosby Company, 1989:817–838

*Lichtenstein JE. Radiologic-pathologic correlation

of inflammatory bowel disease. *Radiol Clin North Am* 1987 Jan;25:3–24

*Marshak RH. Granulomatous disease of the intestinal tract (Crohn's disease). *Radiology* 1975;114:3–22

*Mekhjian HS, Switz DM, Melny KCS, Rankin GB, Brooks RK. Clinical features and natural history of Crohn's disease. *Gastroenterology* 1979;77:898–906

Olmsted WW, Madewell JE. Lymphangiectasia of the small intestine: description and pathophysiology of the roentgenographic signs. *Gastrointest Radiol* 1976;1:241–243

Robbins AH, Schimmel EM, Rao KCVG. Gastrointestinal mastocytosis: radiologic alterations after ethanol ingestion. *Am J Roentgenol* 1972;115:297–299

Shimkin PM, Waldmann TA, Krugman RL. Intestinal lymphangiectasia. *Am J Roentgenol* 1970;110:827–841

### Type IV Folds

#### Hypoproteinemia

Marshak RH, Khilnani M, Eliasoph J, Wolf BS. Intestinal edema. *Am J Roentgenol* 1967;101:379–387

Marshak RH, Wolf BS, Cohen N, Janowitz HD. Protein-losing disorders of the gastrointestinal tract: roentgen features. *Radiology* 1961;77:893–904

### Type V Folds

*Baer AN, Bayless TM, Yardley JH. Intestinal ulceration and malabsorption syndromes. *Gastroenterology* 1980;79:754–765

*Bova JG, Friedman AC, Weser E, Hopens TA, Wytock DH. Adaptation of the ileum in nontropical sprue: reversal of the jejunoileal fold pattern. *AJR* 1985;144:299–302

Caldwell WL, Swanson VL, Bayless TM. The importance and reliability of the roentgenographic examination of the small bowel in patients with tropical sprue. *Radiology* 1965;84:227–239

*Cohen MD, Lintott DJ. Transient small bowel intussusception in adult coeliac disease. *Clin Radiol* 1978;29:529–534

*Herlinger H, Maglinte DDT. Jejunal fold separation in adult celiac disease: relevance of enteroclysis. *Radiology* 1986;158:605–611

Marshak RH, Lindner AE. Malabsorption syndrome: sprue. In: Marshak RH, Lindner AE, eds. *Radiology of the small intestine*, 2nd ed. Philadelphia: WB Saunders, 1976:10–32

Marshak RH, Wolf BS, Adlersberg D. Roentgen

studies of the small intestine in sprue. *Am J Roentgenol* 1954;72:380–400

## Inflammatory Disorders

### Crohn's Disease

Frager DH, Goldman M, Beneventano TC. Computed tomography in Crohn disease. *J Comput Assist Tomogr* 1983;7:819–824

*Glick SN. Crohn's disease of the small intestine. *Radiol Clin North Am* 1987 Jan;25:25–45

Goldberg HI, Gore RM, Margulis AR, Moss AA, Baker EL. Computed tomography in the evaluation of Crohn disease. *AJR* 1983;140:277–282

*Jones B, Fishman EK, Hamilton SR, et al. Submucosal accumulation of fat in inflammatory bowel disease: CT/pathologic correlation. *J Comput Assist Tomogr* 1986;10:759–763

*Keighley MRB, Eastwood D, Ambrose NS, Allan RN, Burdon DW. Incidence and microbiology of abdominal and pelvic abscess in Crohn's disease. *Gastroenterology* 1982;83:1271–1275

Lambiase RE, Cronan JJ, Dorfman GS, Paolella LP, Haas RA. Percutaneous drainage of abscesses in patients with Crohn disease. *AJR* 1988;150:1043–1045

Marshak RH, Lindner AE. Regional enteritis. In: Marshak RH, Lindner AE, eds. *Radiology of the small intestine*, 2nd ed. Philadelphia: WB Saunders, 1976:179–245

*Megibow AJ, Bosniak MA, Ambos MA, Redmond PE. Crohn's disease causing hydronephrosis. *J Comput Assist Tomogr* 1981;5:909–911

Pringot J, Bodart P. Inflammatory diseases. In: Margulis AR, Burhenne HJ, eds. *Alimentary tract radiology*, 4th ed, vol 1. St. Louis: CV Mosby Company, 1989:759–815

*Safrit HD, Mauro MA, Jaques PF. Percutaneous abscess drainage in Crohn's disease. *AJR* 1987;148:859–862

### Others

Bhansali SK. Abdominal tuberculosis: experiences with 300 cases. *Am J Gastroenterol* 1977;67:324–337

*Carrera GF, Young S, Lewicki AM. Intestinal tuberculosis. *Gastrointest Radiol* 1976;1:147–155

*Fisk JD, Shulman HM, Greening RR, McDonald GB, Sale GE, Thomas ED. Gastrointestinal radiographic features of human graft-vs-host disease. *AJR* 1981;136:329–336

Hulnick DH, Megibow AJ, Naidich DP, Hilton S, Cho KC, Balthazar EJ. Abdominal tuberculosis: CT evaluation. *Radiology* 1985;157:199–204

*Jones B, Kramer SS, Saral R, et al. Gastrointestinal

inflammation after bone marrow transplantation: graft-versus-host disease or opportunistic infection? *AJR* 1988;150:277–281

Reeder MM, Palmer PES. Infections and infestations. In: Margulis AR, Burhenne HJ, eds. *Alimentary tract radiology*, 4th ed, vol 2. St. Louis: CV Mosby Company, 1989:1475–1542

Rosenberg HK, Serota FT, Koch P, Borden S IV, August CS. Radiographic features of gastrointestinal graft-*vs*-host disease. *Radiology* 1981;138: 371–374

Schimmelpenninck M, Zwaan F. Radiographic features of small intestinal injury in human graft-versus-host disease. *Gastrointest Radiol* 1982;7: 29–33

## Benign Neoplasms

Abrahamson J, Shandling B. Intestinal hemangiomata in childhood and a syndrome for diagnosis: a collective review. *J Pediatr Surg* 1973;8:487–495

*Bank ER, Hernandez RJ, Byrne WJ. Gastrointestinal hemangiomatosis in children: demonstration with CT. *Radiology* 1987;165:657–658

*Dodds WJ. Clinical and roentgen features of the intestinal polyposis syndromes. *Gastrointest Radiol* 1976;1:127–142

*Dozois RR, Kempers RD, Dahlin DC, Bartholomew LG. Ovarian tumors associated with the Peutz-Jeghers syndrome. *Ann Surg* 1970;172: 233–238

Fernandez MJ, Davis RP, Nora PF. Gastrointestinal lipomas. *Arch Surg* 1983;118:1081–1083

Gentry RW, Dockerty MB, Clagett OT. Vascular malformations and vascular tumors of the gastrointestinal tract. *Int Abstr Surg* 1949;88: 281–323

Good CA. Tumors of the small intestine: Caldwell Lecture, 1962. *Am J Roentgenol* 1963;89: 685–705

Heiken JP, Forde KA, Gold RP. Computed tomography as a definitive method for diagnosing gastrointestinal lipomas. *Radiology* 1982;142:409–414

Hurwitz MM, Redleaf PD, Williams HJ, Edwards JE. Lipomas of the gastrointestinal tract: an analysis of seventy-two tumors. *Am J Roentgenol* 1967;99:84–89

LiVolsi VA, Perzin KH. Inflammatory pseudotumors (inflammatory fibrous polyps) of the small intestine: a clinicopathologic study. *Am J Dig Dis* 1975;20:325–336

Marshak RH, Lindner AE. Benign small bowel tumors and their malignant counterparts. In: Marshak RH, Lindner AE, eds. *Radiology of the small intestine*, 2nd ed. Philadelphia: WB Saunders, **1976**:301–341

Megibow AJ, Redmond PE, Bosniak MA, Horowitz L. Diagnosis of gastrointestinal lipomas by CT. *AJR* **1979**;133:743–745

Mellish RWP. Multiple hemangiomas of the gastrointestinal tract in children. *Am J Surg* **1971**;121:412–417

Ormson MJ, Stephens DH, Carlson HC. CT recognition of intestinal lipomatosis. *AJR* **1985**;144; 313–314

Sheedy PF II, Fulton RE, Atwell DT. Angiographic evaluation of patients with chronic gastrointestinal bleeding. *Am J Roentgenol* **1975**;123: 338–347

### Malignant Neoplasms

Balthazar EJ. Carcinoid tumors of the alimentary tract. I. Radiographic diagnosis. *Gastrointest Radiol* **1978**;3:47—56

*Dragosics B, Bauer P, Radaszkiewicz T. Primary gastrointestinal non-Hodgkin's lymphomas: a retrospective clinicopathologic study of 150 cases. *Cancer* **1985**;55:1060–1073

*Dudiak KM, Johnson CD, Stephens DH. Primary tumors of the small intestine: CT evaluation. *AJR* **1989**;152:995–998

Ghahremani GG, Meyers MA, Port RB. Calcified primary tumors of the gastrointestinal tract. *Gastrointest Radiol* **1978**;2:331–339

Goldstein HM, Beydoun MT, Dodd GD. Radiologic spectrum of melanoma metastatic to the gastrointestinal tract. *Am J Roentgenol* **1977**;129: 605–612

Good CA. Tumors of the small intestine: Caldwell Lecture, 1962. *Am J Roentgenol* **1963**;89: 685–705

Kinkhabwala M, Balthazar EJ. Carcinoid tumors of the alimentary tract. II. Angiographic diagnosis of small intestinal and colonic lesions. *Gastrointest Radiol* **1978**;3:57–61

Koehler RE. Neoplasms. In: Margulis AR, Burhenne HJ, eds. *Alimentary tract radiology*, 4th ed, vol 1. St. Louis, The CV Mosby Company, **1989**:817–838

Marshak RH, Lindner AE. Primary and metastatic carcinoma of the small bowel. In: Marshak RH, Lindner AE, eds. *Radiology of the small intestine*. Philadelphia: WB Saunders, **1976**:358–386

Marshak RH, Lindner AE. Lymphosarcoma, Hodgkin's disease and melanosarcoma. In: Marshak RH, Lindner AE, eds. *Radiology of the small intestine*. Philadelphia: WB Saunders, **1976**: 409–450

McAfee JG, Donner MW. Differential diagnosis of calcifications encountered in abdominal radiographs. *Am J Med Sci* **1962**;243:609–650

McCarthy SM, Stark DD, Moss AA, Goldberg HI. Computed tomography of malignant carcinoid disease. *J Comput Assist Tomogr* **1984**;8:846–850

McLeod AJ, Zornoza J, Shirkhoda A. Leiomyosarcoma: computed tomographic findings. *Radiology* **1984**;152:133–136

Megibow AJ, Balthazar EJ, Hulnick DH, Naidich DP, Bosniak MA. CT evaluation of gastrointestinal leiomyomas and leiomyosarcomas. *AJR* **1985**; 144:727–731

*Meyers MA. Intraperitoneal spread of malignancies and its effect on the bowel. *Clin Radiol* **1981**; 32:129–146

Meyers MA, McSweeney J. Secondary neoplasms of the small bowel. *Radiology* **1972**;105:1–11

Moertel CG. An odyssey in the land of small tumors. *J Clin Oncol* **1987**;5:1503–1522

*Moertel CG, Sauer WG, Dockerty MB, Baggenstoss AH. Life history of the carcinoid tumor of the small intestine. *Cancer* **1961**;14:901–912

Oddson TA, Rice RP, Seigler HF, Thompson WM, Kelvin FM, Clark WM. The spectrum of small bowel melanoma. *Gastrointest Radiol* **1978**; 3:419–423

Pagani JJ, Bernardino ME. CT-radiographic correlation of ulcerating small bowel lymphomas. *AJR* **1981**;136:998–1000.

Picus D, Glazer HS, Levitt RG, Husband JE. Computed tomography of abdominal carcinoid tumors. *AJR* **1984**;143:581–584

Pomerantz H, Margolin HN. Metastases to the gastrointestinal tract from malignant melanoma. *Am J Roentgenol* **1962**;88:712–717

*Reintgen DS, Thompson W, Garbutt J, Seigler HF. Radiologic, endoscopic, and surgical considerations of melanoma metastatic to the gastrointestinal tract. *Surgery* **1984**;95:635–639

*Rubesin SE, Gilchrist AM, Bronner M, et al. Non-Hodgkin lymphoma of the small intestine. *Radiographics* **1990**;10:985–998

Smith SJ, Carlson HC, Gisvold JJ. Secondary neoplasms of the small bowel. *Radiology* **1977**; 125:29–33

Zboralske FF, Bessolo RJ. Metastatic carcinoma to the mesentery and gut. *Radiology* **1967**;88: 302–310

## Miscellaneous

### Malrotation

Ablow RC, Hoffer FA, Seashore JH, Touloukian RJ. Z-shaped duodenojejunal loop: sign of mesenteric fixation anomaly and congenital bands. *AJR* **1983**;141:461–464

Firor HV, Harris VJ. Rotational abnormalities of the gut: re-emphasis of a neglected facet, isolated incomplete rotation of the duodenum. *Am J Roentgenol* **1974**;120:315–321

Fisher JK. Computed tomographic diagnosis of volvulus in intestinal malrotation. *Radiology* **1981**;140:145–146

Jackson A, Bisset R, Dickson AP. Case report: malrotation and midgut volvulus presenting as malabsorption. *Clin Radiol* **1989**;40:536–537

Rabinowitz JG, Moseley JE. The small bowel in infants and children. In: Marshak RH, Lindner AE, eds. *Radiology of the small intestine*, 2nd ed. Philadelphia: WB Saunders, **1976**:451–501

### Gallstone Ileus

Eisenman JI, Finck EJ, O'Loughlin BJ. Gallstone ileus: a review of the roentgenographic findings and report of a new roentgen sign. *Am J Roentgenol* **1967**;101:361–366

*Hudspeth AS, McGuirt WF. Gallstone ileus: a continuing surgical problem. *Arch Surg* **1970**;100:668–672

Safaie-Shirazi S, Printen KJ. Gallstone ileus: review of forty cases. *J Am Geriatr Soc* **1972**;20:335–339

### Duplication Cyst

Bower RJ, Sieber WK, Kiesewetter WB. Alimentary tract duplications in children. *Ann Surg* **1978**;188:669–674

Fitch SJ, Tonkin IL, Tonkin AK. Imaging of foregut duplication cysts. *Radiographics* **1986**;6:189–201

Lamont AC, Starinksy R, Cremin BJ. Ultrasonic diagnosis of duplication cysts in children. *Br J Radiol* **1984**;57:463–467

Livingston PA, Pollock EJ, Renert WA, Seaman WB. A radiological sign in the diagnosis of enterogenous cysts. *Radiology* **1971**;98:543–545

Lo J, Sage MR, Paterson HS, Hamilton DW. Gastric duplication in an adult. *J Comput Assist Tomogr* **1983**;7:328–330

Sieber WK. Alimentary tract duplications. *J Pediatr Surg* **1979**;14:83–85

### Idiopathic Intestinal Pseudo-Obstruction

Schuffler MD, Rohrmann CA Jr, Templeton FE. The radiologic manifestations of idiopathic intestinal pseudoobstruction. *Am J Roentgenol* **1976**;127:729–736

### Pneumatosis Intestinalis

Connor R, Jones B, Fishman EK, Siegelman SS. Pneumatosis intestinalis: role of computed tomography in diagnosis and management. *J Comput Assist Tomogr* **1984**;8:269–275

Ecker JA, Williams RG, Clay KL. *Pneumatosis cystoides intestinalis*—bullous emphysema of the intestine: a review of the literature. *Am J Gastroenterol* **1971**;56:125–136

Kelvin FM, Korobkin M, Rauch RF, Rice RP, Silverman PM. Computed tomography of pneumatosis intestinalis. *J Comput Assist Tomogr* **1984**;8:276–280

Meyers MA, Ghahremani GG, Clements JL Jr, Goodman K. Pneumatosis intestinalis. *Gastrointest Radiol* **1977**;2:91–105

### Diverticulosis

*Dunn V, Nelson JA. Jejunal diverticulosis and chronic pneumoperitoneum. *Gastrointest Radiol* **1979**;4:165–168

*Eckhauser FE, Zelenock GB, Freier DT. Acute complications of jejuno-ileal pseudodiverticulosis: surgical implications and management. *Am J Surg* **1979**;138:320–323

*Giustra PE, Killoran PJ, Root JA, Ward WW. Jejunal diverticulitis. *Radiology* **1977**;125:609–611

Salomonowitz E, Wittich G, Hajek P, Jantsch H, Czembirek H. Detection of intestinal diverticula by double-contrast small bowel enema: differentiation from other intestinal diverticula. *Gastrointest Radiol* **1983**;8:271–278

*Taylor MT. Massive hemorrhage from jejunal diverticulosis. *Am J Surg* **1969**;118:117–120

### Meckel's Diverticulum

Berquist TH, Nolan NG, Stephens DH, Carlson HC. Specificity of 99mTc-pertechnetate in scintigraphic diagnosis of Meckel's diverticulum: review of 100 cases. *J Nucl Med* **1976**;17:465–469

*Dalinka MK, Wunder JF. Meckel's diverticulum and its complications, with emphasis on roentgenologic demonstration. *Radiology* **1973**;106:295–298

*Maglinte DDT, Elmore MF, Isenberg M, Dolan PA. Meckel diverticulum: radiographic demonstration by enteroclysis. *AJR* **1980**;134:925–932

Sfakianakis GN, Conway JJ. Detection of ectopic gastric mucosa in Meckel's diverticulum and in other aberrations by scintigraphy. I. Pathophysiology and 10-year clinical experience. II. Indications and methods—a 10-year experience. *J Nucl Med* **1981**;22:647–654; 732–738

# CHAPTER 5

# Colon

**Case 359**

## PSEUDOTUMOR SPLENIC IMPRESSION

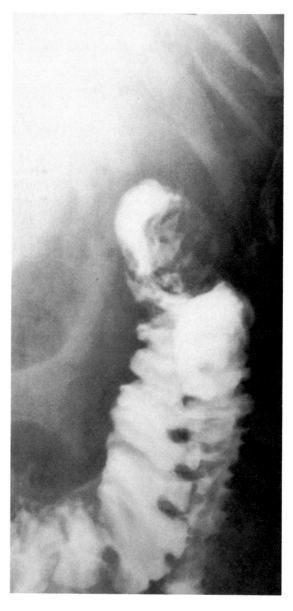

A smooth-surfaced filling defect is present in the splenic flexure of the colon. This is due to the tip of the spleen pressing on the colon.

A filling defect is most often encountered in patients with splenomegaly. The impression is usually broad based, with an associated spleniform soft-tissue mass arising from the left upper quadrant. Distension of the colon is helpful in demonstrating the extraluminal origin of the mass. Equivocal cases could be further evaluated with colonoscopy to exclude a mucosal lesion, or CT may be used to exclude an extraluminal mass and directly visualize the relationship of the colon and spleen.

## Case 360

## INNOMINATE GROOVES

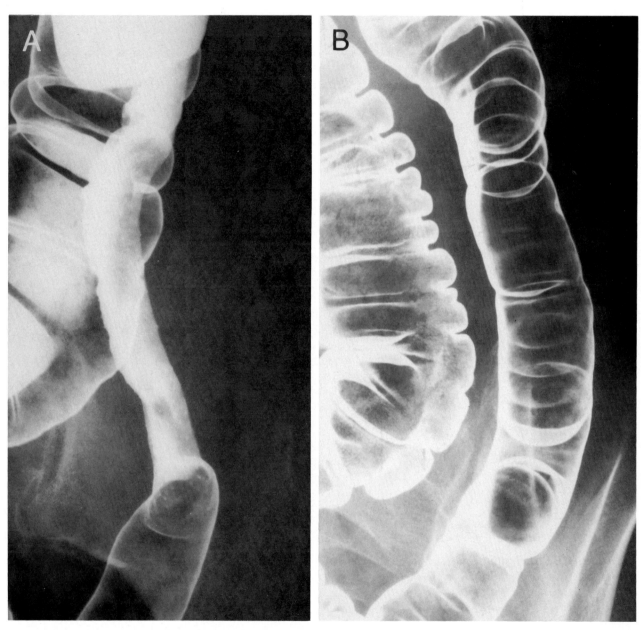

**A.** Multiple spiculations and collections of barium are present in the partially collapsed descending colon.

**B.** Air-distended view of the same colonic segment is normal and without evidence of ulceration.

Innominate lines (grooves) represent collections of barium within the crevices of the normally collapsed colon. The lines are only seen within the partially filled colon and disappear with complete distension (as seen in this case). Their importance lies in differentiating these normal lines from mucosal ulcerations seen in patients with inflammatory bowel disease or infectious colitis. Real mucosal ulcers persist and are well demonstrated on views of the colon with air distension.

## Case 361

## COLONIC SPASM

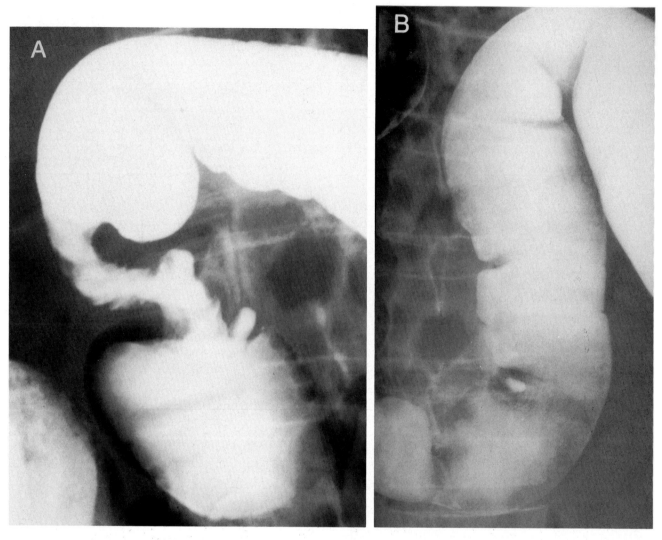

**A.** A focal region of narrowing is present in the colon. Mucosal markings are visible within the narrowed segment.

**B.** The narrowed segment has now relaxed and is completely distended and appears normal. The transient nature of this narrowing is typical of colonic spasm.

Colonic spasm can occur as a focal area of narrowing or as a part of a continuous propulsive contraction ("mass movement"). The contraction usually lasts a variable time, but occasionally it can be quite persistent. These persistent focal areas of spasm can simulate annular cancers. Careful inspection of the mucosa and the use of glucagon can be helpful in equivocal cases.

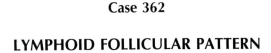

## Case 362

# LYMPHOID FOLLICULAR PATTERN

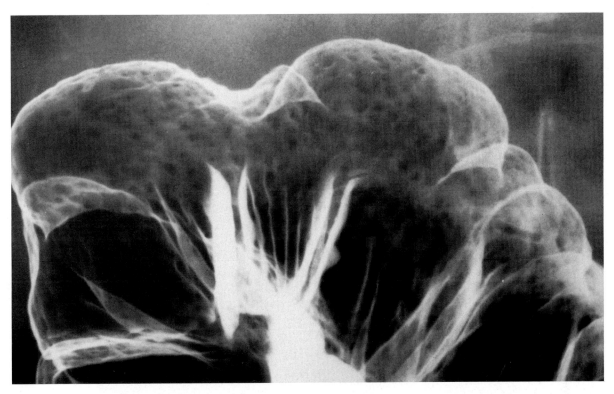

Multiple, tiny, submucosal nodular filling defects are uniformly distributed in the colon. The appearance is typical of a normal lymphoid follicular pattern.

The lymphoid follicular pattern is a common finding in normal children and in 10% to 15% of normal adults (Kelvin et al., 1979). The double-contrast technique is usually required to identify the subtle textural changes of this entity. The key finding is the small size (<4 mm diameter) of the filling defects that are uniformly distributed in the colon. Usually the right side of the colon

is affected more than the left. A polyposis syndrome usually has filling defects of larger and more variable size, and some will be pedunculated (Cases 373, 374, 376, and 377). The lymphoid nodules and aphthous ulcers in Crohn's disease are usually somewhat larger and often in a patchy segmental distribution (Cases 424 and 425). Diffuse lymphoma has submucosal nodules of larger (>4 mm) and variable size (Cases 401 and 402). Retained stool has angular margins whereas lymphoid nodules are smooth and rounded.

**Case 363**

## LYMPHOID FOLLICULAR PATTERN

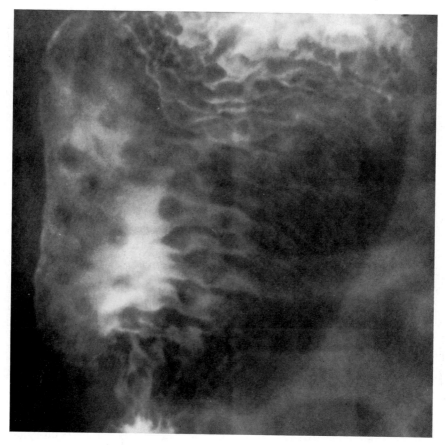

Multiple nodules of uniform size are present in the colon. A central collection of barium is visible within several of these nodules and represents umbilication at the apex of the nodule.

Umbilication of lymphoid nodules can be a normal finding. The main differential consideration is Crohn's colitis with multiple aphthous ulcers (Case 425). Usually the aphthous ulcers of Crohn's disease are nonuniform in distribution and size. Often the ulcers will be seen to coalesce and form transverse ulcerations. It may be impossible to exclude inflammatory bowel disease on the basis of the radiographic findings alone. Clinical correlation is always suggested, and follow-up studies to assess for disease progression or endoscopic biopsy can also be helpful.

**Case 364**

## NORMAL COLON: CT

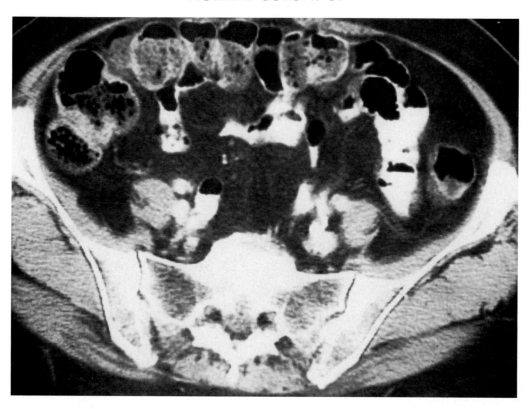

A normal colon is visible on this CT scan. Residual fecal material is nearly always present if there has been no colonic preparation. Bowel-wall thickness is a key observation for detection of colonic abnormalities at CT. Normally, the colonic wall is not more than 3 mm thick (Fisher, 1982). The wall may appear slightly thicker (≤5 mm normally) if the colon is not fully distended. The wall is homogeneously dense and symmetrical, with sharply defined inner and outer contours.

**Case 365**

## NORMAL ILEOCECAL VALVE

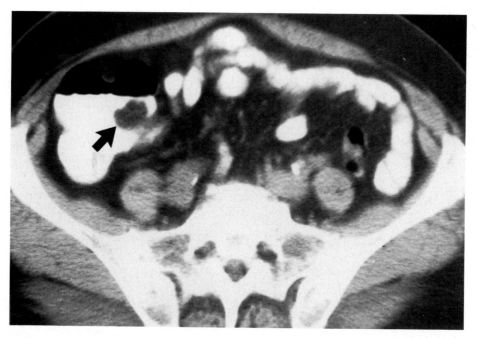

The barium- and air-filled cecum contains a filling defect the density of fat *(arrow)*. This structure represents a normal fatty ileocecal valve. Usually the terminal ileum can be traced to the ileocecal valve. The ho-mogeneous fatty density is characteristic of a normal valve. A lipoma could have a similar appearance, but it would be. in a different location (Case 407).

**Case 366**

## NORMAL APPENDIX

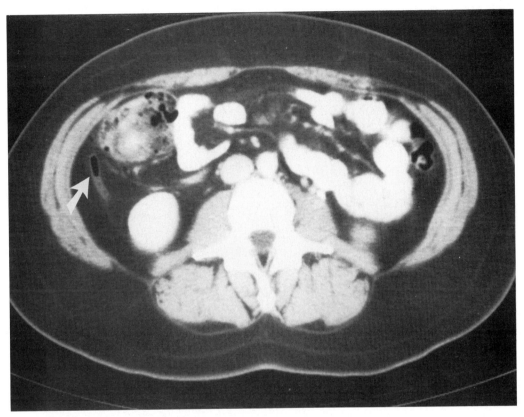

The appendix *(arrow)* is visible as a small air- and fluid-filled tubular structure arising from the base of the cecum. Notice that the appendiceal wall is sharply defined and thin (1–2 mm). The normal periappendiceal fat is of homogeneously low attenuation.

## Case 367

## PEDUNCULATED POLYP

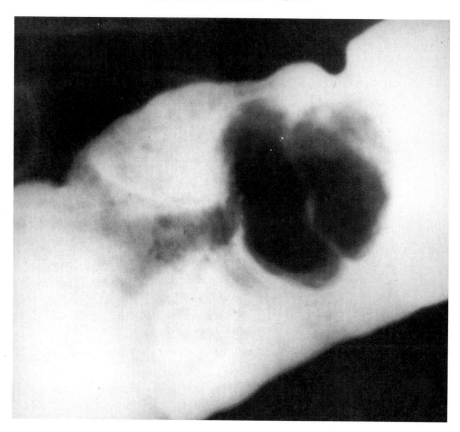

A pedunculated polyp is present in the midtransverse colon.

Polyps of the colon can be classified by histologic type: hyperplastic (retention), adenomatous, and hamartomatous. Hyperplastic polyps are generally small (<1 cm diameter) and are not believed to have malignant potential. Adenomatous polyps can be further classified into three histologic subtypes: tubular, tubulovillous, and villous adenomas. Most authorities now believe that the majority of adenocarcinomas of the colon arise from preexisting adenomas (Muto et al., 1975). Polyps with a higher percentage of villous features are at a higher risk for malignant transformation than are tubular adenomas. Polyp diameter is also an important factor in assessing the risk of malignancy in an adenomatous polyp, because the larger the polyp the higher the risk. Muto et al. (1975) tabulated this data as follows.

Malignant Potential of Colorectal Adenomas*

| Histologic type | Adenomas, % | | |
| --- | --- | --- | --- |
| | <1 cm | 1–2 cm | >2 cm |
| Tubular | 1.0 | 10.2 | 34.7 |
| Tubulovillous | 3.9 | 7.4 | 45.8 |
| Villous | 9.5 | 10.3 | 52.5 |

*From Muto T, Bussey HJR, Morson BC. *Cancer* **1975**;36:2251–2270. By permission of American Cancer Society.

Hamartomatous polyps are associated with Peutz-Jeghers syndrome (Case 376). Retention polyps are found in patients with juvenile polyposis (Case 377).

## Case 368

## SESSILE POLYP

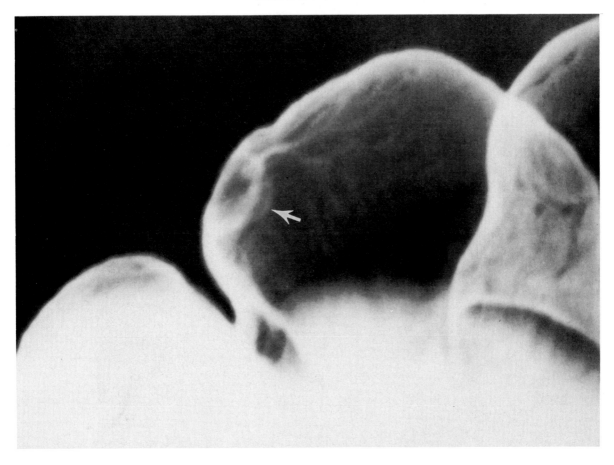

A sessile polyp *(arrow)* is present in the colon. The appearance of this polyp resembles a "bowler hat," with the brim representing the base of the polyp attached to the colonic wall. The intraluminal protrusion is represented by the top of the hat.

There are no radiographic criteria that distinguish adenomatous polyps from the other histologic types. Sessile polyps, those with a broad base, and polyps greater than 1 cm in diameter are generally considered to be more worrisome than pedunculated and small (<1 cm) polyps. Even polyps less than 1 cm in diameter cannot be dismissed as insignificant. The majority of these polyps are adenomatous, and a small percentage of these will grow and eventually undergo malignant transformation (Feczko et al., 1984). Polyps are usually multiple, and synchronous lesions are seen in 25% to 50% of patients (Arminski and McLean, 1964). Nearly half of all polyps are located in the rectosigmoid, 20% in the right colon, and 29% to 35% in the transverse and descending colon (Bernstein et al., 1985).

## Case 369

## PSEUDOPOLYP

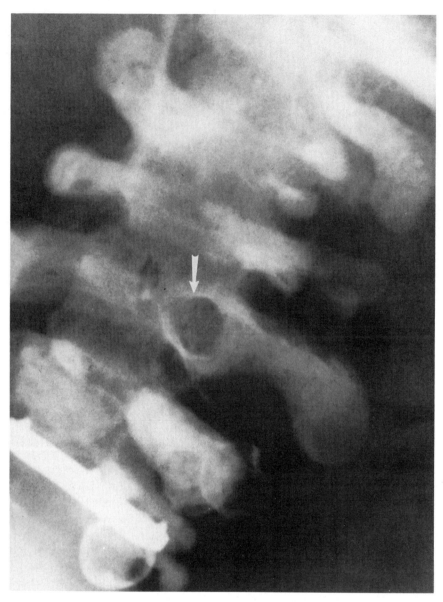

A round filling defect *(arrow)* is present in the sigmoid colon. Sigmoid diverticulosis is present. The filling defect has a bright white ring of barium around it. The last finding indicates barium filling around stool within a diverticulum.

Diverticulosis is a common finding, especially among older individuals. Stool may fill a diverticulum and remain lodged within it despite proper cathartics and cleansing enemas. When viewed en face, the stool-filled diverticulum can simulate a polyp. Identifying the rim of barium around the pseudopolyp is key to excluding a real polyp. If tangential views are possible, stool can often be seen within the diverticulum.

**Case 370**

## VILLOUS ADENOMA

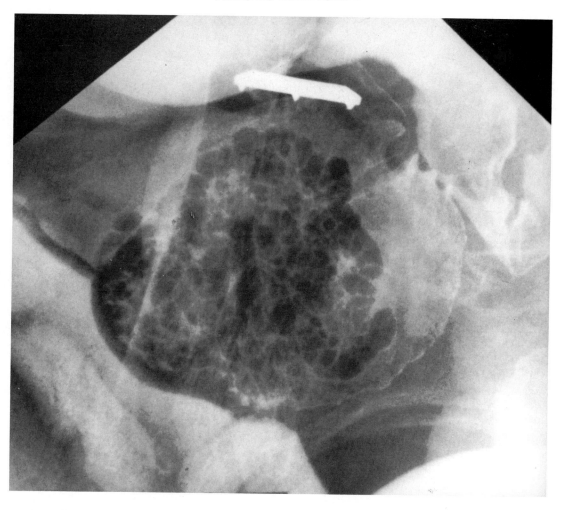

A large polypoid mass is present in the base of the cecum. The "raspberry" or "cauliflower" surface appearance is typical of a villous tumor. A villous adenoma with foci of adenocarcinoma was removed at operation. The metallic measurement marker is 2 cm long.

Villous adenomas can be recognized if the typical surface features are visible. Characteristically, barium fills the interstices of the tumor between the individual fronds. Unfortunately, it is usually not possible to detect villous features within small polyps. Usually, polyps must be nearly 2 cm in diameter before the typical features are recognizable. Villous tumors are usually soft and compressible, and rectal lesions can easily be missed on digital examinations. Because villous tumors have a high risk of malignancy, they should be removed.

## Case 371

## ADENOMA: CARCINOMA TRANSFORMATION

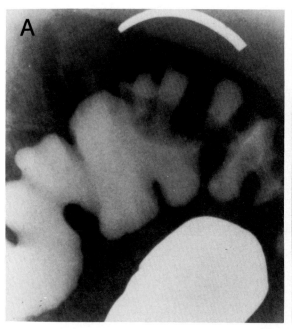 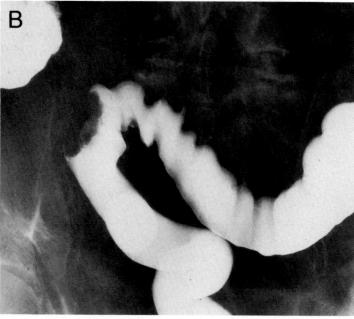

**A.** A large pedunculated polyp is present in the sigmoid colon.

**B.** Eight years later, a large sessile carcinoma has developed at the site of the previous polyp.

Today, most researchers believe that the majority of colon cancers arise from preexisting polyps (Muto et al., 1975). This case supports that hypothesis. The role of radiologists is to detect all polypoid colonic lesions with the hope that they can be successfully removed before malignant degeneration. Risk factors for the development of colorectal polyps include increasing age (10% incidence after age 50 years) (Ott and Gelfand, 1978), history of previous polyps, and family history of colon polyps or carcinoma. Patients with ulcerative colitis also have a higher incidence of colon cancer developing.

## Case 372

## POLYPOSIS SYNDROMES

(See Cases 373–377.)

| Syndrome | Histologic Type | Predominant Organ | Inheritance | Comments/Associated Findings |
|---|---|---|---|---|
| *Hereditary* | | | | |
| 1. Familial | Adenomatous | Colon | Autosomal dominant | Colon cancer, without colectomy |
| Gardner's | | | | Desmoid tumors, osteomas, epidermoid cysts, soft-tissue tumors of the skin, dental abnormalities, periampullary duodenal carcinomas, colon cancer without colectomy |
| 2. Peutz-Jeghers | Hamartomatous | Small bowel | Autosomal dominant | Mucocutaneous melanin pigmentation |
| 3. Turcot's | Benign adenomas | Colon | Autosomal recessive | Central nervous system tumors (supratentorial gliomas) |
| *Nonhereditary* | | | | |
| 4. Juvenile | Inflammatory (hyperplastic) (retention) | Colon | Inherited in some patients (autosomal dominant) | |
| 5. Cronkhite-Canada | Inflammatory (hyperplastic) (retention) | Stomach, colon | None | Ectodermal changes: alopecia, hyperpigmentation of skin, dystrophic changes, changes in nails |

## Case 373

## FAMILIAL POLYPOSIS

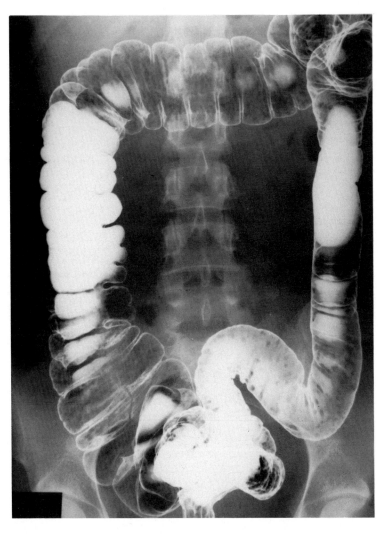

Multiple, polypoid filling defects are present throughout the colon. These findings are characteristic of a polyposis syndrome.

Familial polyposis is the commonest of the polyposis syndromes characterized by large numbers of adenomatous polyps that often carpet the entire colon. There are no extraintestinal manifestations in familial polyposis. Patients often present with rectal bleeding in their early thirties, and if a colectomy is not performed, they will die from adenocarcinoma of the colon in their early forties. Family screening should be performed in sporadic cases.

Radiographically, innumerable polyps are identified throughout the entire colon and may be found in the small bowel and stomach. Occasionally, the polyps

may conglomerate and appear as bizarre filling defects in the colon.

Differential considerations include inflammatory polyps in either ulcerative colitis or Crohn's colitis (Case 414). In patients with ulcerative colitis, there is often a granular background throughout the involved colon (Case 413). Patients with Crohn's colitis often have rectal sparing and skip areas of involvement (Case 426). Peutz-Jeghers syndrome usually has only a few colonic polyps (Case 376); the majority are located in the small bowel. Nodular lymphoma often has thickened haustral folds, and the polyps may not be as sharply marginated due to their submucosal location (Cases 401 and 402).

## Case 374

## GARDNER'S SYNDROME

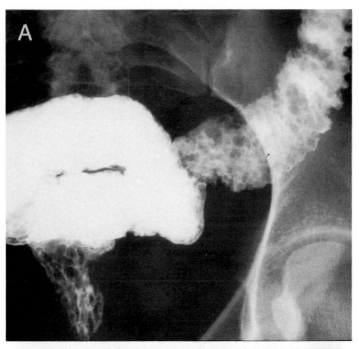

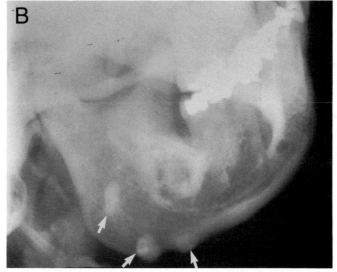

**A.** Innumerable polyps are present throughout the visualized colon. These findings are consistent with a polyposis syndrome.

**B.** Multiple osteomas *(arrows)* are visible arising from the mandible.

Gardner's syndrome is believed to represent a disease identical to familial polyposis, with various extraintestinal manifestations. The colonic polyps do not differ in distribution, growth pattern, number, histologic type, or malignant potential from familial polyposis.

Localized areas of dense bone (osteomas) are commonly present, often involving the skull, mandible, and maxilla. Long bone cortical thickening and dental abnormalities are common.

## Case 375

## GARDNER'S SYNDROME: DESMOID TUMOR

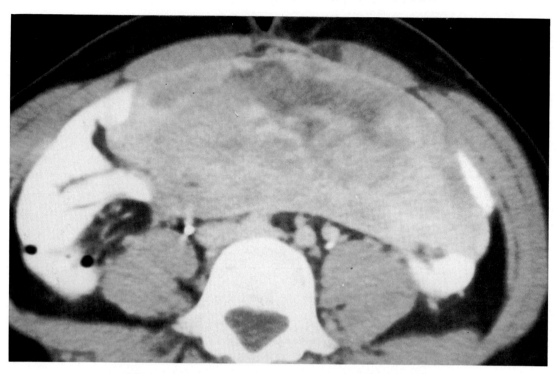

A huge soft-tissue tumor occupies a large portion of the abdomen. At operation, a desmoid tumor was removed in this patient with known Gardner's syndrome.

Soft-tissue tumors in patients with Gardner's syndrome include: (1) sebaceous cysts; (2) benign mesenchymal tumors, such as fibromas, lipofibromas, lipomas, leiomyomas, and neurofibromas; (3) malignant mesenchymal tumors; and (4) fibrous tissue prolifera-

tion producing desmoid tumors, keloids, peritoneal adhesions, and mesenteric and retroperitoneal fibrosis. Large abdominal desmoid tumors (as in this case) usually occur after total colectomy.

Approximately 20% of these patients have the triad of colonic polyps, osteomas, and mesenchymal tumors.

Case 376

# PEUTZ-JEGHERS SYNDROME

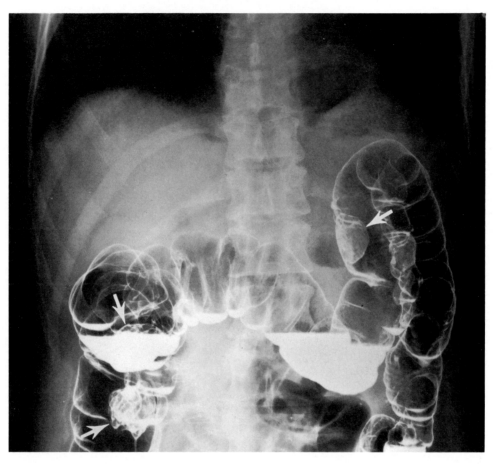

Multiple large polyps *(arrows)* are present in the colon. The diagnosis of Peutz-Jeghers syndrome was made on the basis of the typical mucocutaneous pigmentations found at physical examination.

Peutz-Jeghers syndrome is a disease of mucocutaneous pigmentation and gastrointestinal polyposis. Patients usually present with symptoms of abdominal cramping, rectal bleeding, melena, or anemia. Cramping is often secondary to transient intussusceptions within the small bowel.

Gastrointestinal polyps are most frequently found in the small bowel (95%) (Case 309), but they can also be identified in the colon and rectum (30%) and stomach (25%) (Bartholomew et al., 1962). The polyps can vary in size and are usually less numerous in the stomach and colon. Polyps in the stomach and small bowel are hamartomatous, but colonic polyps are usually adenomatous (and potentially malignant). Alimentary tract malignancies develop in 2% to 3% of patients (Dozois et al., 1969).

**Case 377**

## JUVENILE POLYPOSIS

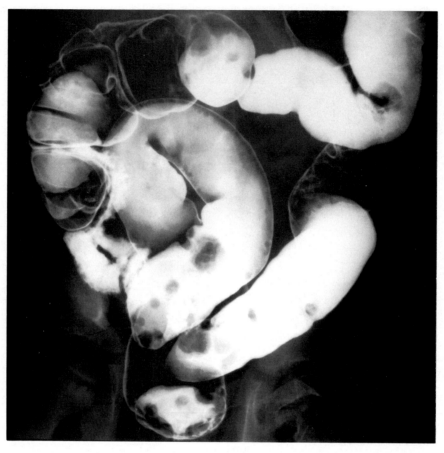

Multiple variable-sized polyps are present in the colon. At biopsy, these polyps were classified as retention or juvenile polyps.

Juvenile polyposis is usually a disorder of children that includes solitary or multiple retention (inflammatory) polyps. Histologically, these polyps have abundant connective tissue stroma containing mucin-filled cystic spaces lined with epithelium. Sporadic cases are usually associated with only a few polyps, whereas the hereditary form is associated with multiple polyps (juvenile polyposis coli). In the latter disease, polyps can be found throughout the alimentary tract. Juvenile polyps may coexist with adenomatous polyps in patients with familial polyposis. The commonest symptoms and signs are rectal bleeding, anemia, and anal prolapse of a polyp.

**Case 378**

## POLYPOID ADENOCARCINOMA

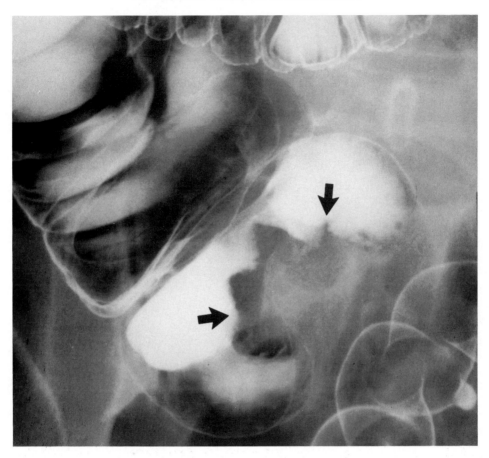

A large polypoid mass *(arrows)* fills the base of the cecum. The contours of the mass are lobulated and angular. These findings are typical of an adenocarcinoma, which was surgically proven in this patient.

Colorectal carcinoma represents a major public health threat. It is one of the commonest (ranked second or third in incidence and frequency) kinds of cancer and causes of cancer-related deaths. Predisposing factors for colon cancer include genetic factors, history of colorectal adenomatous polyps, ulcerative colitis, and Crohn's colitis. A direct descendant of a patient with colorectal cancer has a 3 to 5 times increased risk of colon cancer developing compared to the general population (Macklin, 1960). It is generally agreed that most adenocarcinomas arise from preexisting adenomatous polyps. Detection and removal of benign polyps can eliminate the risk of developing most colon cancers. Patients with ulcerative colitis usually develop multiple regions of dysplasia prior to malignant transformation. Although typical annular carcinomas are often seen in these patients, many cancers will penetrate and grow within the submucosa, mimicking a benign stricture. Generally, cancers complicating ulcerative colitis are higher grade and more aggressive.

The distribution of colon cancers appears to have been shifting toward the proximal colon since the 1940s. Today, approximately 50% to 60% of cancers are located within the rectosigmoid, 25% to 35% in the ascending colon and cecum, and the remaining 5% to 25% in the transverse and descending colon (Kelvin et al., 1988). The reported sensitivity of the barium enema ranges from 18% to 98%, with higher rates associated with polyps larger than 7 mm (Gelfand and Ott, 1981). The mortality rate (secondary to colonic perforation) is estimated at 1/20,000 to 1/50,000 patients examined (Gilbert et al., 1984).

**415**

## Case 379

## ANNULAR ADENOCARCINOMA

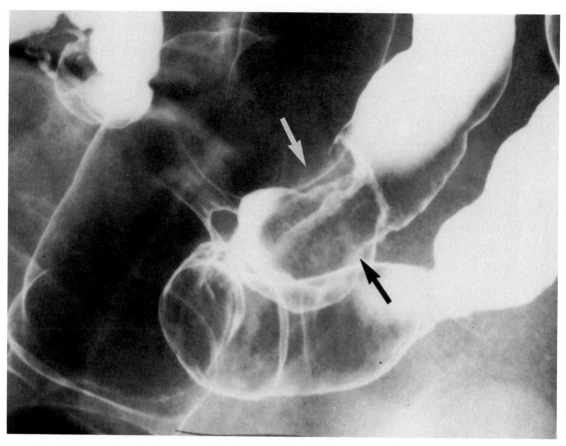

A nearly annular, ulcerative adenocarcinoma *(arrows)* is present in the mid-sigmoid colon. The lesion has margins that are abrupt and shouldered, resembling a napkin ring.

Advanced colon cancers often appear as annular constricting lesions. Most tumors are less than 6 cm long. These tumors are thought to arise from a flat, plaquelike growth which extends circumferentially around the bowel lumen. Most small cancers are indistinguishable from benign polyps. It is for this reason that most polyps ≥1 cm in diameter are removed.

**Case 380**

## OBSTRUCTING POLYPOID ADENOCARCINOMA

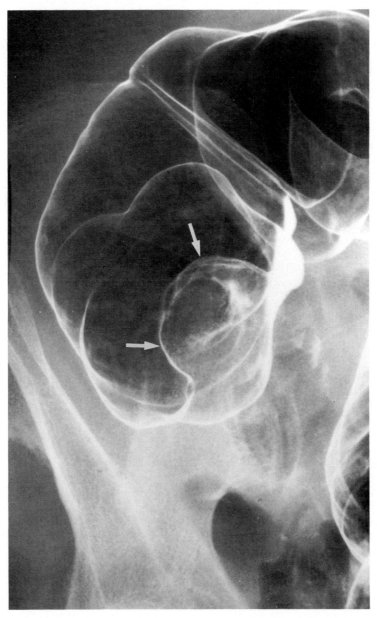

A polypoid mass *(arrows)* is present in the mid-ascending colon. No contrast material has passed proximal to the obstructing mass. A 5-cm Dukes stage B2 adenocarcinoma was removed at operation.

Colon cancer is the most frequent cause of large-bowel obstruction. An enema with contrast material is a rapid and accurate method to determine the cause of the obstruction. Colitis has been reported to occur proximal to an obstructing lesion in some patients. High-grade obstruction and a competent ileocecal valve can also lead to elevated intraluminal pressure, decreased venous flow, and possible colonic ischemia (Whitehouse and Watt, 1977).

**417**

## Case 381

# VILLOUS ADENOCARCINOMA

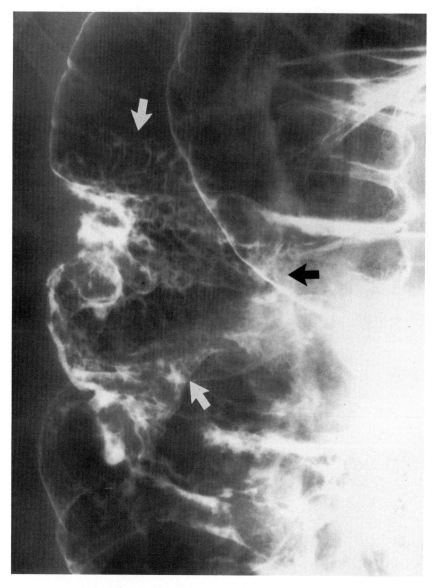

A villous tumor *(arrows)* is present along the lateral wall of the mid-ascending colon. The frondlike nature of the mass indicates its villous nature. Its size suggests a malignancy. At operation, a villous adenoma containing a Dukes stage B1 adenocarcinoma was removed.

Villous adenomas have the highest incidence of malignant transformation of all adenomatous polyps. The villous nature of these lesions can be suspected by identifying a lacelike or raspberrylike surface contour. Usually, lesions are more than 1 cm in diameter before the villous features are visible.

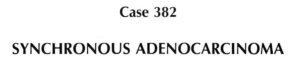

## Case 382

# SYNCHRONOUS ADENOCARCINOMA

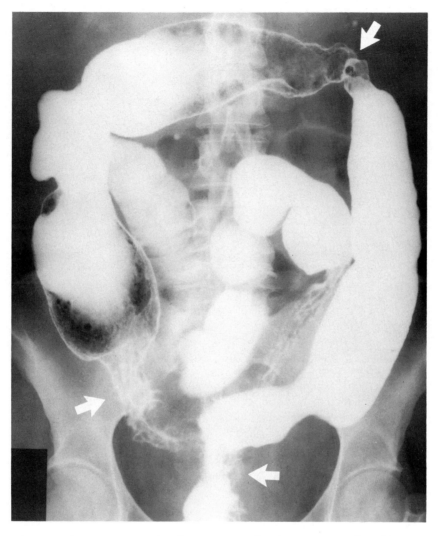

There are at least three regions *(arrows)* of colonic narrowing: cecum, splenic flexure, and rectosigmoid. This patient had a long history of ulcerative colitis. At operation, multiple colon cancers were present as well as peritoneal carcinomatosis.

Patients with long-standing (>10 years) ulcerative colitis have an increased risk of colon cancer developing. These cancers may be multicentric (as in this patient) and appear as either typical annular cancers (Case 420) or regions of tapered narrowing (Case 421).

Approximately 5% of patients with an ordinary colon carcinoma have another synchronous cancer (Abrams and Reines, 1979). Therefore, it is important to examine the entire colon—even after the discovery of an unsuspected lesion. In one series, less than one-third of synchronous lesions were palpable at operation (Heald and Bussey, 1975). Only if the patient has a high-grade obstruction from the cancer should the proximal colon not be examined. Polyps are also more commonly found in patients with either a synchronous polyp or cancer or a history of previous polyp or cancer. Metachronous cancers, those developing at a later date in patients with a previous history of colorectal cancer, occur in about 5% of patients (Morson, 1974).

## Case 383

## COLON CARCINOMA

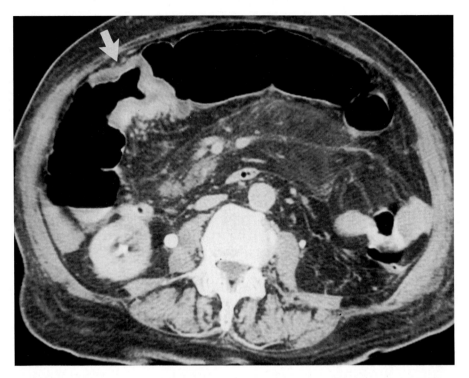

A short segment of circumferential bowel-wall thickening *(arrow)* is present in the hepatic flexure of the colon. The wall thickening abruptly meets the normal colonic wall. An annular carcinoma was later confirmed in this location.

CT is not recommended as a primary diagnostic modality for the detection of colon cancer. The depth of bowel-wall invasion is poorly demonstrated at CT, and it is common for nodal metastases to occur within normal-size lymph nodes. CT does have a moderately high sensitivity (81%) for the detection of distant metastases (Dukes stage D lesions) (Balthazar et al., 1988). Common sites for distant extranodal metastases include liver and peritoneum and local invasion of adjacent organs.

**Case 384**

## RECTAL CANCER

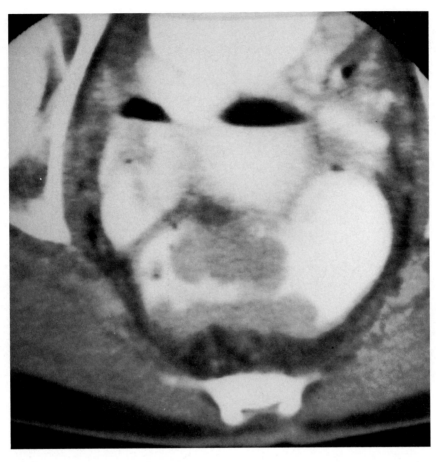

An annular "apple core" or "napkin ring" lesion is causing circumferential bowel-wall thickening of the rectosigmoid. The irregular luminal contours and abrupt shelflike margins are typical of an adenocarcinoma. The tumor was confirmed at operation.

## Case 385

## RECTAL VILLOUS ADENOCARCINOMA

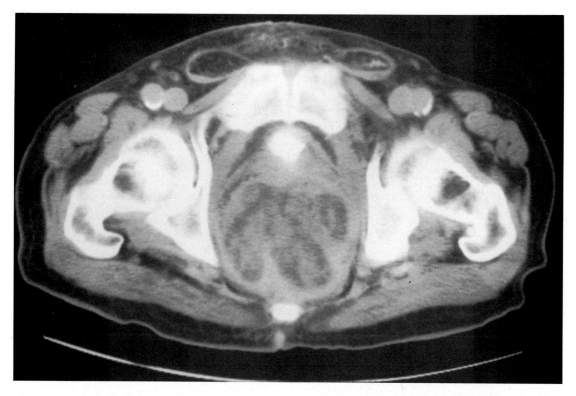

The rectal lumen is markedly distended, and the rectal wall is unevenly thickened. Multiple, intraluminal soft-tissue masses are present within the rectum. These masses have a tree-like appearance, typical of the gross pathologic appearance of a villous tumor. A villous adenocarcinoma was present at biopsy. It is unusual to vi-sualize the villous features of a colonic tumor at CT. Usually, only localized bowel-wall thickening or a focal mass is seen. In this patient the large size and the morphology of the mass were helpful in predicting the histologic type.

## Case 386

## RECTAL CANCER

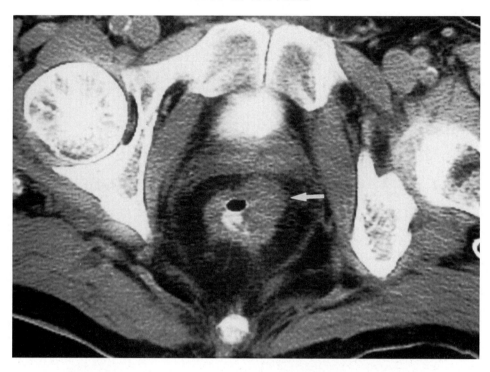

Asymmetric and masslike thickening *(arrow)* is present on the left side of the rectal wall. A rectal cancer was confirmed at endoscopy.

Preoperative staging of rectal tumors has generated considerable interest recently. Tumors that are confined within the bowel wall can be managed with conservative yet curative procedures. Advanced tumors can often benefit from preoperative radiation therapy. Accurate assessment of regional nodes could affect the surgical decision to perform a local or a more aggressive resection. Currently, routine CT is not used in our practice because of its relatively low sensitivity in detecting perirectal fatty infiltration and nodal metastases.

**Case 387**

# INTUSSUSCEPTING COLON CANCER

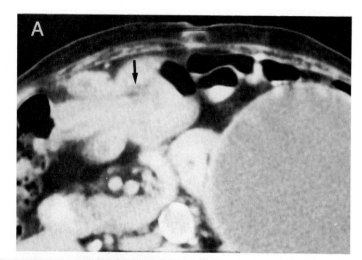

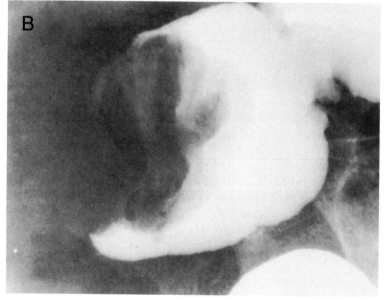

**A.** An intussusception is present within the right transverse colon. A linear band of low-density mesenteric fat is visible within the mass *(arrow)*. A lead point for the intussusception is not seen. There is also a mass the density of water arising from the left kidney and containing several enhancing mural nodules.

**B.** A follow-up barium enema demonstrated a polypoid colon cancer acting as the lead point for the reducible intussusception. At operation, both a colon cancer and a cystic renal adenocarcinoma were removed.

Colon cancer is the most frequent cause of a colo-colic intussusception in adults. The radiographic appearance at barium enema and CT is usually diagnostic. As in the small bowel, a sausage-shaped filling defect is seen within a shortened colon. A "coiled-spring" appearance is often visible at the proximal end of the mass. Sometimes it is possible to fully reduce the intussusception and to identify the offending mass at contrast enema. In many patients the cancer is located in the cecum. Visualization of mesenteric fat and occasionally vessels within the mass is pathognomonic (as in this case) of an intussusception at CT.

## Case 388

## RECTAL CANCER: CONFINED TO BOWEL WALL

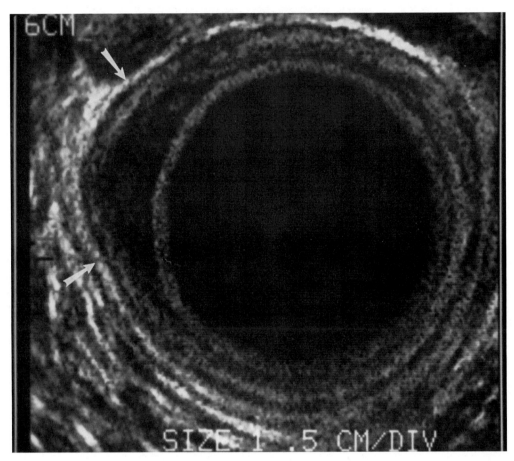

The normal bowel-wall layers are visible except for a localized area of bowel-wall thickening at the 9- to 10-o'clock position. The outermost echogenic layer (muscularis propria and perirectal fat interface) is intact *(arrows)* overlying this mass. This finding indicates that the tumor is confined to the bowel wall (Dukes stage B1 lesion).

Endorectal sonography can routinely display the five

*From Jochem RJ, Reading CC, Dozois RR, Carpenter HA, Wolff BG, Charboneau JW. Mayo Clin Proc* **1990;** *65:1571–1577.*

normal layers of the bowel. The innermost echogenic layer represents the balloon-mucosal interface; the next hypoechoic layer, the muscularis mucosa; the middle echogenic layer, the submucosa; the fourth hypoechoic ring, the muscularis propria; and the outer echogenic ring, the muscularis propria/perirectal fat interface. The outer echogenic layer is the key ring in distinguishing tumors confined to the bowel wall from those extending into the perirectal fat. This technique is also sensitive in detecting perirectal lymph nodes but nonspecific in distinguishing metastatic from inflammatory nodes (Jochem et al., 1990).

## Case 389

## RECTAL CANCER: PERIRECTAL EXTENSION

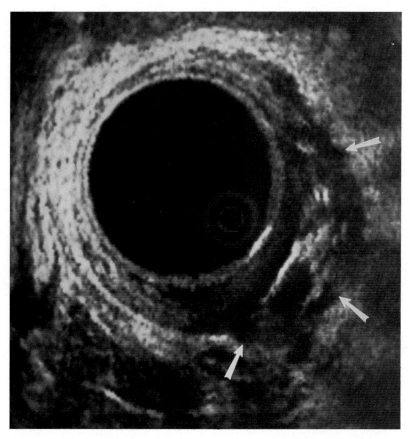

The entire left side of the rectal wall is abnormally

*From Jochem RJ, Reading CC, Dozois RR, Carpenter HA, Wolff BG, Charboneau JW. Mayo Clin Proc **1990;** 65:1571–1577.*

thickened, with loss of the normal echogenic bowel layers. In addition, tumor *(arrows)* can be seen to extend deeply into the perirectal fat (Dukes stage B2) through the muscularis propria/perirectal fat interface.

## Case 390

## PERFORATED COLON CARCINOMA

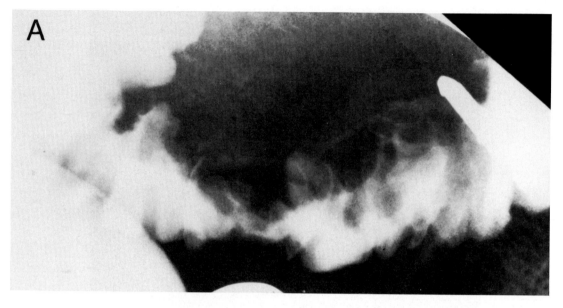

**A.** The sigmoid lumen is narrowed and there is a lobulated mass deforming the superior sigmoid contour. The lobulated contours are worrisome for neoplasm but mucosal destruction or ulceration is not identified.

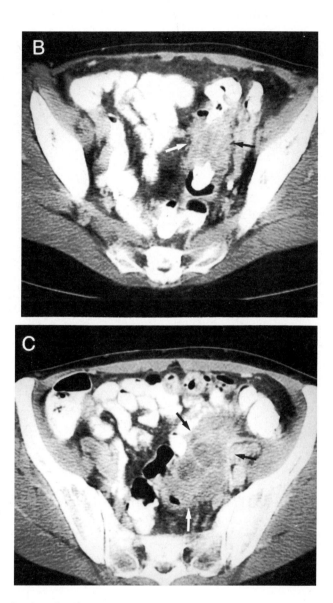

**B** and **C.** A mixed-density (fluid and soft tissue) mass *(arrows)* is present within the perisigmoidal tissues. Radiographically, it is impossible to distinguish diverticulitis from a perforated colon cancer in this patient. At operation, a perforated colon cancer was resected.

Perforated colon cancers are unusual, accounting for 2.5% to 8% of all colorectal cancers (Miller et al., 1966). The importance of this entity lies in the fact that patients may present with signs suggesting diverticulitis and receive suboptimal therapy. In addition, curative resection is less likely and operative mortality is higher. Gross perforation with peritoneal contamination (found in a minority of patients) has only a 7% 5-year survival (Glenn and McSherry, 1971).

A contrast enema usually does not demonstrate the site of colonic perforation. Common findings on contrast enema include a long area of segmental narrowing and extrinsic mass effect or obstruction. Mucosal ulceration can be difficult to evaluate because of the associated inflammatory changes. Findings at CT include a colorectal mass associated with an abscess the density of fluid or phlegmon. Metastatic disease is often identified.

## Case 391

## PERFORATED COLON CANCER

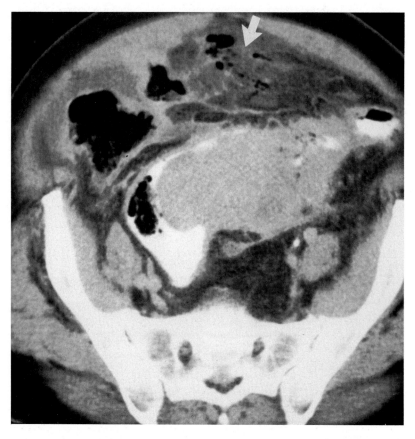

A large soft-tissue mass narrows and deforms the sigmoid colon. Contrast material is visible within the sigmoid lumen. Soft-tissue stranding is present throughout the perisigmoidal fat. Extraluminal gas *(arrow)* is present in the soft tissues anterior to the sigmoid colon.

Differential considerations include either diverticulitis with a phlegmonous inflammatory mass (Cases 439, 440, and 442) or a perforated colon cancer. At operation, a perforated colon carcinoma was removed.

**Case 392**

# COLON CANCER: LOCAL INVASION AND FISTULA

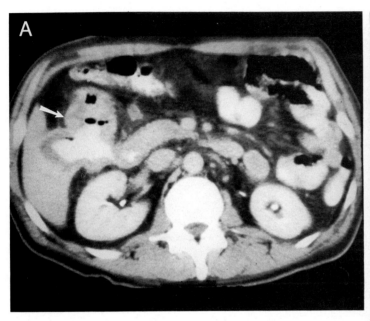

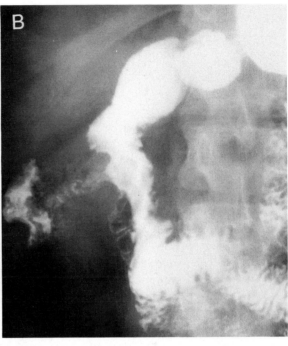

**A.** Circumferential bowel-wall thickening *(arrow)* is present in the hepatic flexure of the colon. The colonic lumen is dilated at the level of the mass, and there is extension into the right lobe of the liver with loss of the normal fat plane between colon and duodenum.

**B.** A fistula is present between the descending duodenum and colon on this upper gastrointestinal examination. At operation, a locally invasive colon cancer was removed.

Local invasion is a relatively common complication of colon cancer. Depending on the organ involved, fistula formation can occur. Common organs to be secondarily involved by colon cancer include the stomach, bladder, and vagina. Other complications include obstruction, perforation (Case 390), intussusception (Case 387), and bleeding. Obstruction is encountered most often.

## Case 393

## RECURRENT COLON CANCER

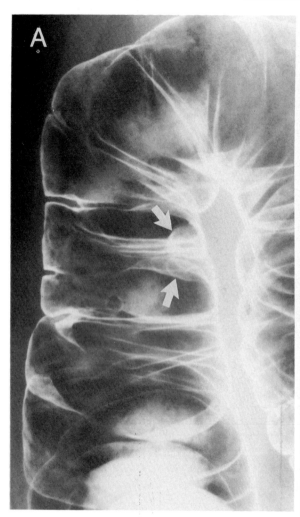

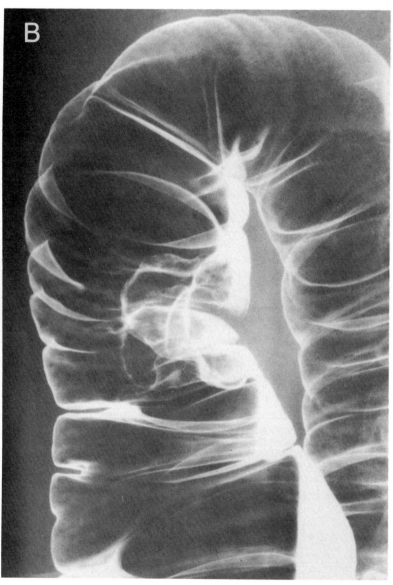

**A.** A sessile polyp *(arrows)* is present along the medial wall of the ascending colon. A tubulovillous adenoma was reported after endoscopic removal.

**B.** Follow-up barium enema 3 years later shows a polypoid carcinoma at the site of the previous polyp. An adenocarcinoma was removed at operation.

Thirty to fifty percent of patients who have undergone curative resection for colon cancer have a recurrence within 2 years (Olson et al., 1980). Locally re-

current colorectal cancers can occur at sites of surgical anastomosis, within pericolic or pelvic fat near the surgical site, or at previous sites of endoscopic removal. Local recurrence developing at the anastomosis is best evaluated by an intraluminal study, i.e., barium enema or endoscopy. Extraluminal and distant disease are best detected at CT. The usual radiographic appearance of an anastomotic recurrence is either a polypoid mass or irregular and eccentric narrowing of the lumen.

### Case 394

## RECURRENT COLORECTAL CARCINOMA

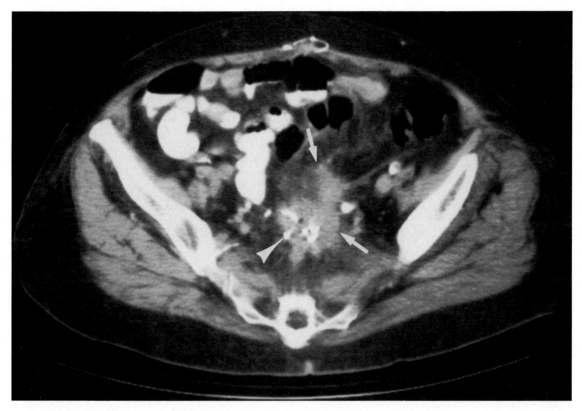

High-density anastomotic surgical clips *(arrowhead)* are present in the region of the rectosigmoid. The bowel wall is thickened and an irregular, poorly defined soft-tissue mass *(arrows)* extends into the pericolic fat. Recurrent carcinoma was confirmed at operation.

Anastomotic recurrences are found most commonly after a low anterior resection for rectal cancer. In this operation, residual tumor may be inadvertently left behind because narrow surgical margins are often necessary. Malignant cells can also be seeded within pericolic tissues at the time of the initial colonic resection. CT is an excellent modality for evaluating the extent and presence of extraluminal disease.

## Case 395

## RECURRENT RECTAL CANCER

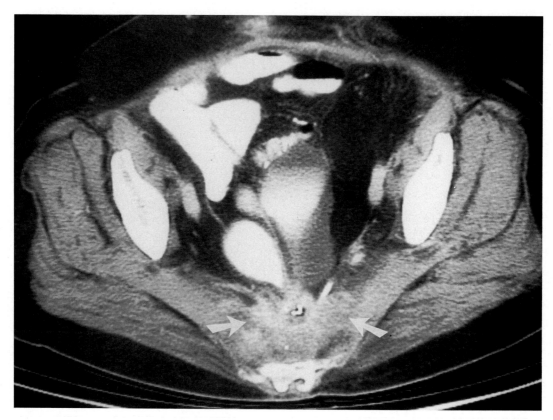

The patient had had an abdominoperineal resection of the rectum for rectal cancer. An enhancing, poorly circumscribed soft-tissue mass *(arrows)* is present in the presacral space. A high-density surgical clip is visible in the superior aspect of the mass near the midline. Recurrent tumor was confirmed by a CT-directed biopsy of the mass.

CT findings of recurrent tumor in the pelvis usually include an expanding presacral soft-tissue mass with indistinct margins. Local invasion and lymphadenopathy can be seen as well as distant metastases (liver, lung, retroperitoneum). Recently, MRI has shown some promise in differentiating postoperative fibrosis (long T1- and short T2-relaxation times) from recurrent tumor (long T1- and T2-relaxation times). The exact role of MRI in evaluating patients for recurrent pelvic tumor is unclear at this time.

Case 396

## POSTOPERATIVE PSEUDOTUMOR

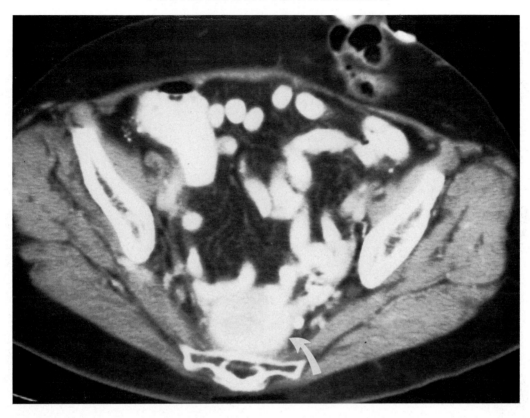

This patient had had an abdominoperineal resection for rectal cancer. The pelvis has a normal postoperative appearance, without evidence of a presacral mass. The uterine fundus *(arrow)* now fills the presacral space and should not be confused with an abnormal mass. In males, often the seminal vesicles and prostate can fill the presacral space. Unopacified bowel loops in this location can also mimic a mass. A colostomy is visible in the left anterior abdominal wall.

A presacral soft-tissue mass generally is visible after an abdominoperineal resection. CT scans are done regularly (baseline scan at 2 to 4 months postoperatively, then every 6 months for 3 years) to assess for local pelvic recurrence (Kelvin et al., 1983). CT findings of benign postoperative fibrosis include: stable or diminished size of the mass, development of distinct margins, and partial separation of the mass from the sacrum. CT findings that suggest recurrent disease should prompt a CT-directed biopsy of the mass to exclude carcinoma.

## Case 397

## COLON METASTASES: PERITONEAL SPREAD

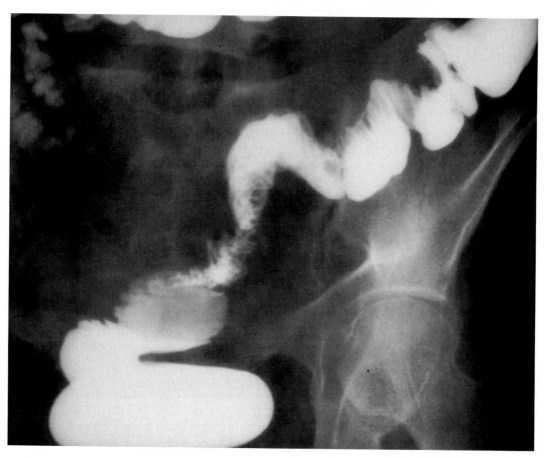

The sigmoid colon is narrowed from mass effect and mucosal tethering is present along its superior surface. These findings are typical of metastatic carcinoma; this patient had ovarian cancer.

Intraperitoneal metastases will implant on peritoneal surfaces in regions where the ascitic flow is arrested. There are four common sites of intraperitoneal seeding: (1) the pouch of Douglas—the most dependent and common location in the abdomen, (2) the ileocecal region—a region where fluid and cells will collect after cascading down the small bowel mesentery into the right lower quadrant, (3) the superior aspect of the sigmoid colon, and (4) the right paracolic gutter—the main channel for fluid traveling from the pelvis into the upper abdomen (Meyers, 1988).

Hematogenous spread to the colon is relatively infrequent. Breast cancer can invade the submucosal tissues and resemble linitis plastica in the affected segment. Narrowing and lack of distensibility are the commonest findings.

Case 398

## PSEUDOMYXOMA PERITONEI

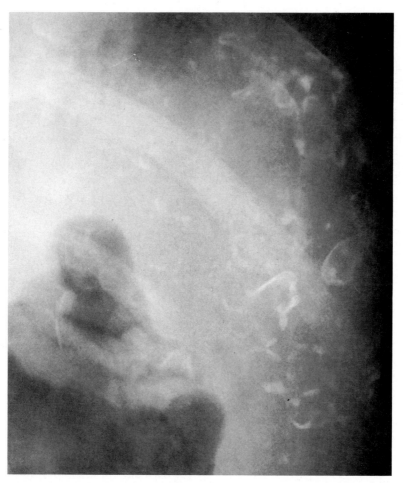

Multiple linear calcifications are seen in the left upper quadrant. Similar findings were present throughout the abdomen in the peritoneal space. This patient had known pseudomyxoma peritonei arising from a mucinous adenocarcinoma of the colon.

Mucinous peritoneal metastases (usually ovary, colon, appendix, stomach) may form masses of mucoidrich tumor (pseudomyxoma peritonei) which may calcify. Calcification of mucinous metastases often appears as fine, amorphous high-density material.

## Case 399

## COLON METASTASES: DIRECT EXTENSION

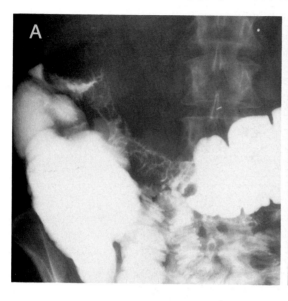 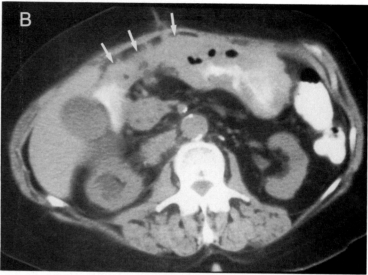

**A.** A long segment of circumferential narrowing is present in the right transverse colon. The mucosa through much of the involved region appears distorted but intact. Multiple calcified gallstones are visible in the right upper quadrant.

**B.** The wall of the gastric antrum is thickened. A contiguous soft-tissue mass *(arrows)* extends from the stomach and engulfs (on lower slices) the colon. The right kidney is obstructed. Metastatic encasement of the colon by direct extension from a gastric primary was found at operation.

Metastatic disease to the colon can occur via several routes: intraperitoneal spread, direct extension, and hematogenous dissemination. Morton Meyers (1988) described the patterns of malignant spread by each route. Understanding these patterns allows the radiologist to make the diagnosis of metastases and to predict the possible origin of the primary tumor.

Direct extension of malignancies is most commonly encountered in patients with ovarian or uterine carcinoma, prostate cancer, and renal carcinoma. Pelvic malignancies often cause a mass effect on the anterior wall of the rectum and on the inferior aspect of the sigmoid. The affected bowel can be narrowed and nodular in contour and contain tethered folds. Prostatic tumors often involve only the anterior aspect of the rectum, but they can also extend circumferentially around the rectum, causing annular narrowing resembling a primary rectal cancer. Renal adenocarcinomas do not usually incite a desmoplastic response as seen in most other metastases. These tumors (either primary or locally recurrent tumors) can invade the colon and appear as a large intraluminal, nonobstructing polypoid mass. Gastric (as in this case) and pancreatic malignancies often invade the transverse colon by extending into the gastrocolic ligament and transverse mesocolon. Classically, gastric malignancies will cause narrowing, mass effect, and tethering of the superior aspect of the transverse colon. Pancreatic malignancies usually involve the inferior aspect of the transverse colon.

## Case 400

## COLON METASTASES: PERITONEAL IMPLANTS

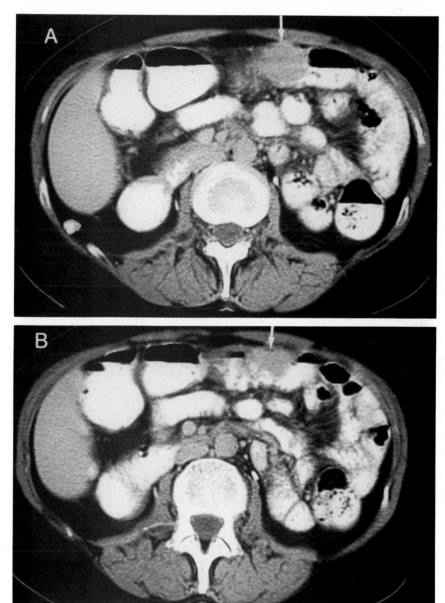

**A** and **B.** A soft-tissue mass *(arrows)* is present along the anterior surface of the transverse colon. At operation, metastatic adenocarcinoma was removed in this woman with known ovarian cancer.

Several abnormalities can be seen at CT in patients with intraperitoneal metastases. Common findings include liver metastases, inhomogeneity and soft-tissue masses within the greater omentum, ascites, small nodular peritoneal soft-tissue densities, mesenteric masses, and soft-tissue masses in dependent regions of the peritoneal space (i.e., pouch of Douglas). In patients with colon cancer, an ovarian metastasis may develop which often appears as a solid and cystic septated mass.

## Case 401

## DIFFUSE LYMPHOMA

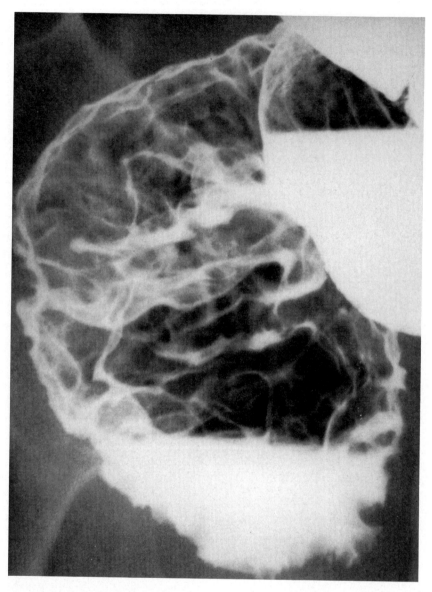

The submucosa of the rectum is diffusely involved with a nodular infiltrative process. This finding is secondary to non-Hodgkin's lymphoma.

The diffuse form of lymphoma begins in the submucosa of the colon. The ileocecal and rectosigmoid regions are most often involved first. As the disease progresses, the entire colon becomes involved. Extension of the tumor into the appendix and terminal ileum is often found. It is unusual for primary colonic lymphoma to extend through the serosa or into the retroperitoneum.

## Case 402

## COLONIC LYMPHOMA

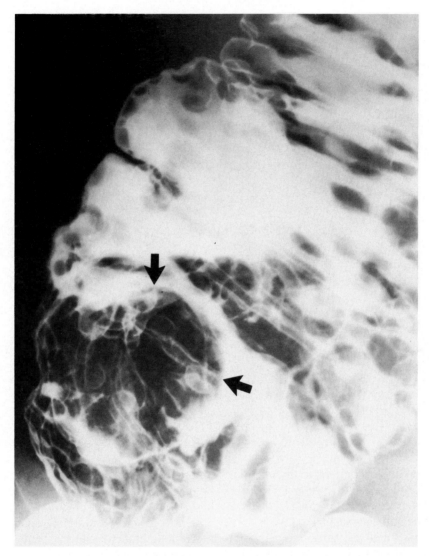

A large filling defect *(arrows)* and multiple, smaller, smooth-surfaced filling defects are present in the cecum. Similar-appearing submucosal nodules were present throughout the rest of the colon. These findings are due to non-Hodgkin's lymphoma.

Primary lymphoma of the colon usually occurs in patients more than 50 years old and most often among men. Symptoms usually include abdominal pain, weight loss, weakness, anorexia, and fever.

Radiologically, early diffuse lymphoma presents with submucosal nodules that involve only a limited portion of the colon. The cecum and rectum are the sites most often involved. Later, innumerable, diffuse filling defects with concomitant haustral thickening are seen.

Differential diagnostic considerations include familial polyposis (haustral folds are usually not thickened) (Case 373), ulcerative colitis (with inflammatory polyps and thickened haustra [Cases 411 and 414]), Crohn's colitis (Case 423), nodular lymphoid hyperplasia (usually seen in children and young adults with tiny [<4 mm] filling defects) (Cases 362 and 363), and schistosomiasis (lacks submucosal nodules and seen in patients from parts of the world in which the disease is endemic).

## Case 403

## LOCALIZED LYMPHOMA

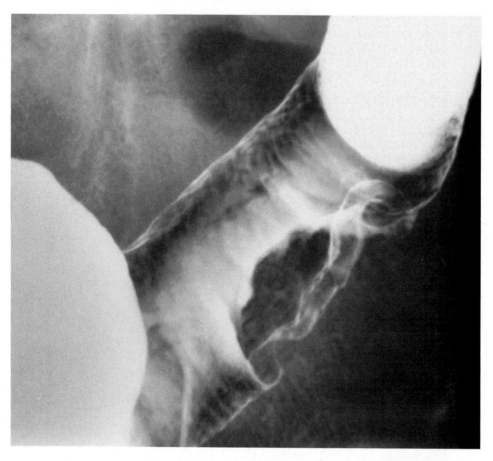

A broad-based sessile mass is present at the junction of the sigmoid and descending colon. The mass resembles a polypoid adenocarcinoma, but localized lymphoma was found at pathologic examination.

Localized lymphomas can have three radiographic presentations: a localized polypoid mass indistinguishable from a polypoid carcinoma (as in this case), a region of narrowing resembling carcinoma (usually without evidence of obstruction), and an aneurysmal segment of colon with luminal dilatation and mucosal ulceration. Intussusception can occur with bulky intraluminal masses.

**Case 404**

## LOCALIZED LYMPHOMA

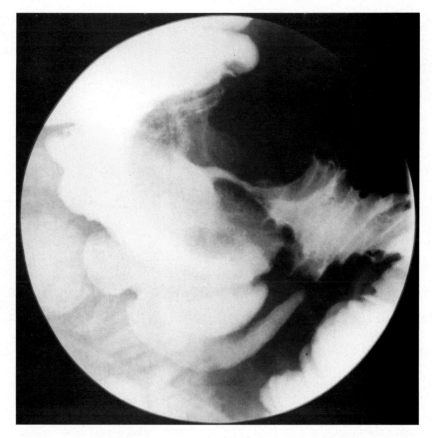

The ileocecal valve is markedly enlarged, and the folds of the terminal ileum are thickened. Localized lymphoma was confirmed later.

## Case 405

## MULTIFOCAL LYMPHOMA

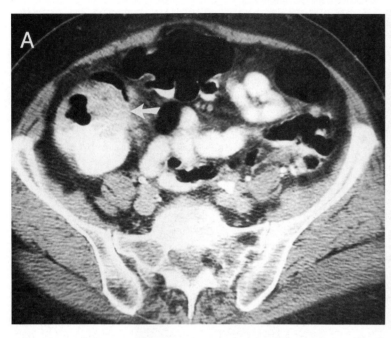 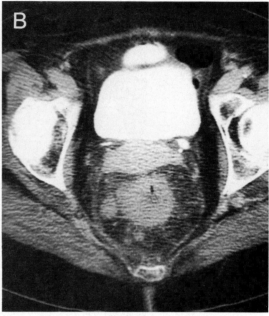

**A.** A localized soft-tissue mass *(arrow)* is present in the medial wall of the cecum. Several small lymph nodes are present within the cecal mesentery.

**B.** The rectal wall is diffusely thickened and several enlarged lymph nodes are visible in the perirectal fat. Multifocal lymphoma was confirmed histologically.

The CT finding of colonic lymphoma is usually focal or diffuse bowel-wall thickening. Perforation is an important complication of this disease that develops be-cause of the lack of the usual desmoplastic reaction encountered with most other tumors. This complication has been reported in 9% to 47% of patients and is often clinically silent (Joseph and Lattes, 1966; Hertzer and Hoerr, 1976). Identification of gas or fluid within a lymphomatous mass may indicate the presence of perforation. CT is an excellent modality for determining the amount of bowel-wall thickening, extent of disease, and presence of associated adenopathy.

# Case 406

## LIPOMA

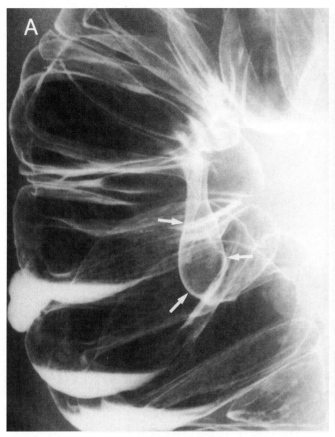 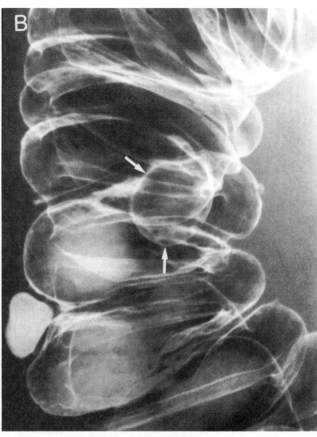

**A.** A pedunculated, smooth-surfaced polyp *(arrows)* is present along the medial aspect of the ascending colon.

**B.** The polyp *(arrows)* has changed shape with a change in position and distension. It now appears as a broad-based submucosal mass. The smooth surface of this lesion indicates its submucosal origin. Its changeable shape favors a lipoma, which was verified histologically.

Colonic lipomas are the most frequent submucosal tumors of the colon. They are slow-growing, benign neoplasms that are most commonly seen in the right side of the colon. Most lipomas are asymptomatic and found incidentally. Occasionally, lipomas can be the lead point for an intussusception, and patients may present with abdominal pain and rectal bleeding (Case 407).

A filling defect (usually >3 cm) with a very smooth surface is most often seen at contrast enema. The tumor is pliable and readily changes shape with compression or with collapse of the colonic lumen. Within the distended colon the mass often will be round, elliptical, or ovoid. It is common for the tumor to elongate and become sausage-shaped within the evacuated colon. The ileocecal valve may also become lipomatous. Often the valve appears enlarged, with a very smooth surface. Pliability and distensibility are key features of a lipomatous tumor which distinguish it from other submucosal lesions.

Case 407

## INTUSSUSCEPTING COLONIC LIPOMA

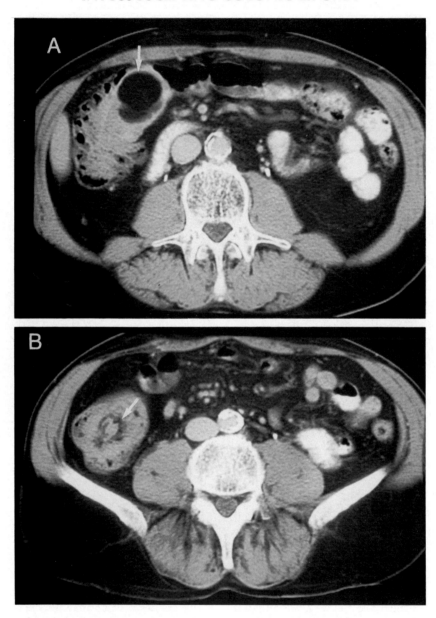

**A.** An intraluminal mass *(arrow)* is present within the right colon. The very low (fatty) density of the mass is pathognomonic of a lipoma.

**B.** At a slightly more caudal level, the characteristic finding of intussuscepting mesenteric fat *(arrow)* is seen within the colon. An intussuscepting lipoma was confirmed at contrast enema.

Most patients with a colonic lipoma are asymptomatic; however, occasionally large intraluminal lipomas cause intussusception, ulceration, or hemorrhage. Lipomas have no risk of malignant degeneration. If the lesion is asymptomatic, no treatment is required. If operation is required, the tumor can be removed by colotomy or myotomy and enucleation.

## Case 408

## MUCOCELE

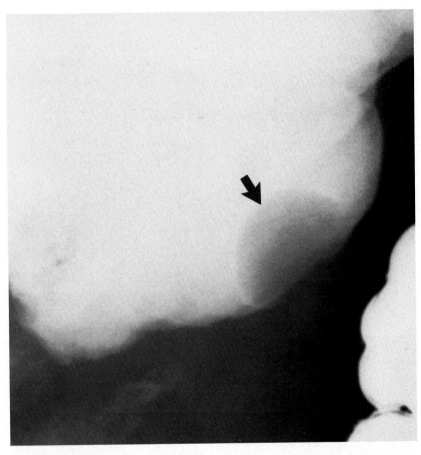

A smooth-surfaced filling defect *(arrow)* is present at the base of the cecum. The appendix is not seen. A mucocele due to an obstructing fecalith was removed at operation.

A mucocele of the appendix is regarded by some authors as a mucous-distended appendix secondary to luminal obstruction by a fecalith, foreign body, adhesion, or volvulus. Other authors include tumorous conditions of the appendix that often obstruct the appendix (Higa et al., 1973). These conditions include focal or diffuse mucosal hyperplasia, mucinous cystadenoma, and mucinous cystadenocarcinoma. Carcinoid tumors of the appendix are not classified with the epithelial-derived adenoma and adenocarcinoma tumors. They are rarely associated with appendiceal mucoceles.

Radiographically, a mucocele usually presents with findings of a smooth filling defect on the base of the cecum. Differential considerations include an appendiceal abscess (Case 430), endometriosis (Case 474), serosal metastases, and abscesses from other locations. Inverted appendiceal stumps are usually smaller and resemble an intraluminal polyp. Cecal carcinomas are usually nodular and have irregular surface contours (Case 378).

## Case 409

## MUCOCELE

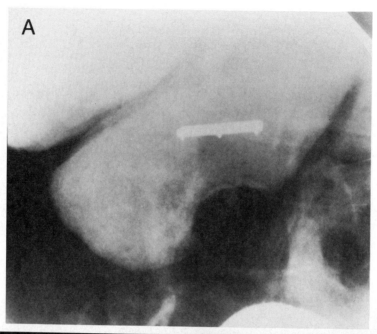

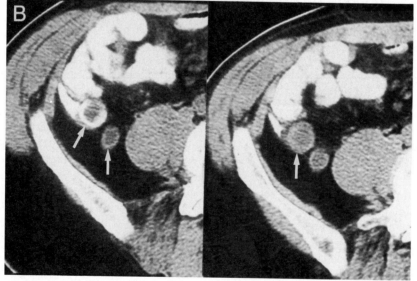

**A.** A smooth-surfaced filling defect is present in the base of the cecum. The appendix is not seen. A compression device containing a 2-cm marker is visible.

**B.** The appendix *(arrows)* is distended and fluid-filled. Linear calcification is present within part of the wall of the appendix. Findings are typical of a mucocele.

CT has improved our ability to diagnose a mucocele. Findings at CT include a thin-walled, cystic, and tubular structure with internal contents of low density. CT is also helpful to assess for metastases in patients with an appendiceal cystadenocarcinoma.

**Case 410**

## APPENDICEAL ADENOCARCINOMA

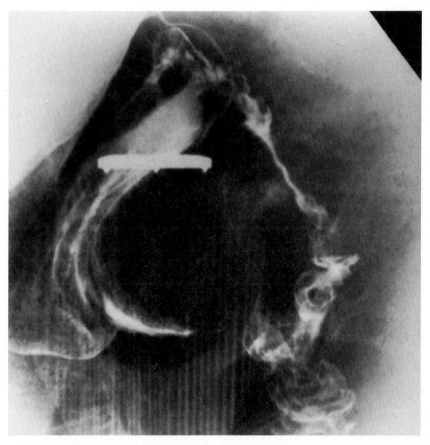

A large, smooth-surfaced filling defect is present in the base of the cecum. At operation, a mucinous cystadenocarcinoma of the appendix was removed. A compression device containing a 2-cm marker is visible.

Patients with appendiceal tumors often (50%) present clinically with symptoms of acute appendicitis. Approximately 15% will be discovered incidentally on histologic examination of the appendix (Otto et al., 1970). Metastatic mucinous cystadenocarcinoma often results in diffuse peritoneal carcinomatosis that pro-

duces large quantities of mucinous material that can calcify. This condition is often referred to as pseudomyxoma peritonei (Case 398).

Differential considerations of large, smooth filling defects in the cecum include lipoma (a soft mass that changes shape on compression) (Case 406), lymphoma (Case 404), appendiceal abscess (Case 430), endometrioma (Case 474), and benign mucocele (Case 408).

## Case 411

## ULCERATIVE COLITIS: TOXIC MEGACOLON

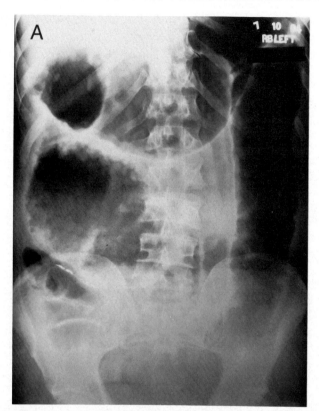

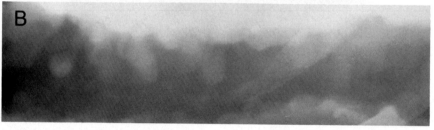

**A.** The colon is distended with gas (adynamic ileus pattern), and there are multiple polypoid masses protruding into the colonic lumen. Findings are typical of toxic megacolon.

**B.** Multiple polyps are seen within the colonic lumen on this close-up view.

Toxic megacolon is a serious complication that can occur in either ulcerative colitis or Crohn's colitis (although it is most frequently seen in patients with ulcerative colitis). This condition occurs in patients during a severe episode of acute inflammation. Dilatation ( > 6 cm) and adynamic ileus often occur because the inflammatory changes have extended into the muscular layers and usually to the serosa of the colon. Extensive mucosal disease can be visualized by identifying nodularity and polypoid changes within the colonic lumen. These polyps usually represent pseudopolyps. Bowel-wall and haustral thickening are secondary to intramural edema and congestion.

Colonic perforation can occur in toxic megacolon, and it has a high morbidity and mortality. Perforation may be suggested by identifying either intramural pneumatosis or pneumoperitoneum. Iatrogenic intervention is a common cause of perforation. In patients with this condition, a contrast enema or colonoscopy should be avoided. Even inflation of a rectal balloon in patients with a fragile, narrowed, and inflamed rectum can easily result in perforation.

Case 412

# ULCERATIVE COLITIS: PANCOLITIS

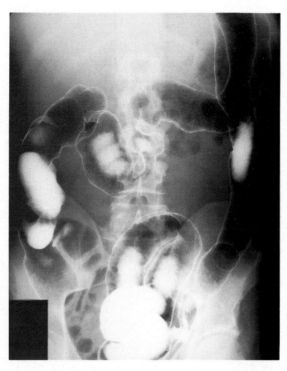

The entire colon is ahaustral, with a diffuse granular-appearing mucosa. The air-filled terminal ileum is dilated. These findings are characteristic of ulcerative colitis.

Ulcerative colitis is a disease of unknown origin that is characterized by an exudative inflammation that predominantly involves the mucosa of the colon. Granulomas are conspicuously absent. Ulceration of the mucosa is nearly always present in patients with active inflammation and is often associated with islands of intervening normal mucosa known as inflammatory polyps or pseudopolyps. Generally, ulcerative colitis begins in the rectum and extends to involve the more proximal colon in a continuous fashion. Inflammatory changes are usually circumferentially similar ("symmetric" bowel-wall involvement).

Clinically, many patients initially experience the sudden onset of bloody diarrhea, abdominal cramping, and fever. Others have an insidious course of vague abdominal pain and frequent stools. Because rectal involvement is common, often the initial diagnosis can be suggested by proctosigmoidoscopy. Extraintestinal manifestations of this disease include erythema no-

dosum, pyoderma gangrenosum, primary sclerosing cholangitis, cholangiocarcinoma, arthritis, sacroiliitis, spondylitis, and iritis. Spondylitis activity has no relationship to the activity of the colon inflammation. Patients with the HLA-B27 histocompatibility antigen are more likely to have spondylitis and iritis develop than patients without the marker.

In order to detect all degrees of disease severity, the double-contrast barium enema should be used in patients with suspected inflammatory bowel disease. Radiologically, three considerations are critical for making the diagnosis of ulcerative colitis.

1. The involved mucosa on an air-contrast barium enema has a granular (sandpaperlike) or stippled appearance.
2. The distribution of the disease is usually one of rectal involvement with disease affecting the more proximal colon in a continuous manner, without skip areas.
3. Circumferential bowel-wall symmetry is maintained. Mucosal ulcerations affect both sides of the bowel with equal severity.

### Case 413

## ULCERATIVE COLITIS: GRANULARITY

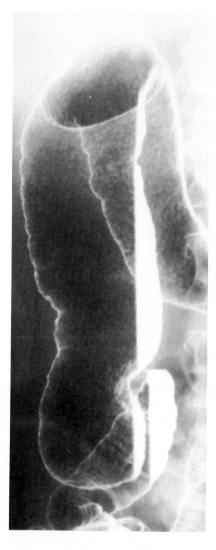

The typical, coarse granular mucosal ulcerations of chronic ulcerative colitis are visible in the right colon of this patient. This patient has pancolitis.

### Case 414

## ULCERATIVE COLITIS: INFLAMMATORY POLYPS

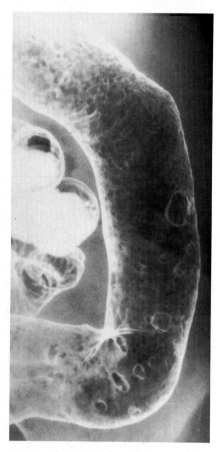

The colon is affected with a coarsely granular mucosal pattern. Numerous polypoid filling defects are also present.

Polypoid changes may develop in any stage of ulcerative colitis. In patients with severe, acute inflammation, pseudopolyps are likely to be present. Pseudopolyps refer to islands of normal colonic mucosa surrounded by denuded ulcerative mucosa. Inflammatory polyps refer to regions of inflamed elevated mucosa surrounded by granular mucosa. These polyps may be sessile or pedunculated, and they more often are found in patients with less severe inflammation than in those with pseudopolyps. Postinflammatory polyps are discussed with Case 415.

**Case 415**

## POSTINFLAMMATORY POLYPS

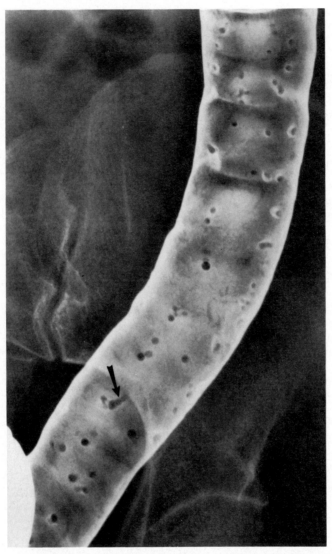

Multiple polypoid filling defects are present in the colon. Some of the polyps are elongated *(arrow)*. The background mucosal pattern is otherwise normal. This is the typical appearance of postinflammatory polyps in this patient with known ulcerative colitis.

Postinflammatory polyps develop during the healing phase in patients with either Crohn's colitis or ulcerative colitis. In the process of epithelial regeneration, true polyps develop (containing submucosa and mucosa). These polyps are often long and thin ("worm-like") and may branch. They are often referred to as fil-iform polyps (from the Latin word *filum* meaning thread).

Postinflammatory polyps are found most often during the healing phase of ulcerative colitis. Polypoid changes are usually multiple and may involve the colon either locally or diffusely. Rarely, a masslike collection of postinflammatory polyps can simulate a villous adenoma or carcinoma. These giant postinflammatory polyps are usually found in the right colon and are associated with other areas of typical filiform polyps.

## Case 416

# ULCERATIVE COLITIS: ATYPICAL MUCOSAL PATTERN

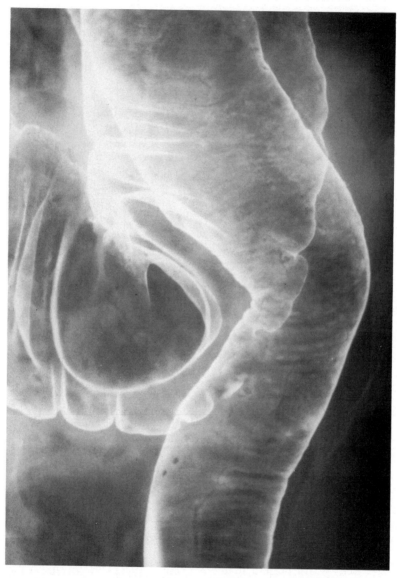

The mucosa in the descending colon has a "stippled" appearance. Many of these ulcerations appear to be isolated and resemble the aphthoid ulcerations of Crohn's colitis (Case 425). Discrete or linear ulcerations are less commonly encountered than diffuse granularity in patients with ulcerative colitis.

Classification of some radiographic changes may be difficult; patients with either ulcerative colitis or Crohn's colitis can occasionally share radiographic findings. Patients with ulcerative colitis and atypical mucosal changes (such as in this case) usually have symmetric and continuous disease that is not found in patients with Crohn's colitis. Generally, variant cases retain enough of the characteristics of either ulcerative colitis or Crohn's colitis to allow proper classification. Symmetry of involvement and mucosal surface changes are usually the most helpful in troublesome cases.

Case 417

# ATYPICAL DISTRIBUTION: HEALING PATTERN IN ULCERATIVE COLITIS

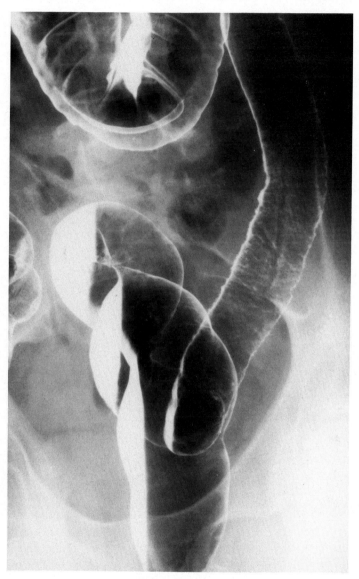

Active ulcerations (stippled and linear) are present in the sigmoid colon. The rectum has a normal featureless mucosa with some mild loss of distensibility. The patient was not using steroid enemas.

Rectal involvement is usually present in patients with ulcerative colitis and can be assumed to have occurred in the past in this patient because of the reduced distensibility of this bowel segment. Patients using steroid enemas may have a normal-appearing rectal mucosa with active disease in the more proximal colon. This distribution of disease can also be seen in patients with ulcerative colitis who have not used steroid enemas because of segmental mucosal healing and repair. The distribution of mucosal healing is the same as active inflammation in patients with ulcerative colitis—beginning in the rectum and progressing proximally in a continuous manner. Therefore, when the healing process begins, the rectum nearly always appears normal first, with variable degrees of inflammation present in the more proximal colon. The most severe disease is usually found proximally in a colonic segment near the leading edge of ascending inflammation.

## Case 418

# CHRONIC ULCERATIVE COLITIS WITH ANKYLOSING SPONDYLITIS

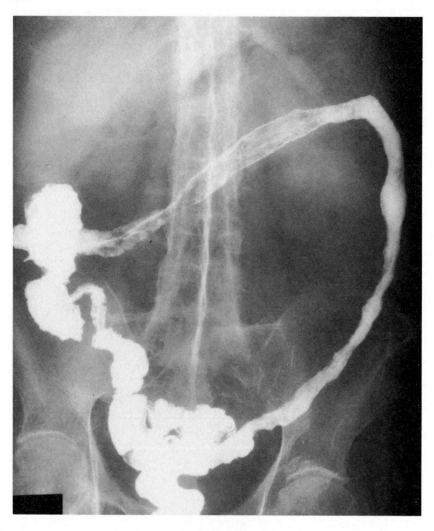

The colon is ahaustral and shortened. These findings are common in patients with long-standing ulcerative colitis. Typical changes of ankylosing spondylitis are also present.

Long-standing ulcerative colitis often results in a colon devoid of the normal haustral markings and a diffusely shortened and often narrowed colonic lumen. The colon usually appears featureless and rigid. Hyper-

trophy of the circular and longitudinal muscle fibers is now believed to be the most frequent cause of these changes.

Spondylitis often precedes the inflammatory bowel disease, whereas the symptoms of peripheral joint disease occur concurrently or following the onset of bowel symptoms.

## Case 419

## ULCERATIVE COLITIS: DYSPLASIA

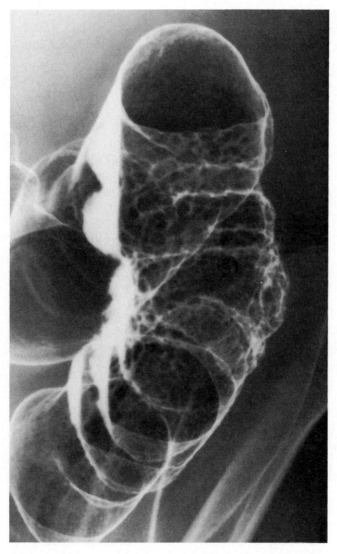

Multiple nodules are present in the descending colon in this patient with a 22-year history of ulcerative colitis. The nodules abut each other and have flattened edges. Endoscopic biopsy demonstrated that the nodules were formed of atypical colonic glands crowded within the lamina propria. This pattern is often encountered in dysplastic nodules.

Patients with ulcerative colitis are at increased risk for developing colon cancer. Those patients at greatest

From Hooyman JR, MacCarty RL, Carpenter HA, Schroeder KW, Carlson HC. AJR *1987;*149:47–51. By permission of the American Roentgen Ray Society.

risk have colonic epithelial dysplasia. Detection of dysplasia in a colitic colon should prompt endoscopic biopsy and possibly prophylactic colectomy. Unfortunately, most mucosal dysplasia is not visible radiographically and requires random endoscopic biopsy for detection.

Radiographically, dysplasia appears as a solitary nodule or multiple nodules. A close grouping of nodules with opposed flattened edges is most commonly (50% of time) associated with dysplasia (Hooyman et al., 1987). Inflammatory polyps may be indistinguishable from dysplastic nodules.

## Case 420

# ULCERATIVE COLITIS: SECONDARY CARCINOMA

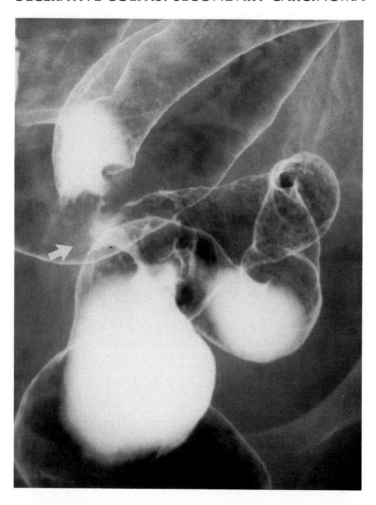

An annular carcinoma *(arrow)* is present in the sigmoid colon. The granular mucosal changes of ulcerative colitis are also present.

Patients with ulcerative colitis have an increased risk of colorectal cancer developing. The risk depends on the extent and duration of inflammation. Patients with pancolitis are at higher risk of colon cancer than patients with only limited disease. The risk of cancer developing begins after a patient has had the disease for 10 years and increases with time. The actual cancer risk varies from study to study—ranging from a 3% to 10% risk of malignancy after 10 years to a 13% to 25% risk after 25 years of ulcerative colitis (de Dombal et al., 1966; Lennard-Jones et al., 1990). The clinical activity of the disease has little effect on the overall cancer risk.

Mucosal dysplasia is the precursor of carcinoma. Most cancers complicating ulcerative colitis are annular constricting lesions (as in this case). Some carcinomas develop as flat, infiltrating tumors—extending into the submucosal tissues and causing either a smooth or an abruptly tapered stricture (Case 421). About one-fourth of all cancers present as strictures (Edwards and Truelove, 1963). Multiple cancers are common. Polypoid masses are rare. Generally, these malignancies are high-grade, aggressive tumors.

Benign strictures can also develop in ulcerative colitis as a result of muscular hypertrophy or as a result of severe inflammation. Because it is impossible to differentiate benign from malignant strictures radiographically, they should all be regarded with suspicion.

Case 421

# ULCERATIVE COLITIS: SECONDARY CARCINOMA

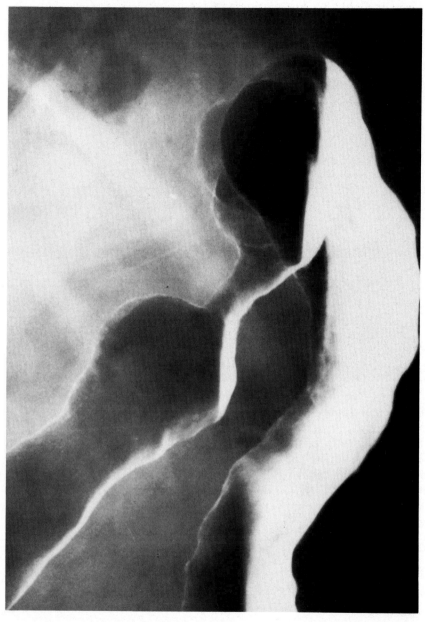

A stricture is present in the region of the splenic flexure of the colon. The lack of haustrations is due to chronic ulcerative colitis. At operation, a submucosal adenocarcinoma was discovered.

Some complicating carcinomas present as benign-appearing strictures. These regions of narrowing may be difficult to detect endoscopically, and a biopsy may not reveal tumor because of its deep submucosal location. All strictures in patients with long-standing ulcerative colitis should be considered potentially malignant.

## Case 422

## SEVERE ULCERATIVE COLITIS: CT

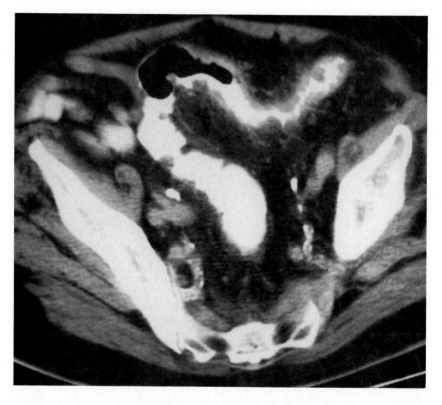

The wall of the sigmoid colon is thickened and there is associated stranding in the pericolonic fat.

Detection of inflammatory diseases of the colon at CT depends on the severity of the disease and the quality of the examination. Usually, mild disease confined to the mucosa is not detectable at CT. Severe disease with inflammatory changes extending to the serosal surface causes bowel-wall thickening and often soft-tissue stranding in the pericolonic fat (as seen in this case). Occasionally, a low-density ring is seen within the bowel wall when viewed in cross section. The low-density changes are believed to represent intramural edema.

Case 423

## CROHN'S DISEASE: ACUTE COLITIS

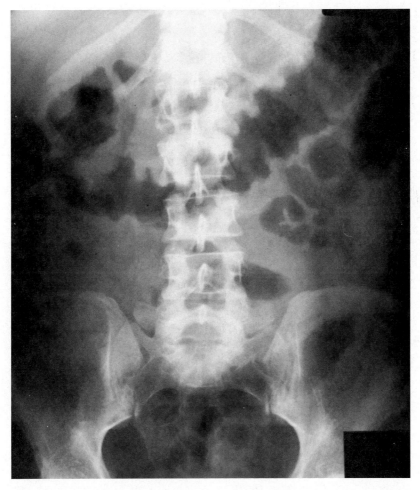

The haustral folds are diffusely thickened throughout the transverse colon. The findings are those of acute colitis that could be due to inflammatory bowel disease (ulcerative colitis or Crohn's colitis), infectious colitis, pseudomembranous colitis, or, less likely, ischemic colitis. This patient had Crohn's colitis.

Most patients with acute colitis will present with similar radiographic findings in the involved portions of the colon. Intramural edema and hemorrhage cause wall and haustral thickening (as seen in this case). Inflammatory polyps can be visible within the gas-filled colon in patients with inflammatory bowel disease (Case 411). The splenic flexure is often an isolated segment of involved colon in elderly patients with ischemic colitis (Case 446). A contrast enema is usually contraindicated in patients with acute colitis because of the risk of perforation. A contrast enema can be performed safely after the acute episode has resolved. Proctoscopy is often useful in revealing the mucosal changes of ulcerative colitis or pseudomembranous colitis.

## Case 424

## CROHN'S COLITIS: EARLY CHANGES

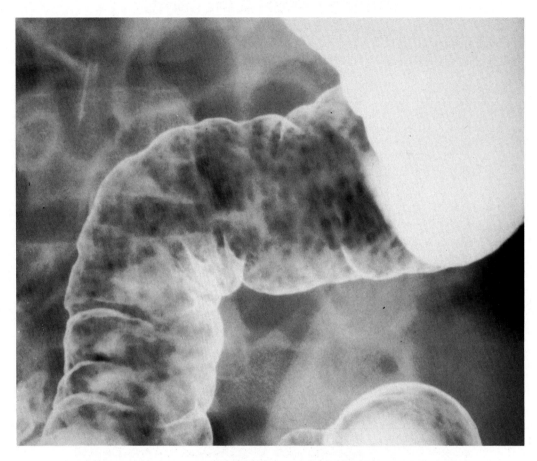

A prominent lymphoid pattern is present in the sigmoid colon. Some of the nodules are mildly enlarged (>4 mm). Typical changes of Crohn's disease developed later in this region.

The earliest change of Crohn's colitis is submucosal granulomatous inflammation. Enlarged lymphoid follicles are often seen radiographically. These mucosal elevations usually have poorly defined borders and may contain a small central umbilication. The early changes of Crohn's colitis are best depicted using the double-contrast technique. A lymphoid pattern can be seen normally in 10% to 15% of adults (Case 362) (Kelvin et al., 1979). These nodules are uniformly small. In some patients it may be impossible to differentiate a normal lymphoid pattern from early Crohn's disease. In these patients, either repeat double-contrast colon examination in several months or endoscopic biopsy is helpful.

Case 425

## CROHN'S COLITIS: APHTHOUS AND CONFLUENT ULCERS

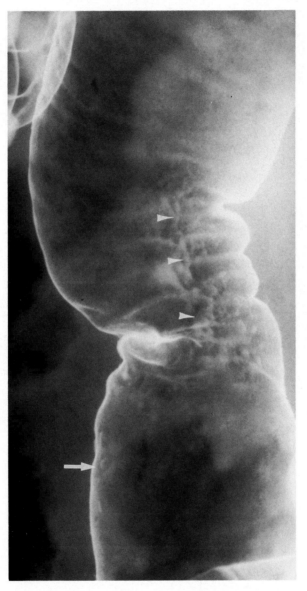

Multiple discrete (aphthous) ulcers *(arrow)* are present within the descending colon. A halo of edema surrounds each ulceration. Many of the ulcers have become confluent, producing a linear ulceration *(arrowheads)*. The intervening mucosa between ulcers appears normal. The distribution of ulcerations is circumferentially asymmetric. All of these findings are characteristic of Crohn's colitis.

Aphthous ulcers develop from enlarged lymphoid follicles that ulcerate centrally. These ulcers are very shallow lesions and usually are not seen in profile. Multiplicity of lesions is common. The central barium collection often varies in size and is always surrounded by a halo of edema. Although the aphthous ulcer is characteristic of Crohn's disease, it is not diagnostic. These lesions have been reported in other infectious colitides, including *Yersinia* and amebic colitis.

## Case 426

## CROHN'S COLITIS: FISTULA

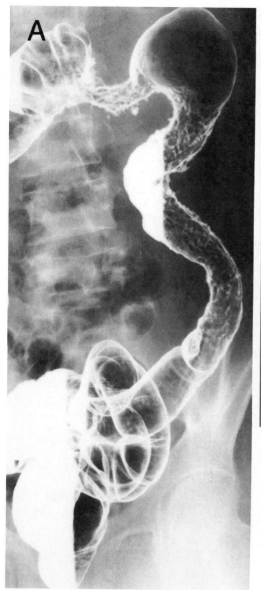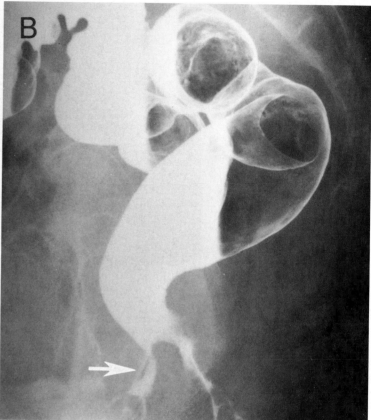

**A.** Segmental regions of narrowing are present in the left transverse and in the descending colon. Polypoid mucosal (inflammatory polyps) changes and deep linear and thornlike ulcers are present in the affected segments. Circumferential asymmetry is present in the splenic flexure due to fibrosis and scarring in the medial wall of the colon.

**B.** The mucosa in the rectum is normal but there is a rectovaginal fistula *(arrow)* arising from the anterior wall of the distal rectum. Findings are characteristic of Crohn's colitis.

Advanced Crohn's colitis is characterized by discontinuous and asymmetric disease (as seen in this case). The rectum is often uninvolved. Deep ulcerations can appear as longitudinal and transverse collections of barium. These ulcers may crisscross, producing a "cobblestone" mucosal appearance. Solitary deep ulcers may appear "thornlike" or as a "collar button." Inflammatory polyps are often present. Colonic strictures are due to transmural inflammation and fibrosis. These strictures do not have the same malignant potential as do those in patients with ulcerative colitis (Case 421).

There is an increased incidence of alimentary-tract malignancies in patients with Crohn's disease; most of these tumors are of colonic origin (Weedon et al., 1973).

Fistulae are common in Crohn's disease and can occur from an involved colonic segment(s) to another bowel loop(s), vagina, bladder, skin, or retroperitoneal organs.

The most important differential consideration is ulcerative colitis. Mucosal granularity, rectal involvement, and continuous and symmetric disease are features of ulcerative colitis that can be helpful in distinguishing it from Crohn's disease (Cases 412–414, 416–418). Ischemic colitis is usually seen in an older population, most commonly affecting the splenic flexure (Cases 446–448). Various infectious colitides (*Actinomyces, Yersinia, Campylobacter, Salmonella, Shigella, Chlamydia, Clostridium, Escherichia coli, Neisseria gonorrhoeae,* and others) can affect the colon. During the acute phase of infection, the changes may be radiologically indistinguishable from those found in patients with ulcerative colitis or Crohn's disease.

## Case 427

# CROHN'S COLITIS: DEEP ULCERATIONS

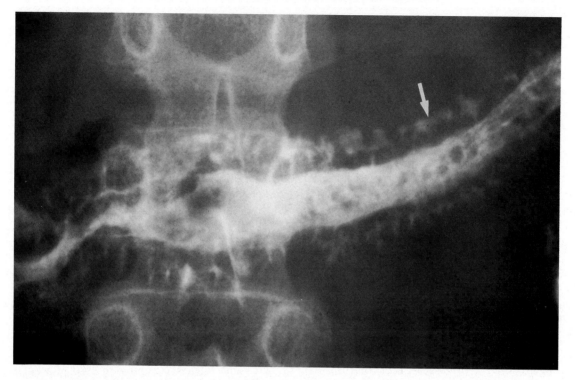

The colonic lumen is narrowed, and there are multiple deep ulcers within the involved segment. A sinus tract *(arrow)* connects some of the ulcers along the superior margin of the colon.

Ulcerations such as in this case can be seen with either Crohn's colitis or ulcerative colitis. They are most frequently encountered in Crohn's disease. In some patients it may be impossible to distinguish ulcerative colitis from Crohn's disease. The distribution, continuity, and symmetry of disease are usually more helpful in distinguishing these diseases than the depth or appearance of the active ulcers.

Crohn's colitis may be accompanied by extraintestinal diseases, including spondyloarthritis, cholelithiasis, sclerosing cholangitis, granulomatous hepatitis, urinary calculi, and amyloidosis.

**Case 428**

## CROHN'S COLITIS: MESENTERIC ABSCESS

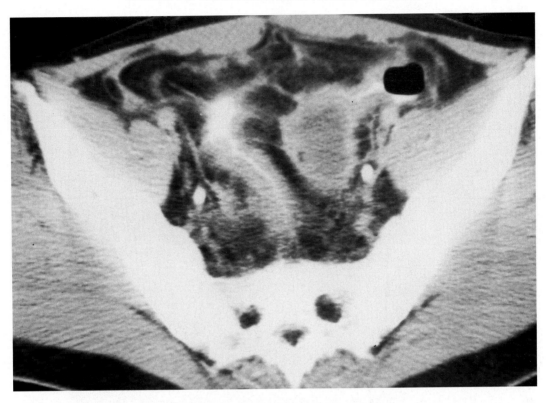

The wall of the rectum and sigmoid colon is thickened. There is associated stranding in the pericolic fat as well as a mass the density of water adjacent to the sigmoid colon. This mass has the appearance of, and was later proven to be, a mesenteric abscess in a patient with known Crohn's colitis.

CT is an excellent tool for visualizing the extraintestinal extent of disease and bowel-wall thickness in patients with inflammatory bowel disease. The typical CT findings of Crohn's colitis include segmental bowel-wall thickening and mesenteric soft-tissue stranding. Generally, the amount of bowel-wall thickening is more marked in Crohn's colitis than in ulcerative coli-

tis. Fatty proliferation of the mesentery (39%) as well as mesenteric lymphadenopathy (18%) can be present (Case 300) (Goldberg et al., 1983). A mesenteric abscess usually appears as an encapsulated fluid collection adjacent to a segment of thick-walled bowel (as seen in this case). In some patients, the adjacent inflammatory changes form a poorly defined soft-tissue mass. These changes are referred to as a phlegmon by some investigators. Percutaneous drainage may be indicated in the treatment of a well-defined mesenteric abscess. The information available at CT is invaluable in determining the feasibility and route for catheter drainage.

## Case 429

## APPENDICOLITH

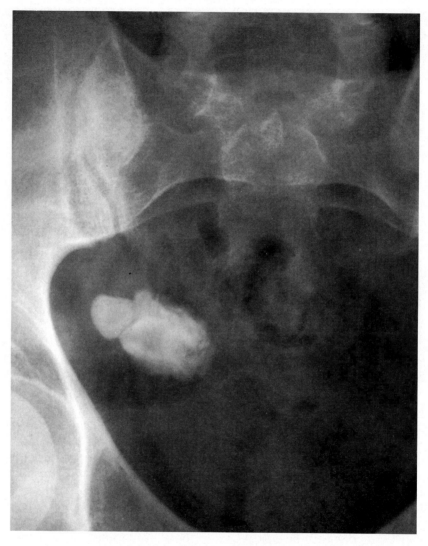

Two laminated calcific densities are present in the right lower quadrant. Findings are typical of appendicoliths.

Appendicoliths develop as a result of calcification about an obstructing nidus of fecal debris within the appendiceal lumen. The calculus often has a lucent center and has an average diameter of 2 cm. Approximately 15% of all patients with appendicitis have a visible calculus (Baker and Elkin, 1983). It is estimated that approximately half of all symptomatic patients with a visible appendicolith already have a perforated appendix (Shimkin, 1978).

Other findings of appendicitis that may be present on an abdominal plain film include an atonic gas-filled terminal ileum or cecum (sentinel loop) or a generalized adynamic ileus if peritonitis has developed.

Differential considerations of abdominal calculi include pelvic phleboliths, ureteral calculi, ectopic gallstones, enteroliths within a Meckel diverticulum, epiploic calcifications, calcified mesenteric lymph nodes (Case 305), bone islands, retained barium, and foreign bodies.

### Case 430

## APPENDICITIS

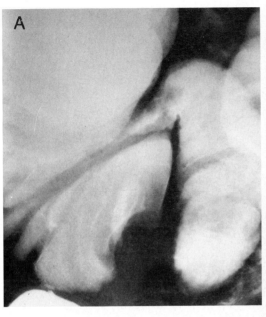
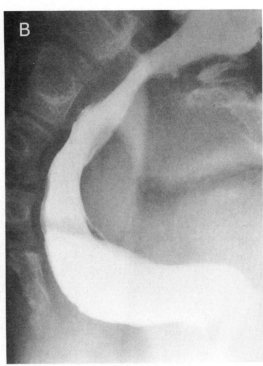

**A.** A smooth-surfaced filling defect is present at the base of the cecum. The appendix did not fill. Diagnostic considerations include an appendiceal abscess, lipoma, mucocele of the appendix, endometrioma, or an abscess secondary to Crohn's disease or pelvic inflammatory disease.

**B.** There is a large mass in the region of the pouch of Douglas that causes anterior compression of the rectosigmoid. At operation, an appendiceal abscess was present as well as a large pelvic abscess in the pouch of Douglas.

Appendicitis is caused by obstruction of the appendiceal lumen, with secondary dilatation, infection, inflammation, ischemia, and possible perforation. Clinically, patients usually complain of generalized abdominal discomfort that localizes to the right lower quadrant. Signs of peritoneal irritation or generalized peritonitis may be present. Early recognition of appendicitis is important because the mortality associated with this disease is low (0.1%) if the appendix is only inflamed but increases to more than 13% with an appendiceal abscess not initially treated with appendectomy (Barnes et al., 1962).

A contrast enema can be helpful in excluding the diagnosis of appendicitis. There is virtually no risk of extravasation of contrast material from the colon or appendix. The enema is performed in the unprepared colon and an attempt is made to fill the appendix with contrast material. Demonstration of the bulbous tip of the appendix is excellent evidence that the entire appendiceal lumen has been filled. Complete filling of the appendix excludes the diagnosis of appendicitis. Normally, the appendix can be completely filled in 80% to 90% of individuals. Patients with appendicitis will have partial or nonfilling of the appendix. A filling defect may be present on the base of the cecum about the appendiceal orifice, particularly if an appendiceal abscess is present (as in this case). Inflammatory changes may be seen on nearby bowel (often terminal ileum) with thickened and edematous folds. The appendix can be located almost anywhere in the abdomen, and the demonstration of the appendix in an unusual location may provide an explanation for confusing clinical signs and symptoms.

## Case 431

## RETROCECAL APPENDICITIS

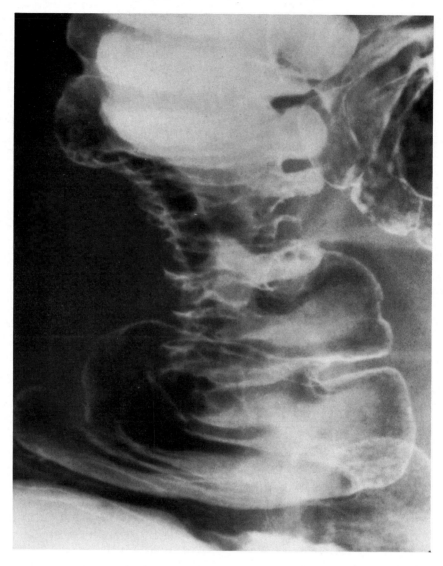

Mass effect is present along the lateral aspect of the mid-ascending colon. There are also thickened and tethered folds in this region. An inflammatory process or serosal metastases could cause this appearance. Retrocecal appendicitis was discovered at operation.

## Case 432

## PERIAPPENDICEAL ABSCESS

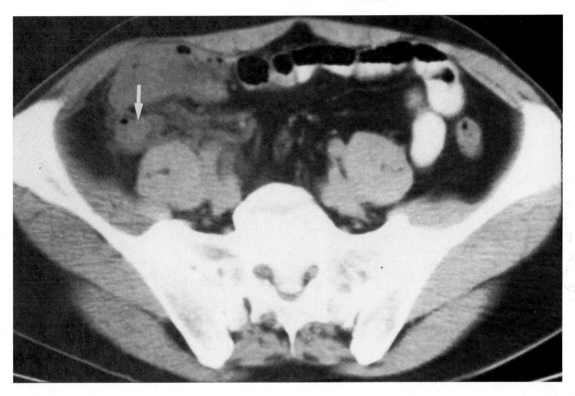

The distended appendiceal lumen is visible in the right lower quadrant *(arrow)* surrounded by a small fluid collection and a single gas bubble. Soft-tissue stranding in the periappendiceal fat is also present. At operation, acute appendicitis with a periappendiceal abscess was present.

CT can directly visualize the appendix and periappendiceal region. CT findings of appendicitis include periappendiceal and mesenteric soft-tissue stranding or a soft-tissue mass, thickening of the wall of the colon, fascial thickening, and a periappendiceal fluid collection (abscess). Direct visualization of the appendix is possible in a majority of patients. Some investigators (Jeffrey et al., 1987) have reported that the size and appearance of an appendiceal abscess can direct proper management. Further study is needed to confirm these findings.

## Case 433

## APPENDICITIS: PELVIC ABSCESS

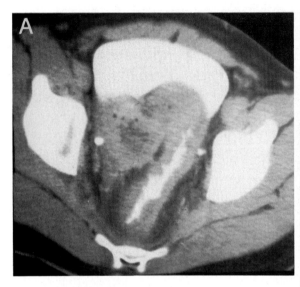

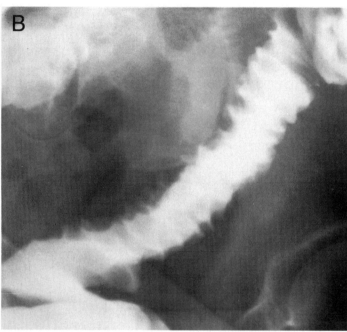

**A.** A large mass is present in the right side of the pelvis; the center is the density of water and has a thick soft-tissue rind. The wall of the sigmoid colon is circumferentially thickened.

**B.** The sigmoid colon is narrowed, contains thickened folds, and has an intact mucosal pattern.

Gangrenous appendicitis and a pelvic abscess were present at operation. The adjacent inflammatory reaction caused the changes in the sigmoid colon.

The operative management of periappendiceal inflammatory masses remains controversial. A periappendiceal abscess is present in a minority of patients with appendicitis. An associated abscess makes a simple appendectomy more difficult, wound closure less successful, abscess recurrence more common, and postoperative complication rate higher. Percutaneous drainage of a well-defined abscess the density of water can be successful in >90% of patients. Poorly defined, phlegmonous abscess collections are generally best treated surgically. Small periappendiceal abscess collections (<3 cm in diameter) have been reported to be cured by antibiotics alone in nearly 90% of patients (Jeffrey et al., 1987).

Case 434

## APPENDICITIS

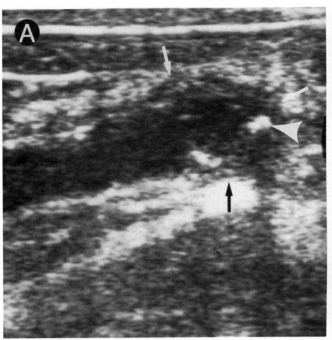
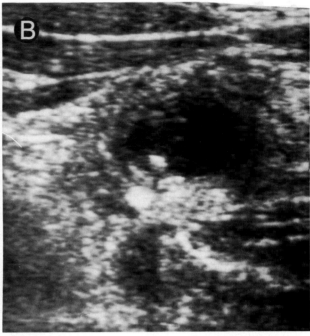

**A.** A distended bulbous-tipped appendix *(arrows)* containing echogenic appendicoliths *(arrowhead)* in its base is visible on this longitudinal sonogram in the right lower quadrant.

**B.** The distended appendix and calculus are also visible on this transverse view of the appendix. The appendix was not compressible.

Ultrasound can be useful for directly visualizing the appendix in patients with equivocal clinical findings. It is estimated that approximately 20% of all laparotomies for appendicitis are negative. The accuracy of sonography has been reported to approach 95% (Jeffrey et al., 1987).

Graded compression of the right lower abdomen is performed in order to empty the cecum and right colon of gas and fluid. The appendix is usually visualized at the base of the cecum. Normally, the appendiceal wall does not exceed 2 mm in thickness. Often the normal appendix is not visible, but an appendix that is abnormally distended (≥6 mm diameter) or has a thickened wall (>2 mm) is considered pathologic (Jeffrey et al., 1988). A periappendiceal fluid collection can often be identified if the appendix is perforated.

Crohn's disease can affect the appendix as part of the spectrum of granulomatous ileocolitis. Occasionally, the disease will be localized solely to the appendix. It is usually not possible to distinguish acute appendicitis from Crohn's appendicitis.

## Case 435

## DIVERTICULOSIS

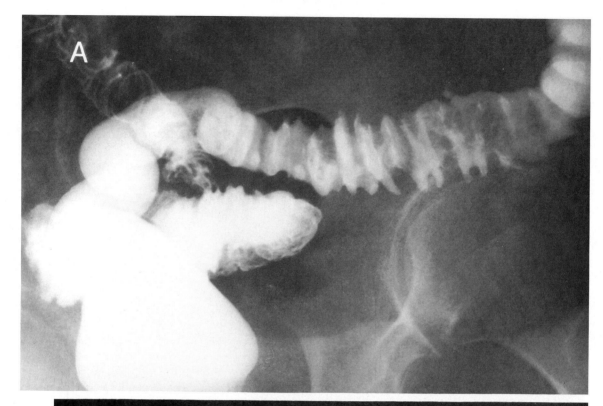

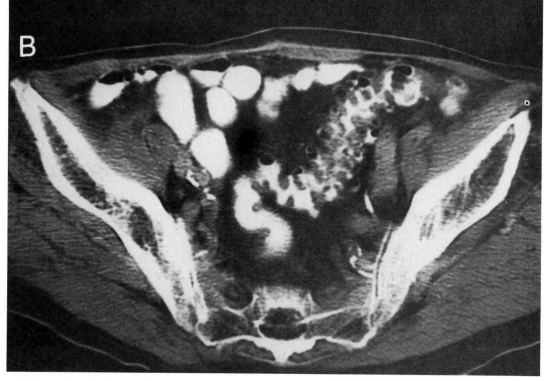

**A.** Multiple sigmoid diverticula are present with associated muscular hypertrophy.

**B.** Diverticulosis and muscular hypertrophy are present in the sigmoid colon. Notice how the diverticula extend beyond the confines of the muscular bowel wall. The normal pericolonic fat is of homogeneously low density.

Diverticula are sac-like outpouchings that extend from the colonic lumen. These protrusions develop as a result of increased intraluminal pressure, with resultant herniation of the colonic mucosa through areas of inherent bowel-wall weakness (where blood vessels penetrate the bowel wall). Many patients have diverticulosis without symptoms, whereas others will have symptoms attributed to irritable bowel syndrome (cramping, pain, and altered bowel habits). Diverticulosis is common and is of clinical importance.

1. Diverticula can be difficult to distinguish from polyps. Polyps can be distinguished from diverticula by demonstrating that the diverticula extend beyond the colonic lumen. No filling defect is encountered on the fluoroscopic single-contrast enema if the diverticula is empty. Double-contrast examinations demonstrate filling of dependently positioned diverticula with contrast material or a ring shadow on the nondependent surface, with a sharp outer margin and blurred inner margin.

2. Residual stool within diverticula can simulate polyps (pseudopolyps). Residual stool can be differentiated from polyps by recognizing that they arise from a diverticula, often requiring that colonic segment to be examined in steep oblique views. Often a dense ring of barium is visible as barium is caught between the wall of the diverticulum and the stool. This is best seen when the diverticulum is viewed en face (Case 369).

3. Gastrointestinal bleeding can develop from erosion of a blood vessel at the base of the diverticulum. Although diverticula more commonly involve the sigmoid colon, bleeding diverticula usually involve the ascending colon and hepatic flexure regions. The severity of bleeding increases with age. Radionuclide-tagged erythrocytes, $^{99m}$Tc-sulfur colloid studies (may detect as little as 0.1 mL/min), or mesenteric angiography (requires at least 0.5 mL/min of bleeding) can be helpful in documenting the cause and location of the bleeding.

4. Inflammation and perforation of a diverticulum result in diverticulitis. Radiographic manifestations of diverticulitis are illustrated in the cases that follow.

## Case 436

## DIVERTICULITIS

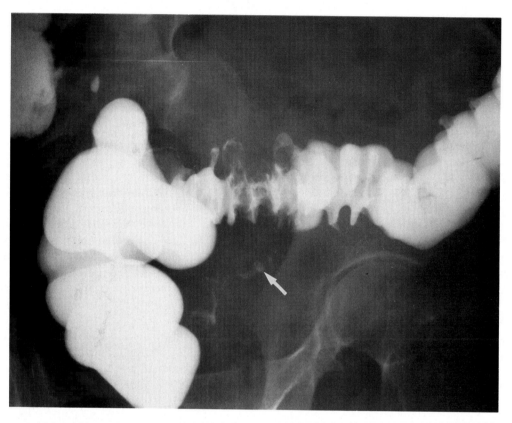

A segmental region of fold thickening is present in the mid-sigmoid colon. A tract *(arrow)* of extravasated barium extends inferiorly from the involved sigmoid within pericolic tissues. The mucosa is intact through the involved region. These findings are typical of diverticulitis.

Diverticulitis occurs as a result of inflammation of a solitary diverticulum and subsequent perforation and extravasation of colonic contents into pericolonic tissues. Usually the pericolonic inflammation or infection is rapidly contained and walled off. Rarely, peritonitis may develop. Diverticulitis may resolve spontaneously, often responding to antibiotic therapy and a soft diet. In some patients, the disease may be more severe; if an intramural or pericolonic abscess develops, it may require percutaneous or surgical drainage. Seeding of the mesenteric veins with microorganisms can result in sepsis, a hepatic abscess, or mesenteric vein thrombosis. Fistulae can develop and communicate with the bladder, vagina, bowel loops, and other locations or organs.

Radiographic findings at contrast enema include: narrowing of the colonic lumen (usually a longer segment is involved compared to colon cancer), thickening of the mucosal folds (from the adjacent inflammation), mass effect with an intact overlying mucosa (secondary to the abscess), and extravasation of contrast material into the abscess cavity. Not all of these findings need to be present to make the proper diagnosis; in fact, contrast extravasation is seen in a minority of patients. The most important differential consideration is carcinoma. Careful assessment of the mucosa is critical for distinguishing these conditions from one another. Other findings besides an ulcerated mucosa in patients with cancer include margins that are abrupt and shouldered and nodularity of the affected colonic segment.

## Case 437

## DIVERTICULITIS

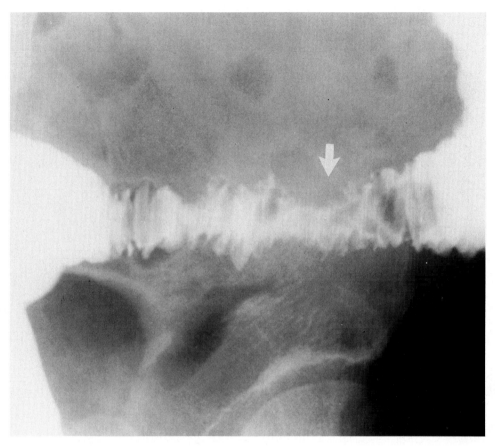

The sigmoid colon is narrowed. Normal mucosal folds are present across this relatively long segment of involved colon. Mass effect *(arrow)* is present along the superior aspect of the sigmoid, and tethered folds are visible inferiorly. Findings are likely due to diverticulitis or serosal metastases. Diverticulitis was confirmed clinically.

This case demonstrates all of the radiographic findings of diverticulitis with the exception of contrast extravasation. Because serosal metastases could have a similar appearance (Case 397), clinical history is often necessary to make the distinction. In addition, patients with diverticulitis often will be focally tender if this region is palpated at fluoroscopy. Careful inspection of the mucosa for the normal, sharply defined, perpendicularly oriented musosal folds is a reliable means of excluding carcinoma.

## Case 438

## DIVERTICULITIS: ATYPICAL

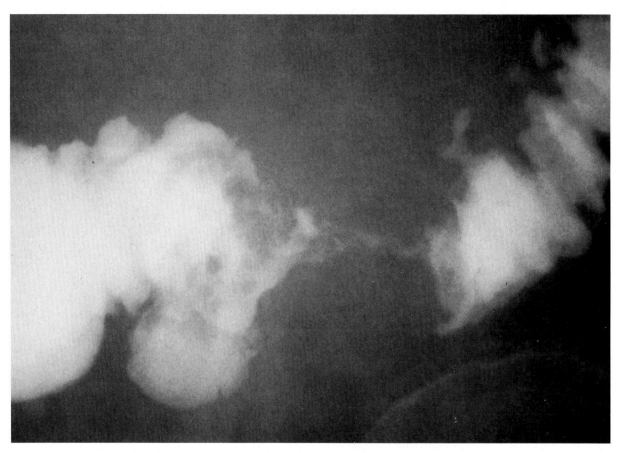

A short focal segment of narrowing is present in the sigmoid colon. The margins of the focal abnormality are abrupt. Normal mucosal markings are difficult to identify throughout the entire segment. The short annular appearance of this abnormality is worrisome for carcinoma. Diverticulitis was found at operation.

This case illustrates that the barium enema may not be able to exclude carcinoma in all patients. It has been estimated that approximately 10% of all contrast enemas performed for diverticulitis will be considered indeterminate, i.e., cancer cannot be excluded (Johnson et al., 1987). Short and nodular segments of narrowed colon as well as the inability to demonstrate normal mucosal folds should be regarded as suggestive of carcinoma. Colonoscopy is often helpful in excluding cancer in equivocal cases if the colonoscope can be passed through the narrowed lumen.

## Case 439

## DIVERTICULITIS: CT

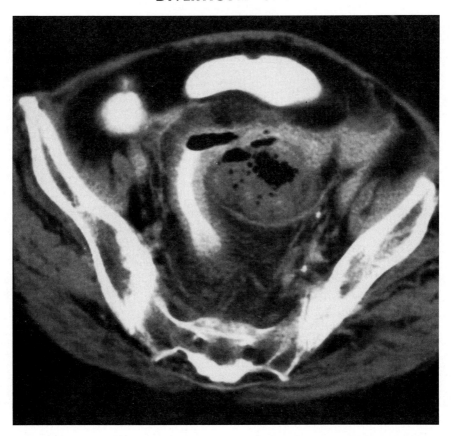

Bowel-wall thickening, mesenteric soft-tissue stranding, and a pericolonic abscess involve the sigmoid colon. These findings were considered diagnostic of diverticulitis. Surgical resection of the sigmoid was performed.

CT can be helpful in evaluating patients with suspected diverticulitis. The advantage of this technique is its ability to directly image the entire bowel wall and extraluminal tissues. CT findings of diverticulitis include bowel-wall thickening, soft-tissue stranding in the pericolonic fat, and a pericolonic abscess (fluid or gas collection). An actual abscess is seen in fewer than half of the patients in our practice. Visualization of the size and location of a pericolonic abscess, a hepatic abscess, or a fistula is helpful information in planning either percutaneous drainage or operation. The major disadvantage of CT is its inability to assess the colonic mucosa and exclude cancer. Most patients with the CT diagnosis of diverticulitis should have a barium enema or endoscopic study to exclude cancer during their follow-up care.

Percutaneous drainage of a diverticular abscess should be considered if a two- or three-stage surgical operation will be required. This generally occurs in patients with large abscess cavities that cannot be removed en bloc at the initial operation. Percutaneous drainage can be helpful by draining and shrinking the abscess preoperatively. After much of the infection and inflammation have subsided, a single-stage sigmoid resection can be safely performed. Obviously, safe access to the abscess must be available for percutaneous drainage. In this particular case, no safe access route was visible. Operation is required if peritoneal signs are present or if there is evidence of peritoneal spillage or abscess rupture.

## Case 440

## DIVERTICULITIS: SMALL MESENTERIC ABSCESS

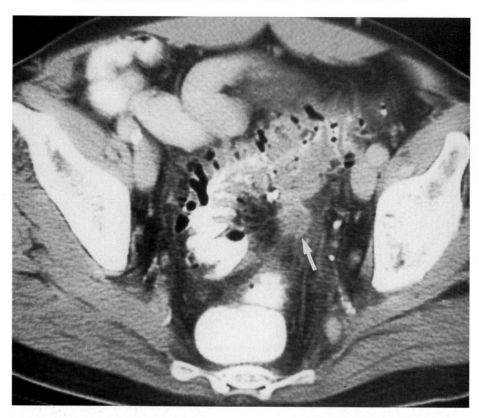

The wall of the sigmoid colon is thickened and a small low-density mass *(arrow)* as well as soft-tissue stranding is present in the sigmoid mesentery. Extensive sigmoid diverticulosis is present. The mesenteric mass represents an abscess, a finding considered diagnostic of diverticulitis at CT.

If operation were to be performed, the size and location of the mesenteric abscess is very favorable for a single-stage sigmoid resection and reanastomosis. The abscess is too small for percutaneous drainage.

**Case 441**

## DIVERTICULITIS: INTRAMURAL ABSCESS

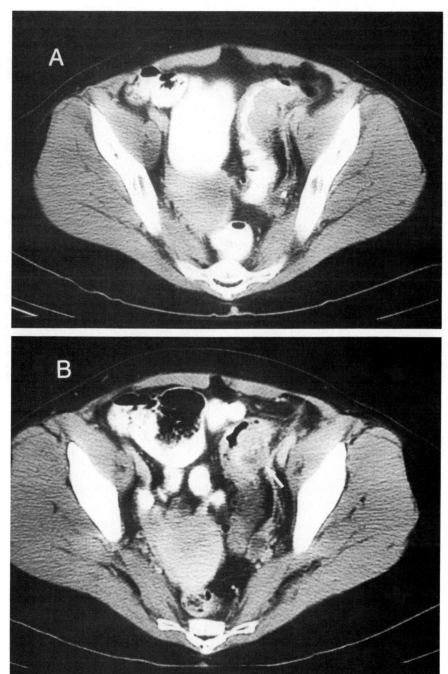

**A.** Near the junction of the sigmoid and descending colon is a focal region of bowel-wall thickening, luminal narrowing, and mesenteric soft-tissue stranding.

**B.** A small low-density mass *(arrow)* is present within the wall of the colon, representing an intramural abscess.

Diverticulitis was confirmed clinically.

## Case 442

# DIVERTICULITIS: INTRAMURAL SINUS TRACT

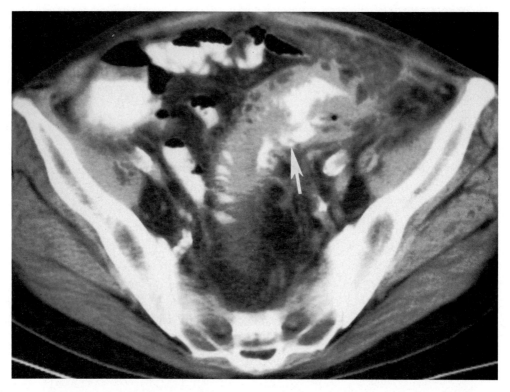

Intraluminal contrast material has extravasated into the bowel wall *(arrow)*. Bowel-wall thickening and mesenteric soft-tissue stranding are also present. These findings are diagnostic of diverticulitis, which was confirmed at operation.

Visualization of an intramural sinus tract or mesenteric abscess is considered diagnostic of diverticulitis at CT. Perforated carcinoma, however, can present with a pericolonic fluid collection (abscess) (Cases 390 and 391). These patients can also have symptoms that mimic diverticulitis. If operation is not performed, it may be prudent to perform a barium enema or colonoscopy to assess the colonic mucosa and exclude carcinoma.

**Case 443**

# SIGMOID CYST

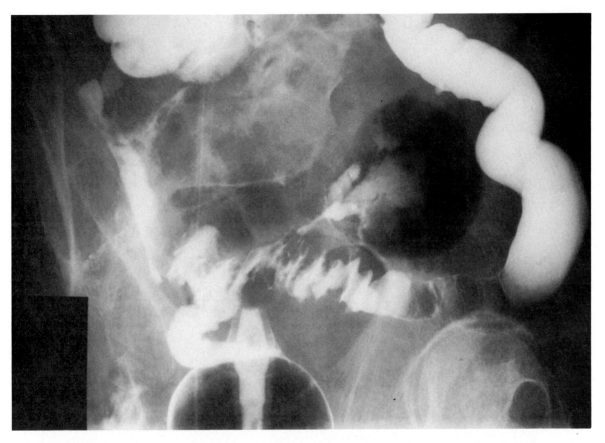

The folds of the sigmoid colon are thickened and tethered. A barium-filled tract arises from the superior aspect of the sigmoid and partially fills a well-defined gas-filled cavity. A fistulous tract was also present between the sigmoid and the destroyed right hip (not pictured). The extraluminal cavity has the typical appearance of a sigmoid cyst. At operation, the sigmoid perforation was found to be caused by a swallowed toothpick.

A sigmoid cyst develops as a result of diverticulitis. A persistent tract forms between the colonic lumen and the abscess cavity. The cavity develops a fibrous well-defined capsule over time. Usually, a ball-valve communication is present which allows air and contrast material into the cyst but incomplete emptying. Sometimes these cysts can reach gigantic proportions, occupying a large volume of the abdomen. Operative resection of the cyst and affected sigmoid is usually performed for cure.

## Case 444

## ACUTE RADIATION COLITIS

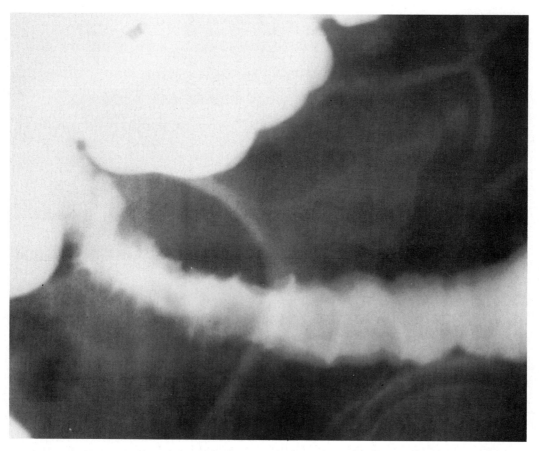

The sigmoid colon is diffusely narrowed. The luminal contour is irregular and the folds are markedly thickened (thumbprinting). This patient had radiation therapy (recently) as treatment for cervical carcinoma. The radiographic findings are consistent with radiation colitis.

Radiation damage to the ileum and colon remains a relatively common occurrence. Most patients have a history of cervical, endometrial, ovarian, or bladder cancer. Symptoms develop in patients after a total of 45 Gy (4,500 rad) has been administered. An occlusive endarteritis is the chief pathologic alteration. Acutely, edema and mucosal ulceration are present. The bowel often has a shaggy appearance, with fold thickening and luminal narrowing.

**Case 445**

## RADIATION-INDUCED STRICTURE

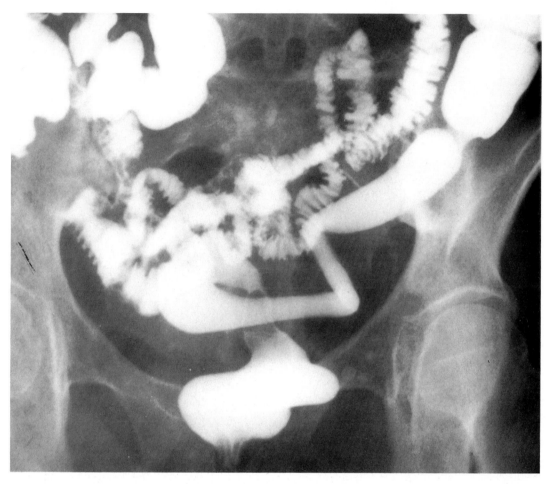

The proximal rectum and sigmoid colon are diffusely narrowed and featureless, devoid of haustral markings. This patient was treated with radiation for cervical cancer 26 years ago. Findings are typical of a radiation-induced stricture.

Radiation-induced strictures are common and of variable lengths. Severe strictures (especially those in the small bowel) can cause luminal obstruction. The normal mucosal markings (haustral folds) are often absent, and there is a gradual tapering of the lumen from normal to abnormal. Patients may complain of diarrhea, cramping, or bleeding. Often the symptoms respond poorly to conservative therapy and operation is required. Surgical treatment can be difficult and associated with a high morbidity due to adherent loops, adhesions, poor tissues, and impaired healing.

## Case 446

# ACUTE ISCHEMIA

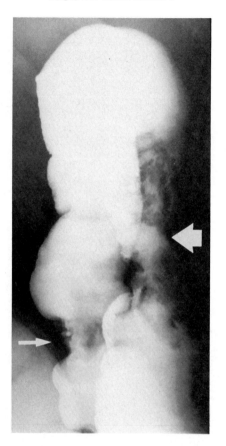

Two segments *(arrows)* of luminal narrowing and mucosal irregularity and ulceration are present in the region of the splenic flexure of the colon. The radiographic findings are consistent with ischemia, but other conditions such as Crohn's colitis, amebiasis, and other infectious causes could have this appearance.

Ischemia of the colon can be caused by various events, including low perfusion states and arterial or venous occlusion. The elderly are at highest risk for this condition, but younger individuals can also be affected—especially those with a vasculitis or a coagulopathy. The splenic flexure is the commonest location for ischemic changes. It represents a watershed region between the inferior and superior mesenteric arterial distributions. This colonic segment would incur the most ischemic damage in patients with low perfusion states. Ischemia is also known to develop proximal to a long-standing (several days or more) colonic obstruction (Senturia and Wald, 1967).

Normally, three events can ensue depending on the degree of ischemia. (1) Mild ischemia—only mucosal sloughing occurs; after the blood supply is reconstituted or collateral blood supply is established, the colon can return to normal. (2) Moderate ischemia affects the deeper layers of the bowel wall with stricture formation after healing. (3) Severe ischemia affects the entire bowel-wall thickness, with transmural necrosis and possible perforation.

Conventional radiographic examination of the ischemic colon is usually limited to plain abdominal radiographs in the severely ischemic patient. Adynamic ileus (Case 460), pneumatosis coli (Cases 467 and 468), pneumoperitoneum (Cases 191–196), and thickened haustral folds (often described as "thumbprinting") can be seen (Cases 423 and 450). Patients with mild and moderate ischemia may also be identified by findings on plain films or barium enema of thickened and edematous haustral folds. After healing, a stricture may develop (Case 449), with gradually tapering margins and a featureless mucosal pattern.

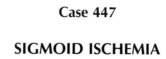

## Case 447

## SIGMOID ISCHEMIA

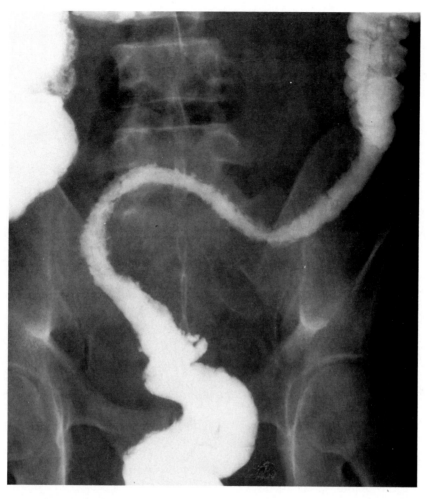

The entire sigmoid colon is narrowed and irregular in contour. These findings could be due to other causes of segmental colitis (inflammatory, infectious, radiation-induced). This patient was found to have idiopathic inferior mesenteric arterial and venous thrombosis.

Patients with localized colonic ischemia often present with colicky pain, diarrhea, and bleeding. Usually the left colon is affected. A low flow state is the commonest underlying predisposing factor.

Chronic intestinal ischemia usually has no radiographic findings on plain films, barium enema, or CT. Patients present with postprandial abdominal pain and weight loss. At angiography there is at least a 50% stenosis affecting two of the three mesenteric vessels. Even with angiographic findings that are consistent with ischemia, the diagnosis is one of exclusion, made after other diseases of the biliary tree and gut have been ruled out.

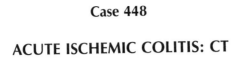

# Case 448

## ACUTE ISCHEMIC COLITIS: CT

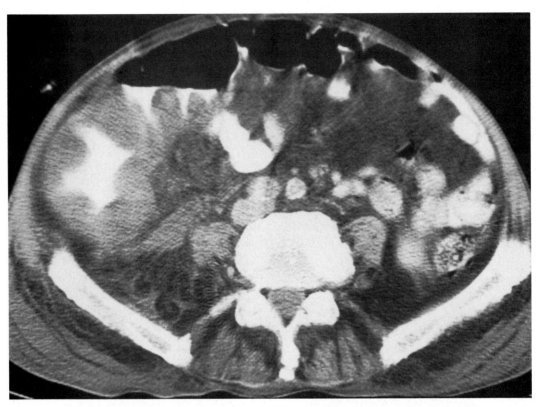

The wall of the right colon is thickened, with enlarged haustra causing "thumbprinting." Soft-tissue stranding is also present within the pericolonic fat. The colon was ischemic and removed at operation.

CT examination of the abdomen is commonly performed to evaluate patients with abdominal pain. Bowel ischemia can present with vague abdominal complaints, and findings at CT can direct the work-up to the appropriate organ.

CT findings are usually nonspecific—segmental bowel-wall thickening and some soft-tissue stranding in the pericolonic fat and mesentery. Occasionally, mesenteric or portal venous gas can be identified (Cases 263–265), a finding that should strongly suggest the diagnosis. Intramural pneumatosis is detected with a high degree of sensitivity at CT, and if it is present, ischemia should be excluded (Cases 257 and 258). Even in the absence of findings on plain abdominal radiographs and on CT, ischemia may be present. Patients with suspicious clinical findings may require further testing with angiography to confirm the diagnosis.

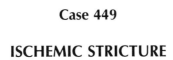

## Case 449

## ISCHEMIC STRICTURE

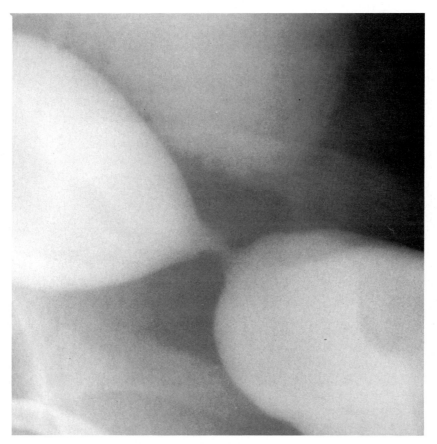

A focal area of narrowing is present in the splenic flexure. The mucosa appears featureless. Tapered margins are present along the proximal limb of the stricture.

Strictures develop after the resolution of moderate or severe colonic ischemia. Fibrosis develops within the colonic wall, with secondary rigidity and narrowing of the lumen. Sometimes sacculations develop. Usually a featureless, narrowed lumen is present. The rectum is an unusual location for a stricture to develop because of the excellent collateral blood supply available to this segment of bowel. The length of the stricture depends on the extent of previous ischemia.

## Case 450

## PSEUDOMEMBRANOUS COLITIS

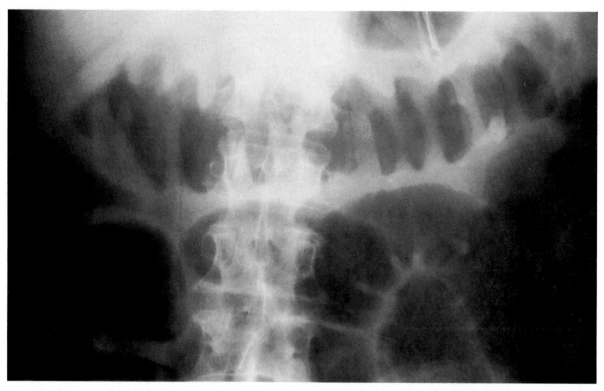

The transverse colon is gas-filled and the haustral markings are diffusely thickened. Findings are those of an acute colitis.

Pseudomembranous colitis is caused by the potent enterotoxins produced by *Clostridium difficile*, a gram-negative bacillus. Infection by this organism usually follows antibiotic therapy (originally described after lincomycin or clindamycin administration). Patients usually present with watery diarrhea. Sigmoidoscopy usually reveals multiple yellowish white plaques covering the colonic mucosa. The diagnosis can be confirmed by performing a stool assay for *C. difficile* enterotoxin.

Radiographically, the disease can often be suggested on the basis of the plain abdominal radiograph. Haustral folds throughout the colon can appear thickened (as in this case). If an intraluminal contrast study is per-

formed, the haustral folds will be thickened and the mucosal surface is often shaggy and irregular in contour (Case 451). The disease can occasionally spare portions of the colon. It is possible for a patient with this disease to have a normal proctoscopic examination, with disease in the more proximal colon.

Other conditions that can present with thickened haustral folds include inflammatory bowel disease (either ulcerative colitis or Crohn's colitis) (Cases 411 and 423), an infectious colitis, and ischemic colitis. Inflammatory polyps may be visible within the colon in patients with inflammatory bowel disease (Case 411). Ischemic colitis usually affects older individuals and involves a segment of bowel (often the splenic flexure) rather than involving the bowel diffusely (Case 446).

Case 451

## PSEUDOMEMBRANOUS COLITIS: CONTRAST ENEMA

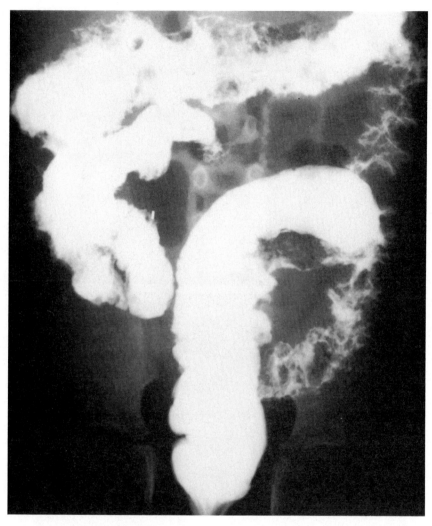

The haustral folds of the colon are diffusely thickened and the mucosa appears shaggy and irregular in contour. Pseudomembranous colitis was diagnosed by a positive stool assay for *Clostridium difficile* enterotoxin.

A barium examination of the colon is usually not necessary in patients with suspected pseudomembranous colitis. In fact, in patients with severe acute colitis, a contrast enema is contraindicated because of the risk of colonic perforation. Some patients have a contrast enema because of confusing or misleading clinical findings. Mild changes of this disease include an irregular or nodular mucosa, sometimes with small, plaque-like filling defects. More severe disease is associated with haustral thickening (Case 450), plaques, and a shaggy contour. Usually the entire colon is affected, but occasionally there may be sparing of the rectosigmoid with proximal colitis.

## Case 452

## PSEUDOMEMBRANOUS COLITIS

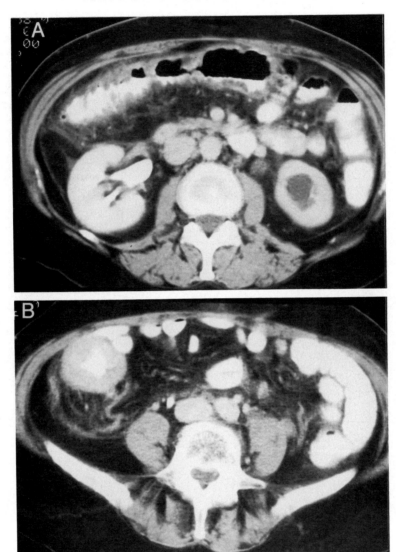

**A** and **B.** The wall of the right and transverse colon is circumferentially thickened. Pericolonic soft-tissue stranding is also present. The findings are nonspecific and could be due to any type of acute colitis. Pseudomembranous colitis was proved by stool assay.

The CT findings in patients with pseudomembranous colitis are usually nonspecific, with colonic wall thickening. The wall thickening may be diffuse or segmental. Patients with inflammatory bowel disease or colonic ischemia could present with identical CT findings (Case 422). Because many patients with pseudomembranous colitis have fever, leukocytosis, and vague abdominal complaints, a CT scan is often done to exclude an intra-abdominal abscess. The findings at CT can be helpful in directing further investigation of the colon, whereas endoscopy and stool assay can reveal the typical yellowish white plaques and the presence of the offending enterotoxin. Once the diagnosis is confirmed, patients are usually treated with vancomycin.

## Case 453

### NEUTROPENIC TYPHLITIS

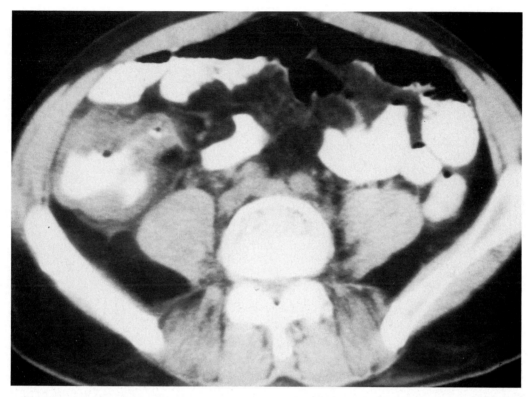

Moderate thickening of the wall of the cecum and terminal ileum is present. These findings are nonspecific and could be due to inflammation, infection, or neoplasm. This patient was being treated for acute lymphocytic leukemia and was severely neutropenic at the time of this examination. Neutropenic typhlitis was suggested in view of the history.

Neutropenic typhlitis is a disease that develops in severely neutropenic patients (usually patients with leukemia or lymphoma who are undergoing chemotherapy) with an associated adynamic ileus. The ileus-induced stasis, distension, and possible ischemia; the direct cytotoxic effect on the mucosa from the medication; and the inability to mount an immunologic defense are important predisposing factors. Pathologically, mucosal and submucosal necrosis, edema, and hemorrhage are present. Perforation can occur.

Radiographically, an adynamic ileus is present on abdominal plain films (Case 460). The haustral folds in the right colon may be thickened. A barium enema is contraindicated if the patient has peritoneal signs suggesting peritonitis. Usually, the barium enema findings confirm the plain film findings of right-sided colonic fold thickening and thumbprinting. Thickening of the colon wall, fascial thickening, and pericolonic soft-tissue stranding are typical findings at CT. Sonography also demonstrates right colonic-wall thickening in these patients.

Several other conditions could present with similar CT findings: inflammatory bowel disease (Case 422), pseudomembranous colitis (Case 452), ischemia, and lymphomatous or leukemic infiltration of the bowel wall.

## Case 454

# NEUTROPENIC TYPHLITIS

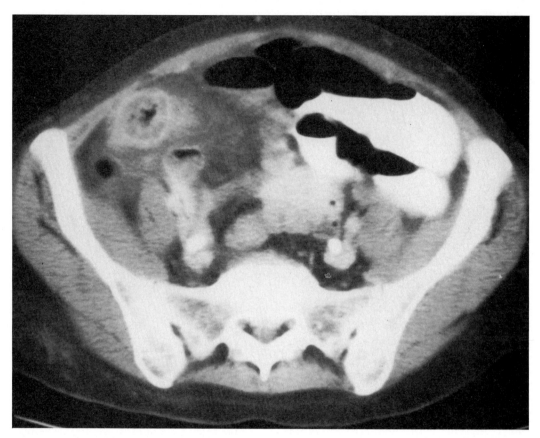

The wall of the right colon is thickened. The submucosal layer of the bowel wall is the density of water. Blurring of the pericolonic fat is present. Findings were due to neutropenic typhlitis.

Patients with neutropenic typhlitis often present with nonspecific complaints and symptoms, including nausea, vomiting, fever, abdominal tenderness, and diarrhea. Findings at CT can be helpful in the appropriate clinical setting to suggest the diagnosis of neutropenic typhlitis. Early diagnosis is important because the mortality has been reported to range from 50% to 100% (Shamberger et al., 1986). Treatment usually involves measures to return neutrophils to the circulation and occasionally operation if perforation, abscess, sepsis, or bleeding has developed.

## Case 455

# PANCREATITIC ABSCESS: COLONIC INFLAMMATION

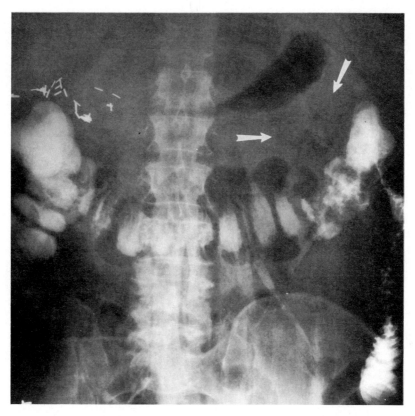

An extraluminal gas *(arrows)* collection (multiple small bubbles) is present in the region of the pancreatic bed. This is the characteristic picture of a pancreatic abscess. Luminal narrowing and thickened folds are present in the descending colon. These findings are secondary to pancreatitis.

Imaging procedures are not necessary in all patients for making the diagnosis of acute pancreatitis. Imaging tests are invaluable for confirming a suggested diagnosis and in detecting a complication of acute pancreatitis (including a pancreatic abscess). CT and sonography have replaced abdominal plain films and intraluminal contrast studies when the diagnosis of acute pancreatitis is suggested. In some patients, however, symptoms may be nonspecific and abdominal plain films are used to assess for the presence of adynamic ileus, obstruction, or tube placements.

A pancreatic effusion is commonly associated with acute pancreatitis. The effusion is located most often within the anterior pararenal space and lesser sac of the retroperitoneum. The mass effect from this fluid can displace the stomach anteriorly and the colon inferiorly. As the volume of the pancreatic effusion increases, it can extend inferiorly, adjacent to the descending colon and along the transverse mesocolon. Inflammatory changes (thickened folds, spasm, narrowing) of the transverse and descending colon can be seen. The splenic flexure of the colon is usually involved with inflammatory changes because of its close proximity to the pancreatic tail. A pancreatic effusion can also dissect within the leaves of the small-bowel mesentery and cause ascites in patients with severe disease. The colon "cut off" sign has been regarded as a classic radiographic finding of acute pancreatitis. Patients with this sign have gaseous distension of the right and transverse colon, with little gas visible beyond the splenic flexure (as seen in this case). It can be impossible to exclude colonic obstruction on plain films, and a contrast enema may be required.

## Case 456

## PANCREATIC ABSCESS: COLONIC FISTULA

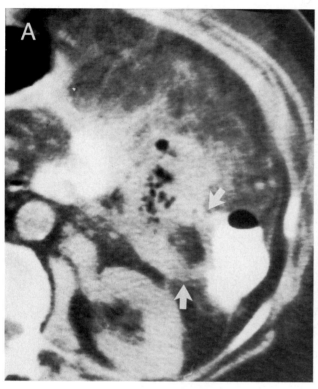 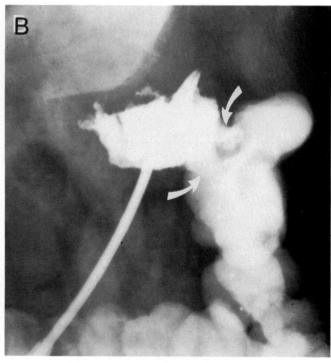

**A.** An abscess is present in the pancreatic bed. An inflammatory reaction and two tracts *(arrows)* can be identified around the splenic flexure of the colon.

**B.** A drainage catheter in the pancreatic abscess cavity is injected with contrast material. A fistula *(arrows)* is present between the abscess and the splenic flexure of the colon.

A pancreatic abscess is a life-threatening complication of acute pancreatitis. CT and sonography are sensitive imaging modalities for detecting peripancreatic fluid—which may or may not be infected. The finding of gas in the pancreatic bed is highly suggestive of in-

fection but not diagnostic. Correlation with clinical information and percutaneous aspiration of fluid are important steps in determining the proper diagnosis. Fistula formation between the pancreatic bed and splenic flexure of the colon is a relatively common complication of pancreatitis and can lead to a pancreatic abscess. Knowledge that a fistula is present is critical in planning proper therapeutic intervention. Colonic resection or percutaneous drainage may be necessary. If the fistula is not repaired operatively, long-term catheter drainage is often required.

Case 457

## SCLERODERMA SACCULATIONS

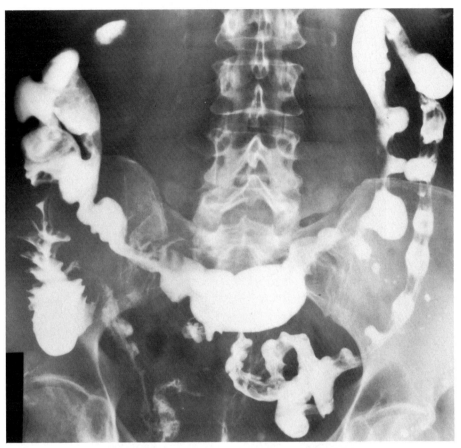

Multiple, wide-mouth sacculations are present along the antimesenteric border of the transverse colon. Findings are typical of scleroderma (progressive systemic sclerosis).

Scleroderma causes patchy replacement of the muscular layers of the colon with collagen and elastic fibers. Intimal proliferation of the feeding arteries with possible ischemia can also occur.

Radiographically, the antimesenteric border of the colon may develop sacculations or pseudodiverticula as a result of the "limp" supporting tissues in the colonic wall. The mesenteric side is not affected because the tissues and vessels in this region continue to sup-

port the bowel wall. Haustral markings may be lost and redundancy (secondary to dilatation and elongation) may be present. Localized areas of narrowing also may be seen as a result of ischemia.

The main differential consideration is Crohn's colitis, with multiple areas of asymmetric bowel-wall involvement and pseudodiverticula (Case 426). The asymmetric changes in Crohn's disease are usually segmental, with normal intervening colon. The pseudodiverticula in patients with Crohn's disease may affect either the mesenteric or antimesenteric border of the colon. The clinical history is often revealing.

## Case 458

## AMEBIASIS

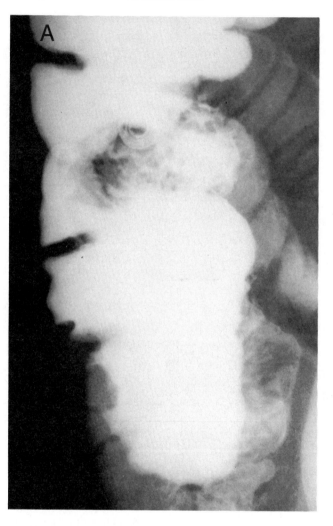

**A.** The cecum is narrowed with an irregular contour due to fine ulcerations.

**B.** The wall of the right colon is thickened. This finding is nonspecific and could be secondary to infectious, inflammatory, or neoplastic disorders.

**C.** A multiloculated, low (fluid)-density mass is present in the right lobe of the liver. This constellation of findings is consistent with amebiasis.

Amebiasis is an infection by the protozoan *Entamoeba histolytica*, which is endemic throughout the world—particularly in tropical climates. Infection occurs by ingestion of the amebic cyst, which in the alkaline environment of the small bowel will shed its inner capsule and release trophozoites. Trophozoites burrow into the intestinal wall—most commonly the cecum and sigmoid colon. Multifocal or confluent ulcerations develop at the site of bowel-wall penetration. Secondary bacterial invasion of the bowel causes marked submucosal edema, bowel-wall thickening, and even hemorrhage (as seen in this case). A focal mass (ameboma) can develop as well as the formation of a hyperplastic granuloma from bacterial invasion. The protozoan infection can spread from the bowel to any part of the body by direct extension and hematogenous and lymphatic dissemination. A hepatic abscess is the usual extraintestinal site for infection (as seen in this case). A liver abscess can erode through the diaphragm and result in pleural, pericardial, bronchial, or lung infection. Penetration of an ulcer through the bowel wall can result in a pericolonic abscess, fistula, peritonitis, or distant intraperitoneal abscess. Long-term changes of amebiasis usually include benign-appearing colonic

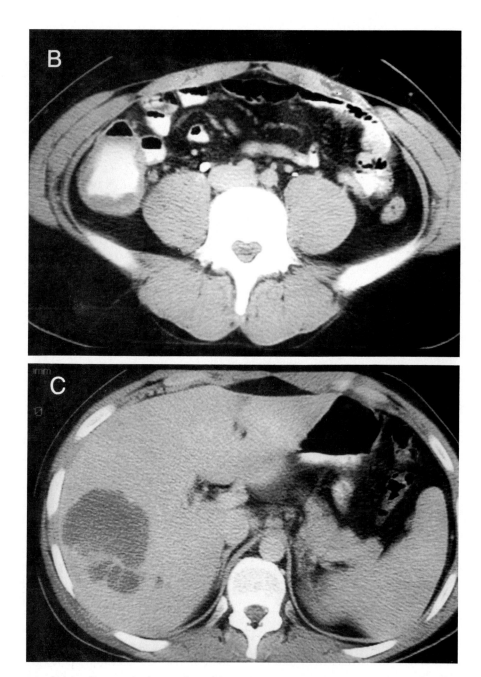

strictures. Treatment of this disease is by antiamebic therapy. Surgical treatment of this disease has a high morbidity and mortality, often without cure.

Radiologically, the cecum and sigmoid colon are affected most often. Involvement of the terminal ileum occurs in a minority of patients. Initially, the patient may have mucosal changes resembling ulcerative colitis (granular-appearing mucosa with fine ulcerations and thickened and edematous haustra). Deeper and more extensive ulcerations may be seen as the disease progresses. The cecum often becomes nondistensible and conical in shape. Amebomas can be indistinguishable from colon cancer. Multiplicity of lesions, ulceration elsewhere in the colon, young age, and travel history may all be helpful in differentiating this disease from carcinoma.

**499**

## Case 459

# MECHANICAL COLONIC OBSTRUCTION

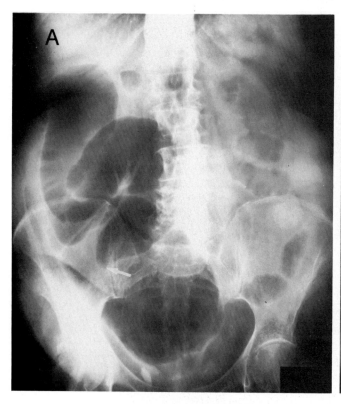

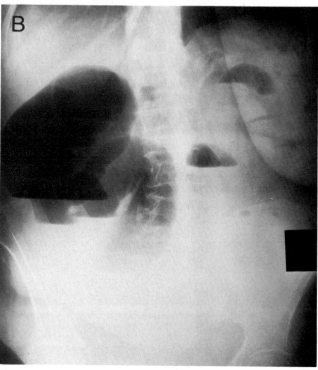

**A.** In this abdominal radiograph, with the patient in the supine position, the cecum and ascending and right transverse colon are distended with gas. No gas is seen distal to the mid-transverse colon *(arrow).* Mildly dilated small-bowel loops are present.

**B.** In this radiograph, with the patient upright, multiple air-fluid levels are seen in the right side of the colon and in two small-bowel loops.

These findings are typical of a mechanical colonic obstruction involving the transverse colon. At operation, an incarcerated loop of transverse colon was found to be obstructed within a midline incisional hernia.

Mechanical colonic obstruction often is due to carcinoma, diverticulitis, volvulus, mass effect from an extracolonic pelvic neoplasm, fecal impaction, and, rarely, a hernia or adhesion. The radiographic findings include dilatation of the colon to the level of obstruction. The colon may be filled with gas (as in this case), fluid, or stool. The small bowel is also often dilated if the ileocecal valve is incompetent. If the valve remains competent, the colon will continue to distend. Perforation can occur with prolonged and marked cecal dilatation. A contrast enema is often necessary to determine the cause of the obstruction. Only a small amount of barium should be passed beyond a high-grade obstruction so that inspissated barium does not cause a problem later (including obstipation and possible obstruction). Chronic obstruction can be recognized by the presence of haustral thickening and the presence of gray and granular-appearing fluid within the colon proximal to the obstruction (Bryk and Soong, 1967).

## Case 460

## ADYNAMIC ILEUS

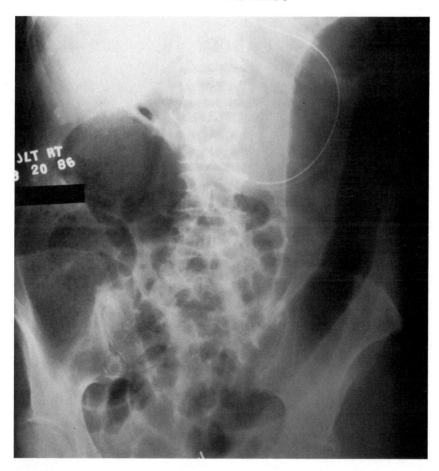

Gas is present in the small bowel and the large bowel. A continuous column of gas fills the colon. The cecum is located normally in the right lower quadrant. Findings are those of an adynamic ileus.

Adynamic ileus of the colon is a condition in which the colon becomes atonic and often dilated. There are numerous causes of this condition, including a postoperative and postanesthesia state, trauma, adjacent inflammation or infection, various medications, various systemic illnesses, and other conditions. Clinically, patients may have poorly localized abdominal distress and pain, a distended abdomen, and diminished bowel sounds.

Radiographically, the colon is usually distended with air and fluid. Often the colon contains most of the visible alimentary gas. The cecum is positioned normally in the right lower quadrant and may be dilated (>9 cm). Gas fills the colon as a "continuous column"; however, often the low descending and sigmoid colon are not air-filled as a result of their dependent location in the peritoneal cavity. Films with the patient decubitus or prone can be helpful in demonstrating the gas-filled portions of the colon in equivocal cases. If a contrast-enema study is performed, no obstruction will be identified.

The main differential consideration is mechanical colonic obstruction (Case 459). If a continuous column of gas throughout the colon is not present, then a limited contrast enema (contrast material is administered up to the level where a continuous air column is present) can be performed to assess for a distal colonic obstruction.

## Case 461

## SIGMOID VOLVULUS

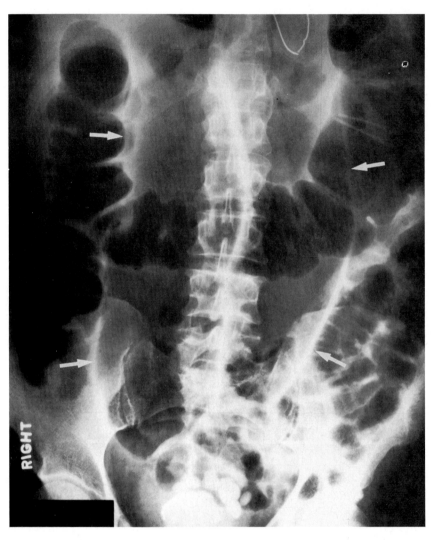

The entire colon is moderately distended with gas, and there is a dilated, inverted U-shaped loop *(arrows)* arising from the pelvis. This appearance is characteristic of a sigmoid volvulus.

Sigmoid volvulus occurs as a result of a redundant sigmoid colon on a loose mesentery that twists on itself and obstructs. Patients are often older individuals with a history of chronic constipation and often they ingest large amounts of bulk in their diet. Acute abdominal pain, distension, and vomiting often occurs.

Radiographically, the diagnosis is usually made by identifying a prominent, "bean-shaped," dilated loop of colon arising from the pelvis on abdominal plain films. Gas is often present in the colon proximal to the sigmoid twist. If the diagnosis is equivocal, the obstruction can be confirmed by a contrast enema (Case 462).

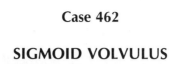

## Case 462

## SIGMOID VOLVULUS

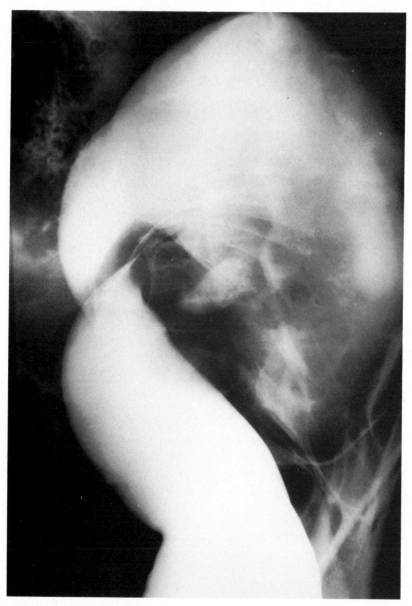

The sigmoid colon gradually tapers and narrows to a region of high-grade obstruction. The colon proximal to the obstruction is dilated. The characteristic "beaking" (twisting) of the colon is visible at the level of the obstruction. This appearance is characteristic of a volvulus—at this location, a sigmoid volvulus.

It is often helpful and possible to pass a rectal tube across the obstruction into the dilated sigmoid loop.

This will decompress the volvulus and provide the opportunity for elective operative repair of the sigmoid (reduction sigmoid colocolostomy). If tube decompression is not possible, then urgent operation is required to prevent sigmoid infarction and perforation. Recurrence of the volvulus is common without operative repair.

## Case 463

## CECAL VOLVULUS

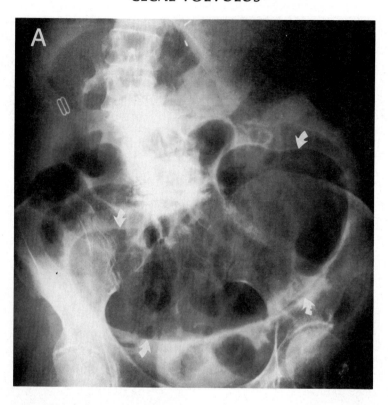

**A.** In this abdominal radiograph with the patient supine, a dilated, gas-filled viscus *(arrows)* fills a large portion of the pelvis and extends slightly into the left upper abdomen. This organ has the shape of an abnormally positioned right colon. Dilated small bowel loops are also present throughout the abdomen. The transverse and left colon are not identified.

**B.** In this radiograph with the patient upright, an air-fluid level is present within the dilated, abnormal colon.

**C.** Obstruction *(arrow)* in the right colon is present on this spot radiograph taken during a contrast enema. There is gradual narrowing of the colon to the point of obstruction. Cecal volvulus was confirmed at laparotomy.

Cecal volvulus occurs as a result of a redundant right colonic mesentery, allowing all or part of the right colon to twist on itself. As the colon twists, it moves into an abnormal location within the abdomen, often in the midline or within the left upper quadrant. The twist causes mechanical obstruction of the colon and often vascular insufficiency of the affected loop. Patients may have a history of intermittent abdominal pain, perhaps due to periodic twisting and untwisting of the colon. Treatment is invariably operative because the risk of

cecal perforation is high, and if perforation has occurred it is associated with a high morbidity and high mortality.

The initial radiologic examination is usually an abdominal plain film. Typically, a dilated (>9 cm) cecum is identified in an abnormal location, often the left upper quadrant. Depending on the duration of symptoms, the colon distal to the obstructing twist has little or no remaining gas within it. Dilated, gas-filled small bowel is often identified. The abdominal film should be scrutinized for evidence of perforation (free air [Cases 190–196] and a rapidly decompressing cecum) as well as evidence of ischemia (portal venous gas [Cases 263–265] and cecal intramural pneumatosis [Cases 256–258, 466–468]). Confirmation of the diagnosis can be rapidly and easily made with a contrast enema. The finding of obstruction in the right colon with a "beaklike" appearance at the site of the twist is typical.

Differential considerations include an obstructing carcinoma in a patient with a mobile cecum and cecal ileus (Case 465). The latter condition always occurs in association with a colonic ileus, and no obstruction exists at the time of the contrast enema. Peritoneal bands or adhesions in association with a mobile right colon could also have a similar presentation.

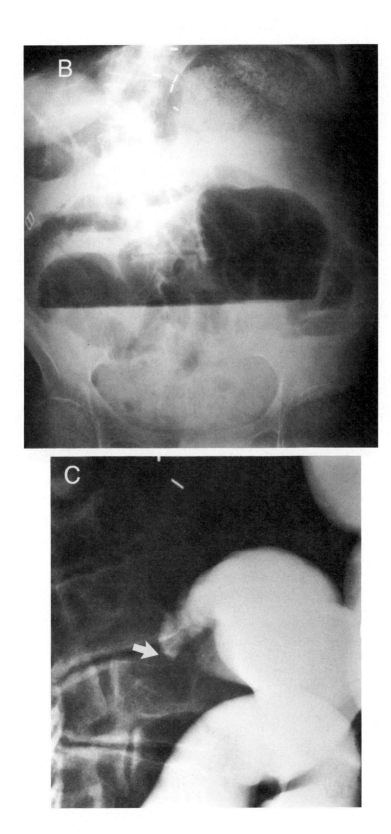

Case 464

# CECAL VOLVULUS: CT

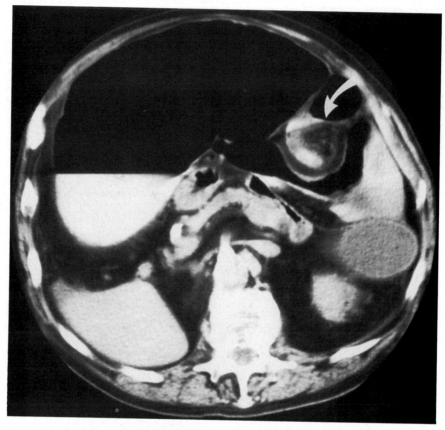

A dilated gas- and contrast-filled viscus (cecum) fills the upper abdomen. A twisted or whorled appearance involving the alimentary tract is present in the right upper abdomen *(arrow)*. Intestines encircle the mesenteric vessels. This appearance is typical of a volvulus.

Usually the diagnosis of volvulus is suggested on the basis of plain abdominal film findings (Case 463) and confirmed with an intraluminal examination with contrast material. A volvulus may be encountered in the course of a CT examination for the evaluation of patients with indeterminate, intermittent abdominal pain. Midgut volvulus can be suspected when a rotational anomaly of the gut is identified (jejunum in the right upper quadrant, colon in the left abdomen) and the superior mesenteric artery is located to the right of the superior mesenteric vein (reversal of the normal anatomic relationships). Cecal volvulus can be more difficult to identify. The cecum is located in an abnormal position in the mid or left abdomen. In the region of the right colon, both bowel and mesentery are twisted and encircle each other (as seen in this case). Equivocal cases may require a contrast enema to confirm the diagnosis.

## Case 465

## CECAL ILEUS

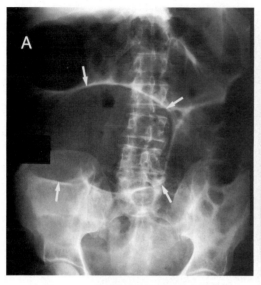 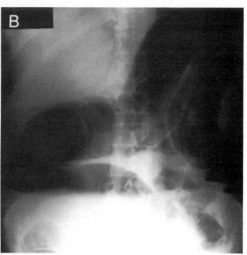

**A** and **B.** In abdominal radiographs with the patient supine **(A)** and upright **(B),** the cecum *(arrows)* is mobile, dilated, and positioned in the right and middle abdomen. Air-fluid levels are present in the cecum and descending colon. Two gas-filled small-bowel loops are visible inferior and lateral to the cecum. There is a continuous column of gas throughout the colon. In the clinical setting of adynamic ileus, these findings are typical of cecal ileus.

Cecal ileus is a condition that can develop in patients with a mobile cecum (10% of the general population) and an underlying colonic adynamic ileus. Most of the patients who have this condition are bedridden, often confined to a supine position (because of medical appliances and infirmity). The mobile cecum rotates anteromedially in the abdomen and gradually distends (to a diameter in excess of 9 cm) as gas enters the cecum from the small bowel. Because of the nondependent cecal location, gas does not empty into the less dilated distal colon. Cecal distension is often worsened by a competent ileocecal valve. Recognition of this entity is important because excessive cecal distension longer than 2 or 3 days has a significant risk of cecal perforation and possible death (Johnson et al., 1985). Cecal perforation occurs more frequently in patients with cecal ileus than with cecal volvulus, mechanical colonic obstruction, or typical colonic ileus. This is probably because patients with obstruction of the colon (cecal volvulus, mechanical colonic obstruction) usually present with symptoms that demand an urgent diagnosis and treatment. Patients with cecal ileus

often have nonspecific abdominal complaints, and cecal distension may go unnoticed for days. The duration of cecal distension (longer than 2 to 3 days) is an important factor in determining the risk of perforation. Actual cecal size (≥9 cm) does not correlate well with risk of perforation (Johnson et al., 1985). If conservative therapy (rectal tubes and cathartics) is not successful, more aggressive therapy using either a surgically placed cecostomy tube or colonoscopic decompression should be instituted. The latter treatment may have to be repeated several times until the ileus resolves.

Radiographically, there is a continuous column of gas throughout most of the colon (colonic ileus) with disproportionate dilatation of the cecum which is abnormally positioned, often in the midabdomen. The ileocecal valve can usually be identified at the 7- or 8-o'clock position on the cecum rather than its normal 4- or 5-o'clock position (as seen in this case). This is due to the rotation of the cecum as it assumes its anteromedial location. If a contrast enema is performed, slow filling of the cecum is often encountered (due to the high intraluminal pressure) *without* obstruction. Care should be taken to avoid filling the colon more than necessary to make the correct diagnosis, because increasing cecal distension can hasten a perforation.

Differential considerations usually include only cecal volvulus (Case 463). Cecal volvulus usually presents radiographically with absence of gas in the colon distal to the twist and obstruction in the right colon at contrast enema.

## Case 466

## PNEUMATOSIS CYSTOIDES COLI

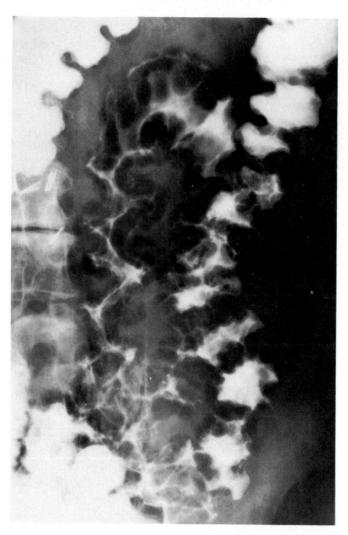

Multiple, intramural, cystic gas collections are present throughout most of the left colon. This appearance is typical of pneumatosis cystoides coli.

Pneumatosis coli refers to intramural air within the colon. Intramural air within the small bowel is referred to as pneumatosis intestinalis or pneumatosis cystoides intestinalis (if the air collections are cystlike). Patients with pneumatosis cystoides coli have endothelial-lined gas-filled cysts within the bowel wall that do not communicate with the lumen. The cysts may vary in size, reaching up to several centimeters in diameter. The cause is unknown but some patients have associated collagen vascular disorders, ischemia, diabetes, and a history of trauma. This condition is often discovered incidentally in patients without symptoms.

The radiologic diagnosis is dependent on recognizing the radiolucent collections of gas within the bowel wall. Often the collections are rounded and grapelike. The left side of the colon is affected more often than the right (excluding the rectum).

Once the gas density of the collections is recognized, no further diagnostic considerations are necessary. The intraluminal protrusions may simulate polyps, lymphoma, segmental colitis (Crohn's colitis), and ischemic colitis. Colitis cystica profunda usually affects the rectum, and the filling defects are not the lucency of gas (Case 470).

## Case 467

## PNEUMATOSIS COLI: LINEAR

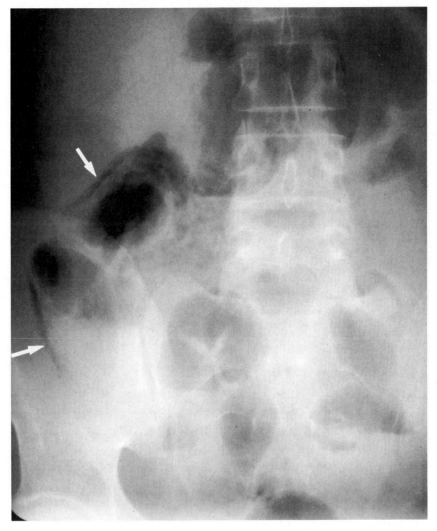

A linear band of intramural gas *(arrows)* is present within the right colon. This patient had recently undergone colonoscopy with biopsy, which was believed to be responsible for the pneumatosis. The patient was treated with antibiotics and dismissed without symptoms.

Pneumatosis coli can be secondary to the same underlying conditions as are found in pneumatosis intestinalis (Cases 259, 260, and 342). The intramural gas may appear cystic (Case 466), but often it is linear in configuration (as in this case). Patients receiving steroid therapy, those with an underlying collagen vascular disease, those who have had a recent mucosal biopsy, or those with a history of chronic obstructive pulmonary disease are most likely to have this condition. These "benign" causes usually do not require any particular treatment. Ischemic colitis is the most important condition to exclude clinically, because emergent operation would be required to prevent perforation.

## Case 468

## PNEUMATOSIS COLI: CT

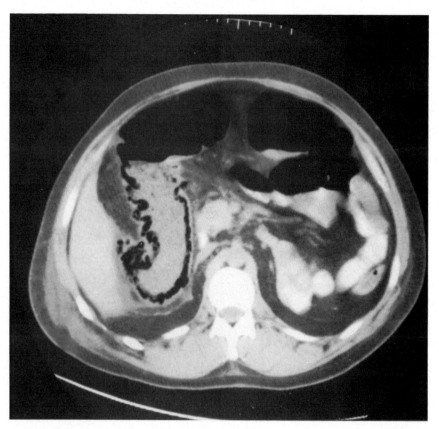

Linear and cystic intramural pneumatosis are present in the right colon. This patient had received a liver transplant and was receiving steroid medication. No treatment was instituted and the patient did well. No-tice how intraluminal gas is always in a nondependent location whereas pneumatosis can be present in any in-tramural location, including the dependent portions of the bowel.

Case 469

## SOLITARY RECTAL ULCER SYNDROME

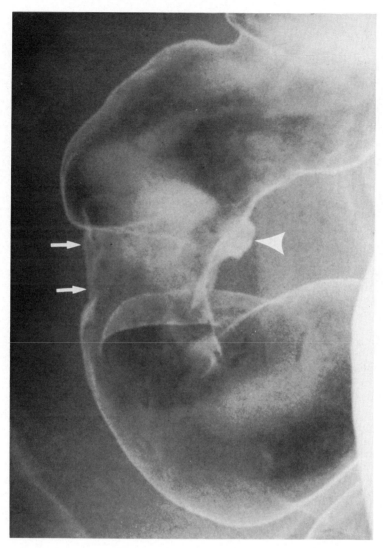

A circumferential ulceration *(arrows)* is present in the midrectum, with a focal ulcer crater *(arrowhead)* anteriorly. At operation, a benign annular ulcer was present.

The solitary rectal ulcer syndrome is a condition found in patients with chronic defecation difficulties and abnormalities of the rectal wall. Patients may also complain of rectal bleeding. Defecation abnormalities include either repeated episodes of rectal intussusception or failure of the puborectalis muscle to relax normally (spastic pelvic floor syndrome). Pathologically, one or more rectal ulcers may be present but are not necessary for the diagnosis. In addition, thickening of the muscularis mucosa and fibroblastic proliferation within the lamina propria are specific features.

Findings at barium enema include: thickened rectal folds, mucosal granularity, rectal stricture, and ulceration. Intussusception, rectal prolapse, failure of the puborectalis muscle to relax, and abnormal perineal descent may be visible at defecating proctography.

Differential considerations include annular neoplasms (Case 379) and inflammatory proctitis (Case 412). The diagnosis of the solitary rectal ulcer syndrome should be considered in patients with a long history of straining at stool. Defecating proctography is the method of choice for making the diagnosis.

**Case 470**

# COLITIS CYSTICA PROFUNDA

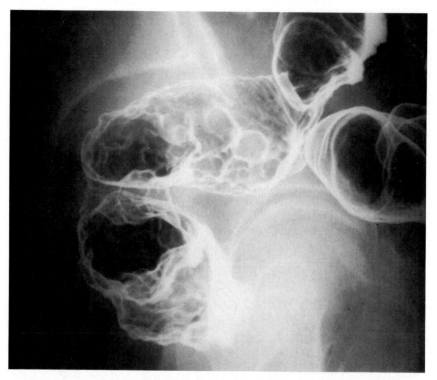

Multiple, round, submucosal filling defects are present within the rectum. The location and appearance are typical of colitis cystica profunda.

Colitis cystica profunda is a disease of unknown cause that is characterized by multiple, mucin-filled cysts within the mucosa and submucosa of the rectum and, rarely, the sigmoid colon. Patients may complain of rectal bleeding, diarrhea, abdominal pain, and prolapse of the rectum. Large cysts can cause obstruction.

Radiographically, multiple, round, submucosal cyst-like filling defects are seen in the rectum. Occasionally the cysts can simulate a large mass and resemble a villous adenoma (Case 381).

Colitis cystica superficialis refers to a condition in which the mucosa is diffusely involved with mucus-filled bullae. It is believed to be of no clinical significance except that it may be associated with pellagra and celiac disease.

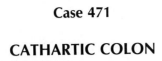

## Case 471

## CATHARTIC COLON

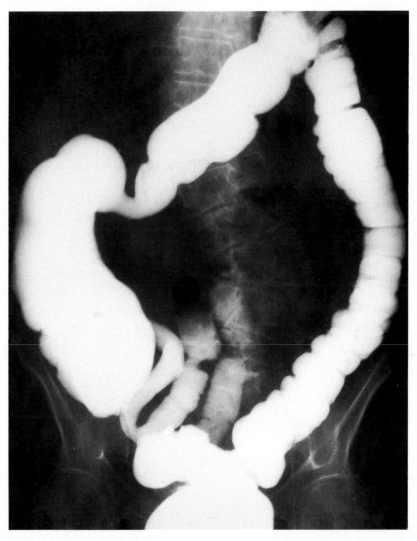

The right and transverse colon are relatively ahaustral; the left colon appears normal. Findings are consistent with cathartic colon.

Cathartic colon is a term used to describe the radiographic changes that occur after prolonged use of irritant cathartics such as cascara, senna, phenolphthalein, and castor oil. The proximal colon is usually affected initially, but left-sided involvement can also be seen.

Findings include lack of haustrations (most common in the right colon), shortening, and inconsistent luminal constrictions. It is believed that the strictures are due to muscular hypertrophy. Observation of these areas at fluoroscopy or on sequential films demonstrates the slow, changeable nature of these narrowed segments. The terminal ileum may appear gaping and resemble "backwash ileitis." Differentiation of this entity from ulcerative colitis can usually be done by obtaining a history. In addition, the distal colon appears to be of normal size and contour in cathartic colon. Shortening of the colon in ulcerative colitis is usually associated with lack of distensibility and narrowing (Case 418). In cathartic colon, the wall remains distensible.

## Case 472

## ENDOMETRIOSIS

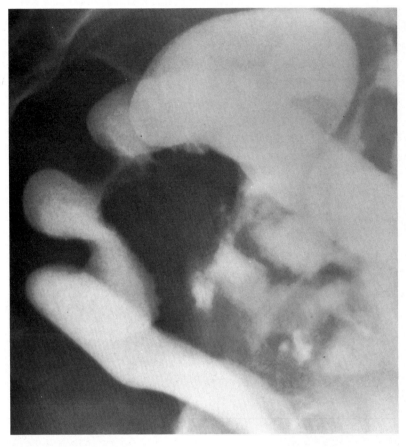

There is an extrinsic mass on the anterior wall of the rectosigmoid. Tethered colonic folds are associated with the mass. Differential considerations include peritoneal implants or drop metastases in the pouch of Douglas, pelvic abscess, and endometriosis. In a woman during the reproductive years without a prior malignancy, endometriosis is an important consideration. Endometriosis was found in this patient at the time of operation.

Endometriosis is the third most common cause of benign filling defects in the colon (after adenomas and lipomas). Intestinal implants are estimated to involve 4% of all women between the ages of 20 and 40 years.

Endometrial tissue extruded from the fallopian tubes can implant on the peritoneal surface, usually in the pouch of Douglas or on the sigmoid colon (most commonly on its inferior surface). The implants invade muscular and submucosal bowel layers and often stimulate local smooth muscle proliferation of the colon, secondary inflammatory changes, and a variable degree of fibrosis. Symptoms include constipation, pelvic pain, diarrhea, and, rarely, rectal bleeding. Typically, the symptoms are cyclical, but not always.

Radiographically, an intramural filling defect is present with an intact overlying mucosa. Sometimes the mucosa may appear pleated or tethered due to the associated desmoplastic reaction (as in this case). Rarely, a constricting lesion is seen with smooth margins and an intact mucosa (Case 473).

## Case 473

## ANNULAR ENDOMETRIOSIS

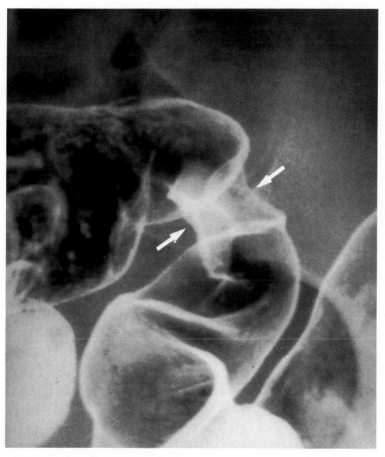

A focal region of annular constriction *(arrows)* is present in the mid-sigmoid colon. A small annular carcinoma could not be excluded. At operation, a circumferential endometrioma was removed.

This is an unusual presentation for endometriosis, but a constricting lesion will be encountered occasionally.

## Case 474

## CECAL ENDOMETRIOSIS

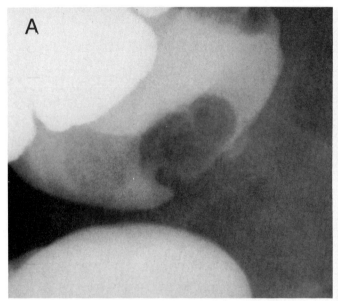

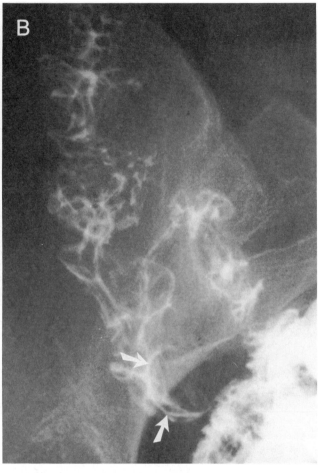

**A.** A small filling defect is present in the base of the cecum.

**B.** The surface of this mass *(arrows)* appeared smooth on the postevacuation film. Common diagnostic considerations include an appendiceal abscess (Case 430 A), mucocele (Case 408), lipoma (Case 406), or lymphoma (Case 404). A cecal polyp was considered less likely because of its smooth surface. The ileocecal region is also a common location for peritoneal implants as well as the pouch of Douglas and sigmoid colon. At operation, an endometrioma was removed.

The radiographic appearance of an endometrioma depends on its anatomic location—serosal, intramuscular, or submucosal. The mucosa is rarely involved. Filling defects usually range from 2 to 7 cm in diameter.

## Case 475

## BIOPSY SITE

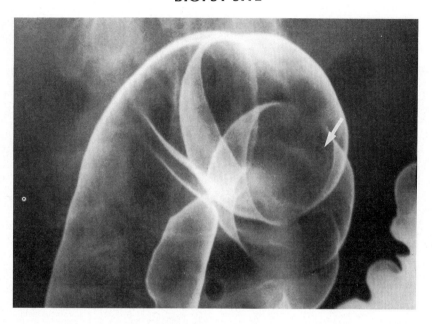

A solitary lesion *(arrow)* is present in the sigmoid colon. The lesion appears "aphthoid," with a central collection of barium surrounded by a symmetric filling defect. This patient had undergone a biopsy in the sigmoid colon recently. The radiographic findings were attributed to the biopsy procedure.

This biopsy defect could be confused with an aphthous ulcer of Crohn's colitis or those associated with an infectious colitis. Discrete ulcers in these patients are almost never solitary. Careful inspection of the colonic mucosa invariably results in additional findings. It is common to delay a barium enema several days after an endoscopic biopsy or polypectomy so as to avoid the possibility of perforation. Deep biopsies have the greatest risk of perforation (Case 478).

## Case 476

## COLONIC PERFORATION

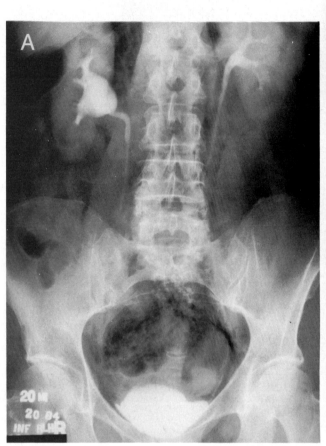

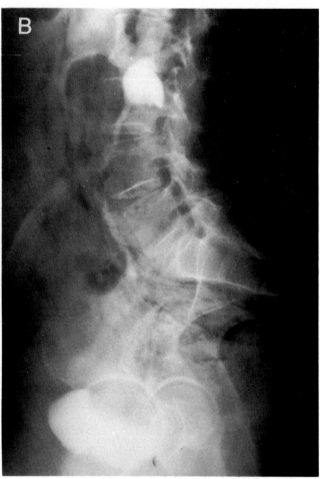

**A.** and **B.** Retroperitoneal gas is present in a perirectal and paraspinal location. Because the majority of the gas resides in the pelvis, it is likely that the source of the gas is also of pelvic origin. This patient had recently had a colonoscopic examination with perforation of the sigmoid. Surgical repair was required. Contrast material is present in the urinary system.

Colonoscopic perforations are reported to occur in approximately 1 in 500 examinations, with a mortality rate between 1/2,000 and 1/5,000 (Rogers et al., 1975; Gilbert et al., 1985). These colonic leaks may not be appreciated at the time of the procedure. Pain often develops and patients seek medical care within a few hours after the examination. Usually, a plain abdominal radiograph will reveal peritoneal, retroperitoneal, or intramural gas (Case 467) if a significant leak has developed. CT is more sensitive than plain films for detecting small amounts of extraluminal gas or pneumatosis. A water-soluble enema is required sometimes to clarify an equivocal finding or to demonstrate the site of the leak.

## Case 477

## RECTAL PERFORATION

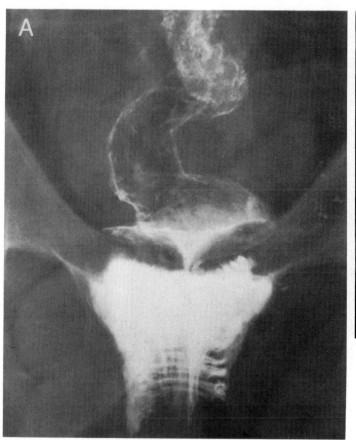

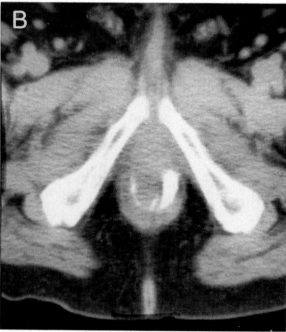

**A.** An unusual collection of contrast material is present around the rectum. Transverse striations represent circular muscles within the rectal wall, indicating that the contrast material resides intramurally. A barium enema tip was improperly placed within the rectum and caused the perforation.

**B.** A linear collection of barium is present within the rectal wall. These findings confirm the findings from the contrast enema.

Perforations after a barium enema are unusual, occurring in 1 in 5,000 to 1 in 10,000 examinations (Ansell, 1987). An improperly placed enema tip or an over-inflated rectal balloon (particularly in patients with an abnormal nondistensible rectum, i.e., ulcerative colitis or a rectal cancer) is the most common cause. If an enema tip is difficult to insert, it is prudent to perform a rectal examination in order to determine the anorectal angle, if a rectal tumor is present, and to lubricate the anal canal. Balloon inflation should be performed so as not to distend the rectum. If patients complain of pain, the balloon should be deflated until it can be retained comfortably.

## Case 478

# COLONIC PERFORATION: INTRAPERITONEAL EXTRAVASATION

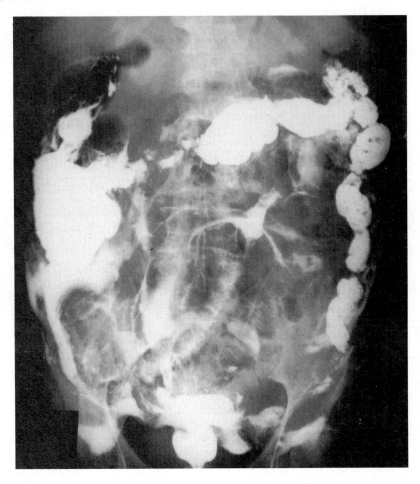

A large amount of extravasated contrast material is present within the peritoneal space. Contrast material is present in the colon and also outlines the serosal surface of many small bowel loops. This patient had a polyp fulgurated on the day before this examination. The colonic defect was surgically repaired.

If a colonic perforation is suspected, a water-soluble agent should be used instead of barium. Barium is difficult to remove surgically and can elicit a granulomatous reaction in the peritoneal cavity.

Case 479

# PELVIC LIPOMATOSIS

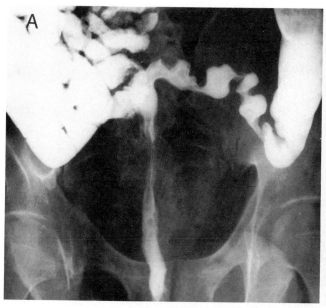

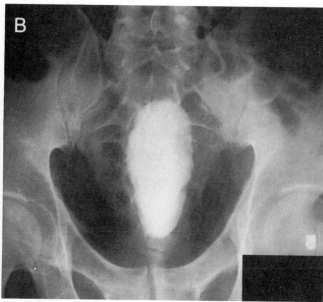

**A.** The rectum is narrowed and straightened. The soft tissues in the pelvis are hyperlucent.

**B.** The bladder is symmetrically narrowed and elevated out of the pelvis. Findings are characteristic of pelvic lipomatosis.

Pelvic lipomatosis is a condition of unknown origin, with fat and fibrous tissue proliferation in the pelvis. The fibrofatty tissue envelops the rectum and bladder. Patients may complain of backache, constipation, or dysuria. Males are affected more often than females.

Abdominal plain films reveal a hyperlucent pelvis. Contrast studies reveal a narrowed and less distensible rectum that resembles a straight tube rising out of the pelvis. The luminal contours and mucosal pattern are otherwise normal. The presacral space is often widened by fat. Similar fatty compression of the bladder is often seen, resulting in a teardrop shape. The ureters may be displaced and mildly to moderately dilated. Clinically, significant ureteral or rectal obstruction is uncommon.

Differential considerations on the basis of the barium enema findings include prostate cancer, which can envelope and narrow the rectum. Radiation proctitis narrows the rectum but does not elongate the rectum or compress the bladder. Pelvic hematomas, postoperative pelvic lymphoceles, and retroperitoneal fibrosis could present with similar plain film findings. CT is a useful examination in differentiating these conditions.

## Case 480

## PELVIC LIPOMATOSIS

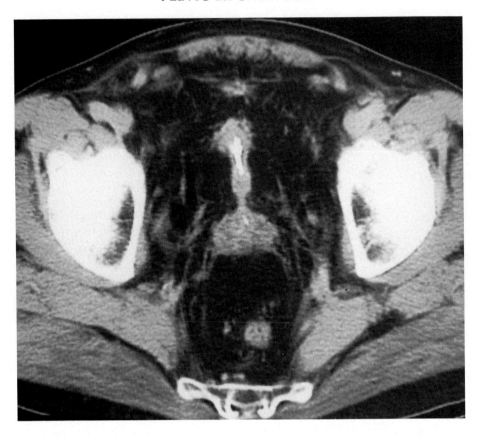

Excessive fatty tissue is present in the pelvis, with associated soft-tissue stranding. The fatty tissue has elevated the prostate anteriorly and narrowed the bladder from side to side.

CT is the most helpful examination in evaluating patients with suspected pelvic lipomatosis and in excluding other soft-tissue abnormalities. The density of the deforming tissues (fat) is diagnostic of this condition.

## Case 481

## FECAL IMPACTION

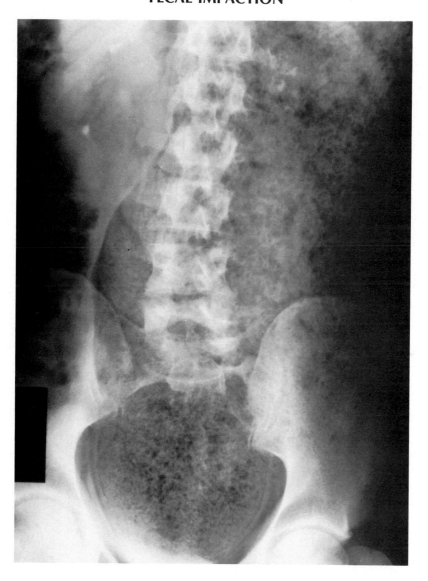

The colon is dilated and filled with a large amount of fecal material. The amount of colonic distension suggests a long-standing process. Residual contrast material is present in the urinary system.

Chronic constipation that may lead to fecal impaction may be caused by various conditions: mechanical obstruction, prolonged bed rest, improper bowel habits, narcotic usage, and various psychogenic or neurenteric disorders.

Radiologically, findings from plain abdominal films include a mottled pattern within a dilated and often redundant colon. A water-soluble enema can be helpful in excluding a mechanical obstruction and in drawing fluid into the colonic lumen that will aid evacuation.

## Case 482

## INTERNAL HEMORRHOID

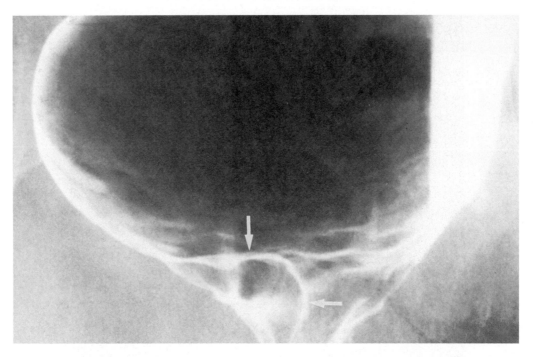

A smooth-surfaced, slightly lobulated filling defect *(arrows)* is present in the distal rectum near the anorectal junction. Internal hemorrhoids were present at endoscopy.

Hemorrhoids are vascular channels that prolapse into the rectum as a result of deterioration of the supporting fibromuscular stroma. Hemorrhoids located above the anorectal junction are classified as internal. Bleeding is a common problem and occurs if the overlying mucosa is eroded. Typical radiographic findings of hemorrhoids include lobulated folds or multiple, small (grapelike) clusters of submucosal nodules within 3 cm of the anorectal junction. It is usually impossible to differentiate a solitary hemorrhoid from a sessile polyp, lipoma, carcinoid, or hypertrophied anal papillae. Because of this it is reasonable to perform endoscopy to further evaluate solitary, distal rectal lesions.

# Case 483

# MASTOCYTOSIS

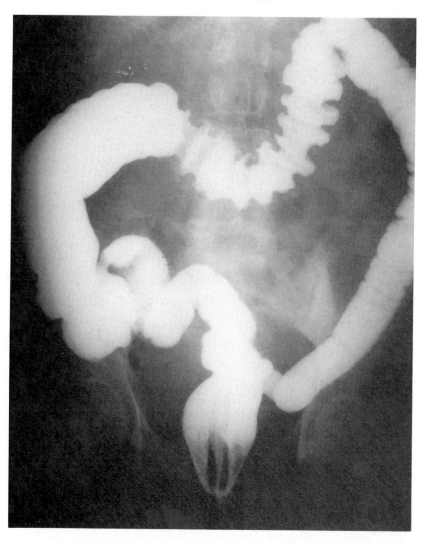

Segmental, haustral fold thickening is present in the transverse colon. This finding is nonspecific and could be the result of several diseases causing bowel wall edema or inflammation or infiltration. This patient was found to have mastocytosis.

Mastocytosis is a rare condition of abnormal deposition of mast cells, often within the skin (urticaria pigmentosa) and less commonly within other organs (liver, spleen, bones, alimentary tract). Gastrointestinal symptoms usually include nausea, vomiting, and diarrhea. There is an increased incidence of peptic ulcer disease in these patients, presumably due to histamine-medi-

ated acid secretion. Malabsorption can also occur with diffuse small-bowel involvement. Many patients experience an intolerance to alcohol which can exacerbate their symptoms.

Pathologically, cellular infiltration (mast cells) and edema are usually present within the bowel wall. The small bowel is most commonly affected, but potentially any portion of the gut can be involved.

Radiographically, fold thickening and distortion are usually present (as seen in this case). Occasionally, a diffuse, fine nodular pattern of sandlike lucencies may be seen. Urticarial lesions have also been described.

## Case 484

## INGUINAL HERNIA

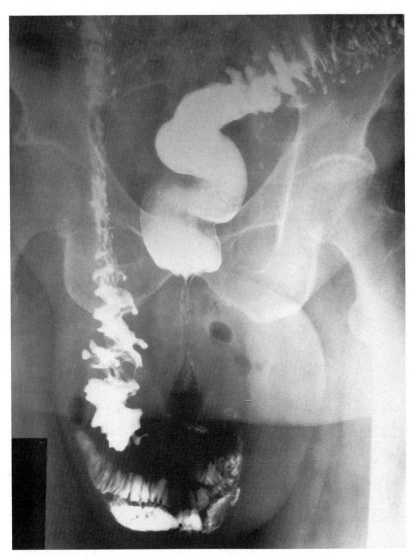

The cecum and distal small bowel are located in the scrotum in this patient with a large inguinal hernia.

Hernias are usually identified when bowel loops are seen to extend beyond the normal contours of the pelvis. Inguinal hernias are common. Left-sided hernias can involve the sigmoid colon, whereas right-sided hernias can contain the cecum and small bowel (as in this case). Hernias can cause bowel obstruction, and bowel strangulation and ischemia are also possible. Inguinal hernias tend to be larger than femoral hernias (Case 485).

**Case 485**

# FEMORAL HERNIA

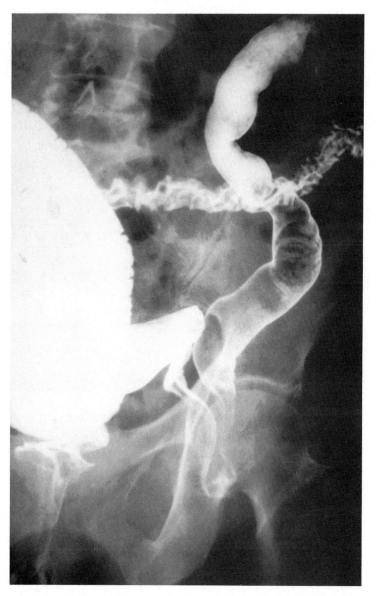

A loop of sigmoid colon is present within a hernia sac in the left inguinal region. At operation, a femoral hernia was found and repaired. Radiographically, it is usually difficult to distinguish an inguinal hernia from a femoral hernia, except that inguinal hernias tend to be larger.

A Richter hernia refers to entrapment of one wall of the bowel in the orifice of the hernia. This is commonly encountered in older women with a femoral hernia. Obstruction is unusual, but strangulation and perforation of the trapped bowel wall can occur.

**Case 486**

## LATERAL ABDOMINAL-WALL HERNIA

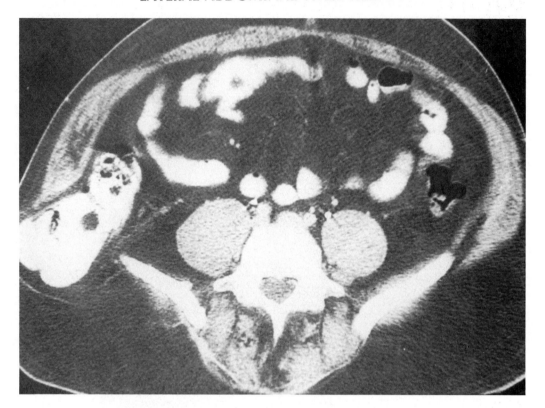

The cecum has herniated through an abdominal-wall defect just posterior to the internal and external oblique muscles.

Case 487

# TRAUMATIC DIAPHRAGMATIC HERNIA

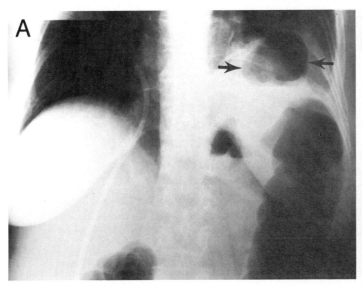

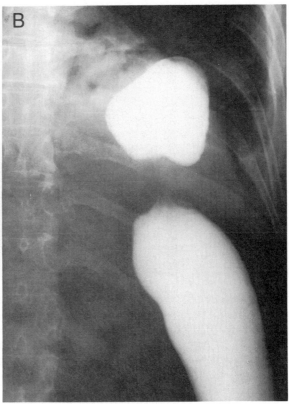

**A.** The abdominal plain film shows a loculated collection of gas in the left upper abdomen *(arrows)*, either in a subdiaphragmatic or intrathoracic location.

**B.** Full-column barium enema shows that the questionable gas collection is the splenic flexure of the colon, which has herniated through a small diaphragmatic defect. The colonic lumen is narrowed as it passes through the diaphragm, and barium could not be advanced into the more proximal colon, indicating obstruction. This patient had a remote history of a splenectomy during a staging operation for lymphoma. At operation, the colon was reduced and infarcted omentum was resected.

Traumatic abdominal hernias are relatively rare conditions due to either blunt external trauma or penetrating wounds. Occasionally, iatrogenic hernias may develop after subdiaphragmatic surgical procedures. The majority of diaphragmatic tears occur on the left, perhaps due to the protective effect of the liver on the right. The stomach is the organ most likely to herniate, followed by colon, small bowel, spleen, and omentum. Complications of obstruction and strangulation occur in the majority of patients if surgical correction is not performed. These complications have a high mortality.

## Case 488

# MORGAGNI HERNIA

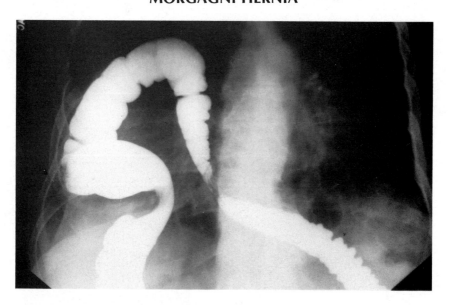

A large segment of transverse colon has herniated into the thorax via a defect in the anterior portion of the diaphragm. This location is characteristic of a Morgagni hernia.

Morgagni hernias are the least common of the diaphragmatic hernias. These occur as a result of a mid-line defect where the right and left pleuroperitoneal folds do not join. The substernal region is always affected, usually near the midline. Omentum often herniates into the thorax, but liver and colon also can be present.

| DIFFERENTIAL DIAGNOSES | CASE NUMBER |
|---|---|
| **SOLITARY FILLING DEFECTS** | |
| Ileocecal valve | 365 |
| Polyp | 367, 368, 370, 371, 393 |
| Adenocarcinoma | 371, 378–381, 383, 385 390, 391, 393 |
| Lipoma | 406, 407 |
| Endometrioma | 474 |
| Lymphoma | 403, 404 |
| Appendicitis | 430, 431 |
| Mucocele | 408, 409 |
| Metastases | 400 |
| **MULTIPLE FILLING DEFECTS** | |
| Stool or bubbles or pseudopolyps | 369 |
| Carcinoma | 382 |
| Polyps | 373, 374, 376, 377 |
| Lymphoid follicular pattern | 362, 363, 424 |
| Inflammatory polyps | 411, 414 |
| Polyposis syndrome | 373, 374, 376, 377 |
| Lymphoma | 401, 402, 405 |
| Metastases | 397 |
| Pneumatosis coli | 466–468 |
| Amebiasis | 458 |
| Colitis cystica profunda | 470 |
| Hemorrhoids | 482 |
| **NARROWING** | |
| Colonic spasm | 361 |
| Carcinoma | 379, 384, 420, 421 |
| Diverticulitis | 436–442 |
| Metastases | 397, 399, 400 |
| Crohn's colitis | 426 |
| Ulcerative colitis | 418, 420 |
| Ischemia | 446–449 |
| Pancreatitis | 455 |
| Radiation enteritis | 444, 445 |
| Endometriosis | 472, 473 |
| Pelvic lipomatosis | 479, 480 |
| **THICKENED FOLDS** | |
| Diverticulitis | 436, 442, 443 |
| Ulcerative colitis | 411, 422 |
| Crohn's colitis | 423 |
| Pseudomembranous colitis | 450, 451 |
| Ischemic colitis | 446–448 |
| Neutropenic colitis | 453, 454 |
| Pancreatitis | 455 |
| Appendicitis | 431, 433 |
| Mastocytosis | 483 |
| Radiation enteritis | 444 |

| DIFFERENTIAL DIAGNOSES | CASE NUMBER |
| --- | --- |
| Crohn's colitis | 426 |
| Scleroderma | 457 |
| Ischemic colitis | 449 |

# SELECTED READINGS

## Normal Anatomy

*Fisher JK. Normal colon wall thickness on CT. *Radiology* 1982;145:415–418

*Kelvin FM, Max RJ, Norton GA, et al. Lymphoid follicular pattern of the colon in adults. *AJR* 1979;133:821–825

## Neoplasms

### Polyps

*Arminski TC, McLean DW. Incidence and distribution of adenomatous polyps of the colon and rectum based on 1,000 autopsy examinations. *Dis Colon Rectum* 1964;7:249–261

*Bartholomew LG, Moore CE, Dahlin DC, Waugh JM. Intestinal polyposis associated with mucocutaneous pigmentation. *Surg Gynecol Obstet* 1962;115:1–11

*Bernstein MA, Feczko PJ, Halpert RD, Simms SM, Ackerman LV. Distribution of colonic polyps: increased incidence of proximal lesions in older patients. *Radiology* 1985;155:35–38

Dodds WJ, Lydon SB. Intestinal polyposis syndromes. *CRC Crit Rev Clin Radiol Nucl Med* 1974;5:295–336

*Dozois RR, Judd ES, Dahlin DC, Bartholomew LG. The Peutz-Jeghers syndrome: is there a predisposition to the development of intestinal malignancy. *Arch Surg* 1969;98:509–516

*Feczko PJ, Bernstein MA, Halpert RD, Ackerman LV. Small colonic polyps: a reappraisal of their significance. *Radiology* 1984;152:301–303

Godard JE, Dodds WJ, Phillips JC, Scanlon GT. Peutz-Jeghers syndrome: clinical and roentgenographic features. *Am J Roentgenol* 1971;113:316–324

Marshak RH, Moseley JE, Wolf BS. The roentgen findings in familial polyposis with special emphasis on differential diagnosis. *Radiology* 1963;80:374–382

Morson BC. The poly-cancer sequence in the large bowel. *Proc R Soc Med* 1974;67:451–457

*Muto T, Bussey HJR, Morson BC. The evolution of cancer of the colon and rectum. *Cancer* 1975;36:2251–2270

*Ott DJ, Gelfand DW. Colorectal tumors: pathology and detection. *AJR* 1978;131:691–695

Sachatello CR, Pickren JW, Grace JT Jr. Generalized juvenile gastrointestinal polyposis: a hereditary syndrome. *Gastroenterology* 1970;58:699–708

Stewart ET, Dodds WJ. Polyps. In: Margulis AR, Burhenne HF, eds. *Alimentary tract radiology*, 4th ed, vol 1. St. Louis: CV Mosby Company, 1989:1017–1049

Veale AMO, McColl I, Bussey HJR, Morson BC. Juvenile polyposis coli. *J Med Genet* 1966;3:5–16

Watne AL, Johnson JG, Chang CH. The challenge of Gardner's syndrome. *CA* 1969;19:266–275

Yonemoto RH, Slayback JB, Byron RL Jr, Rosen RB. Familial polyposis of the entire gastrointestinal tract. *Arch Surg* 1969;99:427–434

Ziter FMH Jr. Roentgenographic findings in Gardner's syndrome. *JAMA* 1965;192:1000–1002

### Adenocarcinoma

*Abrams JS, Reines HD. Increasing incidence of right-sided lesions in colorectal cancer. *Am J Surg* 1979;137:522–526

*Balthazar EJ, Megibow AJ, Hulnick D, Naidich DP. Carcinoma of the colon: detection and preoperative staging by CT. *AJR* 1988;150:301–306

Buy J-N, Moss AA, Ghossain MA, et al. Peritoneal implants from ovarian tumors: CT findings. *Radiology* 1988;169:691–694

Chen YM, Ott DJ, Wolfman NT, Gelfand DW, Karsteadt N, Bechtold RE. Recurrent colorectal carcinoma: evaluation with barium enema examination and CT. *Radiology* 1987;163:307–310

Freeny PC, Marks WM, Ryan JA, Bolen JW. Colorectal carcinoma evaluation with CT: preoperative staging and detection of postoperative recurrence. *Radiology* 1986;158:347–353

*Gelfand DW, Ott DJ. Single- vs. double-contrast gastrointestinal studies: critical analysis of reported statistics. *AJR* 1981;137:523–528

*Gilbert DA, Hallstrom AP, Shaneyfelt SL, Mahler AK, Silverstein FE, and 674 Members of the ASGE. The national ASGE colonoscopy survey —complications of colonoscopy (abstract). *Gastrointest Endosc* 1984;30:156

*Glenn F, McSherry CK. Obstruction and perforation in colo-rectal cancer. *Ann Surg* 1971;173:983–992

*Heald RJ, Bussey HJR. Clinical experiences at St. Mark's Hospital with multiple synchronous cancers of the colon and rectum. *Dis Colon Rectum* 1975;18:6–10

Hulnick DH, Megibow AJ, Balthazar EJ, Gordon RB, Surapenini R, Bosniak MA. Perforated colorectal neoplasms: correlation of clinical, contrast enema, and CT examinations. *Radiology* 1987;164:611–615

*Jochem RJ, Reading CC, Dozois RR, Carpenter HA, Wolff BG, Charboneau JW. Endorectal ultrasonographic staging of rectal carcinoma. *Mayo Clin Proc* 1990;65:1571–1577

Kelvin FM. Radiologic approach to the detection of colorectal neoplasia. *Radiol Clin North Am* 1982 Dec;20:743–759

*Kelvin FM, Korobkin M, Heaston DK, Grant JP, Akwari O. The pelvis after surgery for rectal carcinoma: serial CT observations with emphasis on nonneoplastic features. *AJR* 1983;141:959–964

*Kelvin FM, Maglinte DDT, Stephens BA. Colorectal carcinoma detected initially with barium enema examination: site distribution and implications. *Radiology* 1988;169:649–651

Krestin GP, Steinbrich W, Friedmann G. Recurrent rectal cancer: diagnosis with MR imaging versus CT. *Radiology* 1988;168:307–311

*Macklin MT. Inheritance of cancer of the stomach and large intestine in man. *J Natl Cancer Inst* 1960;24:551–571

*Meyers MA. *Dynamic radiology of the abdomen: normal and pathologic anatomy*, 3rd ed. New York: Springer-Verlag, 1988:91–178

*Miller LD, Boruchow IB, Fitts WT Jr. An analysis of 284 patients with perforative carcinoma of the colon. *Surg Gynecol Obstet* 1966;123:1212–1218

*Morson B. The polyp-cancer sequence in the large bowel. *Proc R Soc Med* 1974;67:451–457

*Olson RM, Perencevich NP, Malcom AW, Chaffey JT, Wilson RE. Patterns of recurrence following curative resection of adenocarcinoma of the colon and rectum. *Cancer* 1980;45:2969–2974

Rifkin MD, Ehrlich SM, Marks G. Staging of rectal carcinoma: prospective comparison of endorectal US and CT. *Radiology* 1989;170:319–322

Walkey MM, Friedman AC, Sohotra P, Radecki PD. CT manifestations of peritoneal carcinomatosis. *AJR* 1988;150:1035–1041

Weilbaecher D, Bolin JA, Hearn D, Odgen W II. Intussusception in adults: review of 160 cases. *Am J Surg* 1971:121:531–535

Whalen E. Colon cancer: diagnosis in an era of cost containment. ACR conference, November 8, 1989. *AJR* 1990;154:875–881

*Whitehouse GH, Watt J. Ischemic colitis associated with carcinoma of the colon. *Gastrointest Radiol* 1977;2:31–35

**Other**

Castro EB, Stearns MW. Lipoma of the large intestine: a review of 45 cases. *Dis Colon Rectum* 1972;15:441–444

Heiken JP, Forde KA, Gold RP. Computed tomography as a definitive method for diagnosing gastrointestinal lipomas. *Radiology* 1982;142:409–414

*Hertzer NR, Hoerr SO. An interpretive review of lymphoma of the stomach. *Surg Gynecol Obstet* 1976;143:113–124

*Higa E, Rosai J, Pizzimbono CA, Wise L. Mucosal hyperplasia, mucinous cystadenoma, and mucinous cystadenocarcinoma of the appendix. A re-evaluation of appendiceal "mucocele." *Cancer* 1973;32:1525–1541

Jeffrey RB Jr, Berk RN. Radiology of the appendix. In: Taveras JM, Ferrucci JT, eds. *Radiology: diagnosis—imaging—intervention*, vol 4. Philadelphia: JB Lippincott, 1986:chap 41, 1–10

*Joseph JL, Lattes R. Gastric lymphosarcoma: clinicopathologic analysis of 71 cases and its relation to disseminated lymphosarcoma. *Am J Clin Pathol* 1966;45:653–669

Marshak RH, Lindner AE, Maklansky D. Lymphosarcoma. In: Marshak RH, Lindner AE, Maklansky D, eds. *Radiology of the colon*. Philadelphia: WB Saunders Company, 1980:367–385

Megibow AJ, Balthazar EJ, Naidich DP, Bosniak MA. Computed tomography of gastrointestinal lymphoma. *AJR* 1983;141:541–547

O'Connell DJ, Thompson AJ. Lymphoma of the colon: the spectrum of radiologic changes. *Gastrointest Radiol* 1978;2:377–385

*Otto RE, Ghislandi EV, Lorenzo GA, Conn J Jr. Primary appendiceal adenocarcinoma. *Am J Surg* 1970;120:704–706

Zornoza J, Dodd GD. Lymphoma of the gastrointestinal tract. *Semin Roentgenol* 1980;15:272–287

**Inflammatory Bowel Disease**

Bartram CI, Laufer I. Inflammatory bowel disease. In: Laufer I, ed. *Double contrast gastrointestinal radiology with endoscopic correlation*. Philadelphia: WB Saunders Company, 1979:601–688

Bartram CI, Walmsley K. A radiological and pathological correlation of the mucosal changes in ulcerative colitis. *Clin Radiol* 1978;29:323–328

*de Dombal FT, Watts JM, Watkinson G, Goligher JC. Local complications of ulcerative colitis: stricture, pseudopolyposis, and carcinoma of the colon and rectum. *Br Med J* 1966;1:1442–1447

*Edwards FC, Truelove SC. The course and prognosis of ulcerative colitis. Part I. Short-term prognosis. Part II. Long-term prognosis. Part IV. Carcinoma of the colon. *Gut* 1963;4:299–308; 309–315; 1964:5:15–22

*Goldberg HI, Gore RM, Margulis AR, Moss AA,

Baker EL. Computer tomography in the evaluation of Crohn disease. *AJR* **1983**;140:277–282

Gore RM, Marn CS, Kirby DF, Vogelzang RL, Neiman HL. CT findings in ulcerative, granulomatous, and indeterminate colitis. *AJR* **1984**;143:279–284

Goulston SJM, McGovern VJ. The nature of benign strictures in ulcerative colitis. *N Engl J Med* **1969**;218:290–295

*Hooyman JR, MacCarty RL, Carpenter HA, Schroeder KW, Carlson HC. Radiographic appearance of mucosal dysplasia associated with ulcerative colitis. *AJR* **1987**;149:47–51

*Kelvin FM, Max RJ, Norton GA, et al. Lymphoid follicular pattern of the colon in adults. *AJR* **1979**;133:821–825

Laufer I, Costopoulos L. Early lesions of Crohn's disease. *AJR* **1978**;130:307–311

*Lennard-Jones JE, Melville DM, Morson BC, Ritchie JK, Williams CB. Precancer and cancer in extensive ulcerative colitis: findings among 401 patients over 22 years. *Gut* **1990**;31:800–806

Lichtenstein JE, Madewell JE, Feigin DS. The collar button ulcer: a radiologic-pathologic correlation. *Gastrointest Radiol* **1979**;4:79–84

Marshak RH. Granulomatous disease of the intestinal tract (Crohn's disease). *Radiology* **1975**;114:3–22

Marshak RH, Korelitz BI, Klein SH, Wolf BS, Janowitz HD. Toxic dilation of the colon in the course of ulcerative colitis. *Gastroenterol* **1960**;38:165–180

Marshak RH, Lindner AE, Maklansky D. Crohn's disease of the colon (granulomatous colitis). In: Marshak RH, Lindner AE, Maklansky D, eds. *Radiology of the colon.* Philadelphia: WB Saunders Company, **1980**:120–188

Thoeni RF, Margulis AR. Inflammatory diseases. In: Margulis AR, Burhenne HJ, eds. *Alimentary tract radiology,* 4th ed, vol 1. St. Louis: CV Mosby Company, **1989**:963–1015

*Weedon DD, Shorter RG, Ilstrup DM, Huizenga KA, Taylor WF. Crohn's disease and cancer. *N Engl J Med* **1973**;289:1099–1103

*Appendicitis*

Abu-Yousef M, Bleicher JJ, Maher JW, Urdaneta LF, Franken EA Jr, Metcalf AM. High-resolution sonography of acute appendicitis. *AJR* **1987**;149:53–58

Balthazar EJ, Megibow AJ, Hulnick D, Gordon RB, Naidich NP, Beranbaum ER. CT of appendicitis. *AJR* **1986**;147:705–710

*Baker SR, Elkin M. *Plain film approach to abdominal calcifications.* Philadelphia: WB Saunders Company, **1983**

*Barnes BA, Behringer GE, Wheelock FC, Wilkins EW. Treatment of appendicitis at the Massachusetts General Hospital (1937–1959). *JAMA* **1962**;180:122–126.

Jeffrey RB Jr, Berk RN. Radiology of the appendix. In: Taveras JM, Ferrucci JT, eds. *Radiology: diagnosis—imaging—intervention,* vol 4. Philadelphia: JB Lippincott, **1986**:chap 41, 1–10

Jeffrey RB Jr, Laing FC, Lewis FR. Acute appendicitis: high-resolution real-time US findings. *Radiology* **1987**;163:11–14

*Jeffrey RB Jr, Laing FC, Townsend RR. Acute appendicitis: sonographic criteria based on 250 cases. *Radiology* **1988**;167:327–329

*Jeffrey RB Jr, Tolentino CS, Federle MP, Laing FC. Percutaneous drainage of periappendiceal abscesses: review of 20 patients. *AJR* **1987**;149:59–62

McAfee JG, Donner MW. Differential diagnosis of calcifications encountered in abdominal radiographs. *Am J Med Sci* **1962**;243:609–650

Mindelzun RE, McCort JJ. Acute abdomen. In: Margulis AR, Burhenne HJ, eds. *Alimentary tract radiology,* 4th ed, vol 1. St Louis: CV Mosby Company, **1989**:291–361

Rice RP, Thompson WM, Fedyshin PJ, Merten DF, Kelvin FM, Williford ME. The barium enema in appendicitis: spectrum of appearances and pitfalls. *Radiographics* **1984**;4:393–409

*Shimkin PM. Radiology of acute appendicitis (commentary). *AJR* **1978**;130:1001–1004

Soter CS. The contribution of the radiologists to the diagnosis of acute appendicitis. *Semin Roentgenol* **1973**;8:375–388

*Diverticulitis*

Hulnick DH, Megibow AJ, Balthazar EJ, Naidich DP, Bosniak MA. Computed tomography in the evaluation of diverticulitis. *Radiology* **1984**;152:491–495

*Johnson CD, Baker ME, Rice RP, Silverman P, Thompson WM. Diagnosis of acute colonic diverticulitis: comparison of barium enema and CT. *AJR* **1987**;148:541–546

Marshak RH, Lindner AE, Maklansky D. Diverticular disease. In: Marshak RH, Lindner AE, Maklansky D, eds. *Radiology of the colon.* Philadelphia: WB Saunders Company, **1980**:401–466

Mueller PR, Saini S, Wittenberg J, et al. Sigmoid diverticular abscesses: percutaneous drainage as an adjunct to surgical resection in 24 cases. *Radiology* **1987**;164:321–325

Schnyder P. Diverticula. In: Margulis AR, Burhenne HJ, eds. *Alimentary tract radiology,* 4th ed, vol 1. St. Louis: CV Mosby Company, **1989**:943–961

Wolf BS, Khilnani M, Marshak RH. Diverticulosis and diverticulitis: roentgen findings and their interpretation. *Am J Roentgenol* **1957**;77:726–743

### Other

Eisenberg RL, Montgomery CK, Margulis AR. Colitis in the elderly: ischemic colitis mimicking ulcerative and granulomatous colitis. *AJR* **1979**;133:1113–1118

Frick MP, Maile CW, Crass JR, Goldberg ME, Delaney JP. Computed tomography of neutropenic colitis. *AJR* **1984**;143:763–765

Gore M, Calenoff L, Rogers LE. Roentgenographic manifestations of ischemic colitis. *JAMA* **1979**; 241:1171–1173

Marshak RH, Lindner AE, Maklansky D. Ischemia of the colon. *Mt Sinai J Med* **1981**;48:180–190

Mason GR, Dietrich P, Friedland GW, Hanks GE. The radiological findings in radiation-induced enteritis and colitis. A review of 30 cases. *Clin Radiol* **1970**;21:232–247

Megibow AJ, Streiter ML, Balthazar EJ, Bosniak MA. Pseudomembranous colitis: diagnosis by computed tomography. *J Comput Assist Tomogr* **1984**;8:281–283

Reeder MM. Parasitic diseases. In: Marshak RH, Lindner AE, Maklansky D, eds. *Radiology of the colon.* Philadelphia: WB Saunders Company, **1980**:189–231

Rogers LF, Goldstein HM. Roentgen manifestations of radiation injury to the gastrointestinal tract. *Gastrointest Radiol* **1977**;2:281–291

Rubesin SE, Levine MS, Glick SN, Herlinger H, Laufer I. Pseudomembranous colitis with rectosigmoid sparing on barium studies. *Radiology* **1989**;170:811–813

*Senturia HR, Wald SM. Ulcerative disease of the intestinal tract proximal to partially obstructing lesions: roentgen appearance. *AJR* **1967**;99:45

*Shamberger RC, Weinstein HJ, Delorey MJ, Levey RH. The medical and surgical management of typhlitis in children with acute nonlymphocytic (myelogenous) leukemia. *Cancer* **1986**;57:603–609

Shimkin PM, Link RJ. Pseudomembranous colitis: a consideration in the barium enema differential

diagnosis of acute generalized ulcerative colitis. *Br J Radiol* **1973**;46:437–439

Smerud MJ, Johnson CD, Stephens DH. Diagnosis of bowel infarction: a comparison of plain films and CT scans in 23 cases. *AJR* **1990**;154:99–103

Stanley RJ, Melson GL, Tedesco FJ. The spectrum of radiographic findings in antibiotic-related pseudomembranous colitis. *Radiology* **1974**;111:519–524

Taylor AJ, Dodds WJ, Gonyo JE, Komorowski RA. Typhlitis in adults. *Gastrointest Radiol* **1985**;10:363–369

Teefey SA, Montana MA, Goldfogel GA, Shuman WP. Sonographic diagnosis of neutropenic typhlitis. *AJR* **1987**;149:731–733

Wittenberg J, Athanasoulis CA, Williams LF Jr, Paredes S, O'Sullivan P, Brown B. Ischemic colitis: radiology and pathophysiology. *Am J Roentgenol* **1975**;123:287–300

### Obstruction and Ileus

Anderson JR, Mills JOM. Caecal volvulus: a frequently missed diagnosis. *Clin Radiol* **1984**;35:65–69

Andersson A, Bergdahl L, van der Linden W. Volvulus of the cecum. *Ann Surg* **1975**;181:876–880

*Bryk D, Soong KY. Colonic ileus and its differential roentgen diagnosis. *Am J Roentgenol* **1967**;101:329–337

Fisher JK. Computed tomographic diagnosis of volvulus in intestinal malrotation. *Radiology* **1981**;140:145–146

Johnson CD. Gross cecal distention. In: Thompson WM, ed. *Common problems in gastrointestinal radiology.* Chicago: Year Book Medical Publishers, **1989**:71–75

*Johnson CD, Rice RP, Kelvin FM, Foster WL, Williford ME. The radiologic evaluation of gross cecal distention: emphasis on cecal ileus. *AJR* **1985**;145:1211–1217

Love L. Large bowel obstruction. *Semin Roentgenol* **1973**;8:299–322

Shaff MI, Himmelfarb E, Sachs GA, Burks DD, Kulkarni MV. The whirl sign: a CT finding in volvulus of the large bowel. *J Comput Assist Tomogr* **1985**;9:410

### Miscellaneous

*Pneumatosis Coli*

Marshak RH, Lindner AE, Maklansky D. Pneumatosis cystoides coli. *Gastrointest Radiol* **1977**;2:85–89

Williams SM, Harned RK. Multiple filling defects in

the colon. In: Thompson WM, ed. *Common problems in gastrointestinal radiology.* Chicago: Year Book Medical Publishers, **1989**:378.

*Solitary Rectal Ulcer Syndrome*

Goei R, Baeten C, Arends JW. Solitary rectal ulcer syndrome: findings at barium enema study and defecography. *Radiology* **1988**;168:303–306

Goei R, Baeten C, Janevski B, van Engelshoven J. The solitary rectal ulcer syndrome: diagnosis with defecography. *AJR* **1987**;149:933–936

*Endometriosis*

Spjut HJ, Perkins DE. Endometriosis of the sigmoid colon and rectum: a roentgenologic and pathologic study. *Am J Roentgenol* **1959**;82:1070–1075

Zimmer G, Kurzban JD, Maklansky D, Marshak RH. Colonic endometriosis: roentgen studies with a five-year follow-up. *Am J Gastroenterol* **1975**;64:410–413

*Iatrogenic Disorders*

*Ansell G. Alimentary tract. In: Ansell G, Wilkins RA, eds. *Complications in diagnostic imaging,* 2nd ed. Oxford: Blackwell Scientific Publications, **1987**:218–246

*Gilbert DA, Hallstrom AP, Shaneyfelt SL, Mahler AK, Silverstein FE, and 674 Members of the ASGE. The national ASGE colonoscopy survey —complications of colonoscopy (abstract). *Gastrointest Endosc* **1984**;30:156.

*Rogers BHG, Silvis SE, Nebel OT, Sugawa C, Mandelstam P. Complications of flexible fiberoptic colonoscopy and polypectomy. *Gastrointest Endosc* **1975**;22:73–77

*Pelvic Lipomatosis*

Church PA, Kazam E. Computed tomography and ultrasound in diagnosis of pelvic lipomatosis. *Urology* **1979**;14:631–633

Farman J, Faegenburg D, Dallemand S, Keohane MF. Pelvic lipomatosis. *Am J Gastroenterol* **1973**;60:640–648

Fogg LG, Smyth JW. Pelvic lipomatosis: a condition simulating pelvic neoplasm. *Radiology* **1968**;90:558–564

Werboff LH, Korobkin M, Klein RS. Pelvic lipomatosis: diagnosis using computed tomography. *J Urol* **1979**;122:257–259

*Hemorrhoids*

Levine MS, Kam LW, Rubesin SE, Ekberg O. Internal hemorrhoids: diagnosis with double-contrast barium enema examinations. *Radiology* **1990**;177:141–144

*Hernias*

Holder LE, Schneider HJ. Spigelian hernias: anatomy and roentgenographic manifestations. *Radiology* **1974**;112:309–313

Meyers MA, Grandone CH. Internal hernias. In: Thompson WM ed. *Common problems in gastrointestinal radiology.* Chicago: Year Book Medical Publishers, **1989**:309–319

# Index